T0228602

Prevention and Management of Dyslipidemia

Prevention and Management of Dyslipidemia

Edited by **Donna Thompson**

New Jersey

Published by Foster Academics,
61 Van Reypen Street,
Jersey City, NJ 07306, USA
www.fosteracademics.com

Prevention and Management of Dyslipidemia
Edited by Donna Thompson

International Standard Book Number: 978-1-63242-331-3 (Hardback)

Printed in the United States of America.

Contents

Preface   VII

Chapter 1   **Liver Sinusoidal Endothelial Cells
            and Regulation of Blood Lipoproteins**   1
            Dmitri Svistounov, Svetlana N. Zykova,
            Victoria C. Cogger, Alessandra Warren,
            Aisling C. McMahon, Robin Fraser and David G. Le Couteur

Chapter 2   **Dyslipidemia and Cardiovascular Disease**   17
            Hossein Fakhrzadeh and Ozra Tabatabaei-Malazy

Chapter 3   **Dyslipidemia and Cardiovascular Risk:
            Lipid Ratios as Risk Factors for Cardiovascular Disease**   35
            Telmo Pereira

Chapter 4   **Dyslipidemia Induced by Stress**   59
            Fernanda Klein Marcondes, Vander José das Neves,
            Rafaela Costa, Andrea Sanches, Tatiana Sousa Cunha,
            Maria José Costa Sampaio Moura, Ana Paula Tanno
            and Dulce Elena Casarini

Chapter 5   **Dyslipidemia and Mental Illness**   83
            D. Saravane

Chapter 6   **Cardiovascular Risk in Tunisian
            Patients with Bipolar I Disorder**   101
            Asma Ezzaher, Dhouha Haj Mouhamed,
            Anwar Mechri, Fadoua Neffati, Wahiba Douki,
            Lotfi Gaha and Mohamed Fadhel Najjar

Chapter 7   **Cholesterol and Triglycerides
            Metabolism Disorder in Malignant Hemopathies**   129
            Romeo-Gabriel Mihăilă

Chapter 8   **Dyslipidemia in Patients with
Lipodystrophy in the Use of Antiretroviral Therapy**   149
Rosana Libonati, Cláudia Dutra, Leonardo Barbosa,
Sandro Oliveira, Paulo Lisbôa and Marcus Libonati

Chapter 9   **Lipids in the Pathogenesis of Benign Prostatic Hyperplasia:
Emerging Connections**   169
Ajit Vikram and Poduri Ramarao

Chapter 10   **Predictors of the Common Adverse
Drug Reactions of Statins**   185
Hadeer Akram AbdulRazzaq, Noorizan Abd Aziz,
Yahaya Hassan, Yaman Walid Kassab and Omar Ismail

Chapter 11   **Fenofibrate: Panacea for Aging-Related Conditions?**   195
Makoto Goto

Permissions

List of Contributors

Preface

In my initial years as a student, I used to run to the library at every possible instance to grab a book and learn something new. Books were my primary source of knowledge and I would not have come such a long way without all that I learnt from them. Thus, when I was approached to edit this book; I became understandably nostalgic. It was an absolute honor to be considered worthy of guiding the current generation as well as those to come. I put all my knowledge and hard work into making this book most beneficial for its readers.

Dyslipidemia has intricate physiopathology, often due to genetic, diet and lifestyle factors. It has various adverse impacts, especially in the development of chronic non-communicable diseases. The growing cases of obesity, changes in lifestyle and environmental factors will make dyslipidemia a global medical and public health hazard, not only for adults but also for children. Important ethnic differences exist due to the prevalence and types of lipid ailment, while elevated serum total and LDL-cholesterol are the main concern in the developed countries, in other countries hypertriglyceridemia and low HDL-cholesterol are more widespread. Various experimental and clinical researches are going on related to the basic mechanisms and treatment of dyslipidemia. This book will deliver an overview of dyslipidemia from distinct facets of prevention, health hazards and treatment.

I wish to thank my publisher for supporting me at every step. I would also like to thank all the authors who have contributed their researches in this book. I hope this book will be a valuable contribution to the progress of the field.

Editor

Liver Sinusoidal Endothelial Cells and Regulation of Blood Lipoproteins

Dmitri Svistounov[1], Svetlana N. Zykova[1,2], Victoria C. Cogger[1],
Alessandra Warren[1], Aisling C. McMahon[1],
Robin Fraser[3] and David G. Le Couteur[1]
[1]*Centre for Education and Research on Ageing and ANZAC Research Institute,
University of Sydney and Concord RG Hospital, Sydney,*
[2]*Department of Nephrology, University Hospital of Northern Norway, Tromsø,*
[3]*University of Otago, Christchurch,*
[1]*Australia*
[2]*Norway*
[3]*New Zealand*

1. Introduction

Dyslipidaemia is a well-described major independent risk factor for cardiovascular disease (Lin et al.). It is well established that the liver plays the central role in lipid metabolism and liver malfunction is one of the main sources of dyslipidemia (Watson et al., 2003). However, most of the studies so far have focused on the role of hepatocytes in lipid turnover. Indeed, hepatocytes do play a central role in liver lipid metabolism, but they are not alone. Hepatocytes do not have direct contact with the circulation. Any blood-borne lipoprotein particle must first pass through a filter comprised of a layer of endothelial cells, lining the walls of liver sinusoids, before it can contact the liver parenchyma. Likewise, lipoproteins remodelled or synthesized by the liver encounter the same barrier before they reach systemic circulation.

2. The structure of the hepatic sinusoid

The hepatic sinusoids are small blood vessels, comparable to capillaries in size, that perfuse the hepatocytes. However, unlike the capillaries in other tissues, sinusoids are formed by a discontinuous endothelium that lacks any significant underlying basement membrane. Walls of sinusoids are formed by the liver sinusoidal endothelial cells (LSECs). LSECs are separated from liver parenchyma by the perisinusoidal extravascular space, known as the space of Disse (Figure 1A). LSECs contribute only 15-20% of all liver cells but comprise 70% of the population of sinusoidal cells in the liver (Arias, 1990; Arii and Imamura, 2000; Blouin et al., 1977; Knook and Sleyster, 1976).

The LSECs are perforated by trans-cytoplasmic pores called fenestrae, which do not have any intervening diaphragmatic membrane, and thus are fully patent holes through the cell (Figure 1A-B). This specialized lace-like morphology of the LSECs minimizes any barrier to the bi-directional transfer of solutes and particulate substrates between the sinusoidal blood and hepatocytes, whilst retaining the capacity and substantial surface area to undergo interactions with circulating blood cells including immune cells (Cogger and Le Couteur, 2009; Fraser et al., 1995; Wisse et al., 1996). Fenestrae are not uniformly distributed over the LSEC surface but are aggregated into groups of tens to hundreds in gossamer thin areas of cytoplasm and towards the periphery of the cell. These areas of fenestral aggregations are termed sieve plates (Figure 1B). Between 60-75% of fenestrae are found within sieve plates in rats (Vidal-Vanaclocha and Barbera-Guillem, 1985) but isolated fenestrae are also frequently observed on the LSEC surface.

The LSEC becomes fenestrated at an early gestational stage (Enzan et al., 1997; Martinez-Hernandez and Amenta, 1993; Nonaka et al., 2007; Smedsrod et al., 2009). The porosity of the sinusoids depends on the number and especially the size or diameter of the fenestrae. The diameter of fenestrae has a normal distribution curve of about 50-200nm (Cogger and Le Couteur, 2009). Gaps larger than about 200nm are regarded as artifacts formed during specimen preparation for electron microscopy (Akinc et al., 2009; Fraser et al., 1978; Fraser et al., 1980; Hilmer et al., 2005a).

Fenestrae have been found in many species including such diverse species as man, rat, mouse, guinea pig, sheep, goat, rabbit, fowl, monkey, baboon, bat, kitten, dog, turtle and fish (Cogger and Le Couteur, 2009).

The fenestrated endothelium was first suggested as a filter of chylomicrons by Wisse in 1970 (Wisse, 1970) from their reported diameters (Fraser et al., 1968) and termed the "liver sieve" once sieving was confirmed (Fraser et al., 1978; Naito and Wisse, 1978). Fenestrae allow the transfer of a wide range of substrates including plasma and plasma molecules, such as plasma proteins, some lipoproteins and colloidal particles (Le Couteur et al., 2005). The latter also include artificial chylomicron-like nanospheres such as Intralipid, but also small viruses leading to hepatitis, viral vectors for DNA manipulation of hepatocytes.

The fenestrated LSEC can be defined as an ultrafiltration system because it is a low pressure system with pores approximately 100nm in diameter. Specifically, the liver sieve can be described as a Loeb–Sourirajan ultrafiltration system, with the LSECs providing the thin porous layer (Baker, 2004). The transfer of fluid across an ultrafiltration system can be calculated using the Hagen Poiseuille equation for ultrafiltration where the flux of fluid is proportional to the number of pores and the radius of the pores to the power of four (Baker, 2004; Le Couteur et al., 2006; Warren et al., 2005). Therefore small changes in the size of fenestrae has profound effects on the size and number of substrates and macromolecules that can gain passage into the space of Disse. Indeed, manipulation of fenestrae diameter might have a role in regulating the transfer of substrates in response to physiological changes, such as feeding and fasting (O'Reilly et al., 2010).

The space of Disse is the extravascular space lying between the hepatocytes and LSECs. It contains some components of extracellular matrix and most components of blood plasma filtered through LSEC's sieve plates. Extracellular matrix in the space of Disse contains fibronectin and collagen type I ,III, V, and VI. Collagen type IV is also present but unlike its sheet-like polymeric presentation in typical basement membranes, here it appears in the form of discontinuous aggregates (Martinez-Hernandez and Amenta, 1993). Of note, basement membrane has not been identified in liver sinusoids in any non-pathological state or developmental stage until old age (Enzan et al., 1997; Martinez-Hernandez and Amenta, 1993; Nonaka et al., 2007; Smedsrod et al., 2009), where its appearance is believed to be a sign of age-related degeneration and – possibly – a cause of pathology.

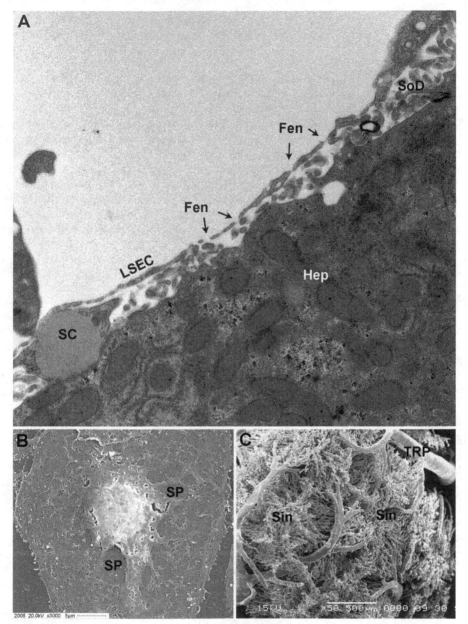

Fig. 1. A: Transmission electron micrograph showing liver sinusoidal endothelial cell (LSEC) perforated by fenestrae (Fen). (Hep) – hepatocyte, (SoD) - space of Disse, (SC) - stellate cells with lipid droplet in space of Disse. B: Scanning electron micrograph of an isolated liver sinusoidal endothelial cell showing fenestrae clustered into sieve plates (SP). C: Scanning electron micrograph of a vascular cast showing branches of the portal vein (TPV) with surrounding sinusoidal network (Sin). (Preparations performed by A Warren).

Multiple microvilli from the the sinusoidal surface of the hepatocytes protrude into the space of Disse and increase the available surface area for the recognition, transport and diffusion of substrates to and from the liver (Cogger and Le Couteur, 2009; Fraser et al., 1995; Wisse et al., 1996).

There are three other cell types residing in the liver sinusoids apart from the LSECs: Kupffer cells (resident liver macrophages), stellate cells and pit cells. Kupffer cells represent only 20% of all the population of liver sinusoidal cells but 80-90% of all tissue macrophages in the body (Knook and Sleyster, 1976). They generally reside within the lumen of the liver sinusoids and take up bacteria and other large particles, such as cell debris, from the circulation by phagocytosis. In response to bacterial infection, Kupffer cells produce cytokines and a number of soluble pro-inflammatory factors that promote influx and activation of neutrophils (Smedsrod et al., 1994; Smedsrod et al., 2009) and may alter the porosity of the sinusoids to promote cirrhosis (Dobbs et al., 1994). Together, LSECs (pinocytosis) and Kupffer cells (phagocytosis) constitute the hepatic reticuloendothelial system (RES), the most powerful scavenger system of mammals and other terrestrial vertebrates (Aschoff, 1924; Kawai et al., 1998).

3. The normal function of the LSEC in regulation of blood lipids

Because of the LSECs fenestrae, all lipoproteins except large chylomicrons have unimpeded access to the hepatocytes. After delivering triglycerides to peripheral tissues, chylomicrons become processed into so-called "chylomicron remnants" that carry significant amounts of cholesterol and are highly pro-atherogenic (Fujioka and Ishikawa, 2009; Karpe et al., 1994). At the same time they become small enough to pass through LSECs fenestrae (Fujioka and Ishikawa, 2009) and can be taken up by hepatocytes, which allows liver parenchyma to be the major site for removal of pro-atherogenic chylomicron remnants from the blood (Cooper, 1997; Dietschy et al., 1993) under normal circumstances. However, fast and efficient blood clearance of highly atherogenic chylomicron-remnants by hepatocytes requires well fenestrated LSECs.

4. Ageing of the LSEC and regulation of blood lipids

Many important diseases, particularly cardiovascular diseases, that result in disability and death, occur late in life, indicating that aging itself is a key risk factor. Old age is associated with significant changes in the cells of the hepatic sinusoid. Previously, it has been considered that the liver does not undergo significant aging changes because of its large functional reserve, regenerative capacity and dual blood supply (Popper, 1986). Only a few descriptions of the aging liver have been generally established, such as an increase in the number of polyploid and binucleate hepatocytes (Schmucker, 1998) and "brown atrophy", which is a reduction in liver mass accompanied by the deposition of the aging pigment, lipofuscin (Popper, 1986). Today it has become clear that age-related changes in hepatic structure and function are significant and influence systemic exposure to xenobiotics, endogenous substances associated with disease and medications (McLean and Le Couteur, 2004). Thus, such changes in the liver have implications for many diseases of aging and the aging process itself.

It has now been reported that old age is associated with substantial ultrastructural changes in the LSECs and space of Disse in intact livers of the rat (Jamieson et al., 2007; Le Couteur et al., 2001), human (McLean et al., 2003), the mouse (Ito et al., 2007; Warren et al., 2005) and the non-human primate, *Papio hamadryas* (Cogger et al., 2003). The findings have been replicated in at least three separate centres around the world (Furrer et al.; Ito et al., 2007; Le Couteur et al., 2001; Stacchiotti et al., 2008). These changes have been termed 'pseudocapillarization' because the aging sinusoids become similar to capillaries seen in other non-fenestrated vascular beds (Le Couteur et al., 2001). Unlike 'capillarization' seen in the hepatic sinusoid in cirrhosis of the liver, aging is not associated with any of the typical changes apparent on light microscopy, such as bridging fibrosis and nodular regeneration (Le Couteur et al., 2001; Le Couteur et al., 2008). In old age, LSEC thickness is increased by approximately 50% and there is a similar reduction of about 50% in the porosity and number of fenestrae (Figure 2). These changes are associated with perisinusoidal basal lamina deposition in many old livers and some scattered collagen in the space of Disse. The effect of aging on the diameter of fenestrae has been inconsistent between species, however there is a trend towards a reduction in diameter of around 5-10% (Le Couteur et al., 2008). Isolated LSECs typically retain some of these ultrastructural changes. Fenestrae diameter was reduced in old age from 194±1 nm to 185±1 nm in isolated rat LSECs (O'Reilly et al., 2009).

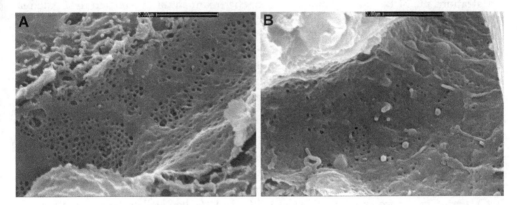

Fig. 2. Scanning electron micrographs of the liver sinusoid of a young (A) and old (B) rat. The loss of fenestrae perforating the endothelial cell surface in the old liver is apparent. (Preparations performed by A Warren).

Fenestrations have a role in the transfer of lipoproteins from blood to the hepatocyte, therefore it is likely that pseudocapillarization of sinusoids will impair lipoprotein clearance by the liver and contribute to dyslipidaemia in older people (Le Couteur et al., 2002). Atherosclerosis increases dramatically with old age and its complications affect most older people (Lakatta and Levy, 2003). The clearance of chylomicron remnants is significantly impaired in older people (Borel et al., 1998; Krasinski et al., 1990) and in those aged 65 years and older, remnant-like lipoprotein cholesterol is associated with the development of coronary artery disease (Simons et al., 2001). To determine whether age-related defenestration impairs the transfer of lipoproteins across the LSECs, the multiple indicator dilution method was used to study lipoprotein disposition in perfused rat livers (Hilmer et al., 2005b). In young livers, lipoproteins (approximately 50 nm diameter) entered the entire extracellular space whereas in old livers, the lipoproteins were confined to the vascular space. These results strongly suggest that age-related pseudocapillarization impairs the hepatic disposition of lipoproteins and thus plays a role in age-related dyslipidaemia.

Matrix heparan sulfate proteoglycans bind and sequester lipoprotein remnants (Williams, 2008). In old age, formation of basal lamina beneath LSECs leads to a change in the proportions of extracellular matrix components and may result in impaired passage of lipoproteins across the space of Disse. However, the importance of this pathway in lipoprotein turnover has not been studied sufficiently, especially in connection to aging.

A reduction in caloric intake by about 40% increases maximum life expectancy and is associated with a delay in the onset of most age-associated disorders and pathology (Everitt et al., 2005). It has also been demonstrated that caloric restriction delays the onset of pseudocapillarization in rats. In the old caloric restricted rats, endothelial thickness was significantly less and fenestrae porosity was significantly greater than in the old ad libitum fed rats. Moreover, caloric restriction prevented the age-related increase in perisinusoidal collagen IV staining (Jamieson et al., 2007). The finding that caloric restriction influences pseudocapillarization suggests that the latter is secondary to the aging process and thus potentially reversible. As a consequence, modulation of LSEC fenestrations might be a therapeutic target for the treatment of age-related dyslipidemia and prevention of vascular disease. On the other hand, early onset of pseudocapillarization and dyslipidemia occur in a transgenic mouse model of Werner syndrome, a rare premature aging syndrome in humans.

Another hallmark of old age - the reduction in liver size as a fraction of body weight - is usually in the order of 25-35% (Le Couteur and McLean, 1998) and is associated with a decrease in the number of hepatocytes. In addition, several studies have shown that the total hepatic blood flow is reduced by about 30-50% (Le Couteur and McLean, 1998). Liver perfusion, which is the blood flow per mass of liver, is also reduced in old age but to a lesser extent than total blood flow. Mechanisms for these changes remain unclear; however, a recent study using high resolution *in vivo* microscopy has shown how pseudocapillarization might contribute to these phenomena. There was a 14% reduction in the numbers of perfused sinusoids with old age and a 35% reduction in sinusoidal blood flow (Ito et al., 2007). Narrower sinusoids with thickened LSECs and swollen stellate cells with abundant lipid droplets were also observed. It was concluded that these changes caused age-related reduction in hepatic perfusion and hepatic blood flow by blocking the sinusoids (Ito et al., 2007). The clearance of highly extracted substrates from the circulation is dependent on blood flow, therefore the age-related reduction in hepatic blood flow has a dramatic effect on the liver's overall function (Le Couteur and McLean, 1998), including the clearance of lipoproteins.

It is reasonable to conclude that pseudocapillarization, in combination with a reduction in hepatic blood flow, are two major factors contributing to age-related dyslipidemia.

5. Scavenger function of LSEC in clearance of oxidized lipoproteins

Another unique feature of LSECs is extraordinary endocytic activity. LSECs are rich in coated pits and vesicles and other organelles associated with endocytosis. Although LSECs constitute only 2.8 % of the total liver volume, they contain about 15% of the total lysosomal volume and about 45% of the pinocytic vesicle volume of the liver (Blouin et al., 1977). Moreover, specific activities of several lysosomal enzymes are higher in LSECs than in other liver cells (Knook and Sleyster, 1980). LSECs express a set of high-affinity endocytic receptors for soluble macromolecular waste products, generated during normal tissue turnover, blood clotting, inflammatory processes and pathological conditions (McCourt et al., 1999; Skogh et al., 1985; Smedsrod, 2004; Smedsrod et al., 1994; Smedsrod et al., 2006; Smedsrod et al., 1997; Smedsrod et al., 1990). Connective tissue macromolecules including hyaluronan, chondroitin sulphate, collagen α-chain, Procollagen Propeptides (PICP, PINP and PIIINP), products released during cell death such as lysosomal enzymes and metabolic byproducts including oxidized low density lipoproteins (oxLDLs), advanced glycation end products, and immune complexes and microbial CpG motifs are exclusively cleared from the blood circulation by mannose receptor-mediated or scavenger receptor-mediated endocytosis in LSECs (Elvevold et al., 2008; Malovic et al., 2007; Martin-Armas et al., 2006; Skogh et al., 1985; Smedsrod, 2004; Smedsrod et al., 1997; Smedsrod et al., 1990).

LSECs express several different scavenger receptors including scavenger receptors –A, scavenger receptors-B, and scavenger receptors-H (Hughes et al., 1995; Malerod et al., 2002). However, stabilin-1 and stabilin-2 have been recognised as the main scavenger receptors on LSECs (Hansen et al., 2005; Hansen et al., 2002; McCourt et al., 1999; Politz et al., 2002; Zhou et al., 2000). Following receptor mediated endocytosis in LSECs most of the ligands are rapidly degraded intra-lysosomally. Thus, LSECs represent a major site of scavenging and degradation of harmful waste macromolecules from the circulation and have therefore been termed 'scavenger endothelial cells' (Seternes et al., 2002).

LSEC endocytosis of oxLDL may also be implicated in the development of atherosclerosis. Atherosclerosis begins as a progressive, chronic inflammatory condition characterized by thickening of the arterial intima through proliferation of intimal smooth muscle cells, which has been shown to be precipitated by cholesterol-rich LDL and triglycerides derived from chylomicron remnants (Fischer-Dzoga et al., 1976). This may then advance to a complex plaque, which can ultimately lead to serious cardiovascular complications, such as myocardial infarction and stroke from occluded arteries. The oxidative modification of LDL has been suggested to play an important role in the development of these events (Steinberg, 1997, 2009). LDL can undergo *in vivo* oxidation in the arterial walls (Yla-Herttuala et al., 1989) and in plasma (Avogaro et al., 1988; Holvoet et al., 1998b). The process starts within the LDL particle with oxidation of polyunsaturated fatty acids which generates a great number of various intermediate and end-products. Formation of free and organic radicals launches a chain reaction that causes fragmentation of both lipid and protein constituents of LDL. Formation of reactive aldehydes, such as malondialdehyde, 4-hydroxynonenal and glyoxal results in chemical modification of side chain amino groups of the lysine residues of apoB-100, which in turn leads to an increased net negative surface charge of the molecule (Baynes and Thorpe, 1999; Fu et al., 1996; Jialal and Devaraj, 1996; Oorni et al., 2000; Witztum and Steinberg, 1991; Young and McEneny, 2001). Therefore, the oxidative modification of LDL involves changes in both the protein and the lipid components of the LDL-particle. This in turn induces changes in surface charge and conformation, which renders LDL a ligand for scavenger receptors, and reduces or abolishes its affinity to the LDL receptor (Berliner and Heinecke, 1996; Li et al., 2011).

In arterial intima, oxLDLs are taken up by macrophages via scavenger receptors. This induces foam cell formation and subsequent atheroma development (Henriksen et al., 1981, 1983; Steinbrecher et al., 1984). Oxldls are commonly present in atherosclerotic lesions of experimental animals and humans (Palinski et al., 1989; Yla-Herttuala et al., 1989). OxLDL has also been identified in plasma of healthy individuals (Avogaro et al., 1988; Ehara et al., 2001; Itabe and Takano, 2000). In patients with cardiovascular disease, plasma levels of oxLDL have been reported to be approximately fourfold higher than in healthy subjects (Ehara et al., 2001; Holvoet et al., 1998b). In addition to cardiovascular disease, increased levels of oxLDL are associated with ageing (Brinkley et al., 2009) and certain age-related pathologies, such as Alzheimer's disease (Kankaanpaa et al., 2009), glomerulosclerosis (Lee, 1999), and diabetes mellitus (Lopes-Virella et al., 1999).

Therefore, timely clearance and maintenance of low circulatory levels of oxLDLs appear to be important for the prevention of atherosclerosis (Holvoet et al., 1998b; Itabe, 2003). Previously, it has been shown that intravenously injected radiolabeled oxLDLs are rapidly removed from blood by uptake in Kupffer cells and LSECs (Ling et al., 1997; Van Berkel et al., 1991). However, a recent study demonstrated that Kupffer cells are only active in uptake of heavily oxidized LDL (Li et al., 2011). which is mainly present in atherosclerotic plaques (Yla-Herttuala et al., 1989) or formed as an artifact during in vitro oxLDL preparation. At the same time, LSECs hold an exclusive role in the uptake of mildly oxidized LDL from the circulation (Li et al., 2011). Mildly oxidized LDL is the major form of oxLDL found in the blood (Chang et al., 1997; Holvoet et al., 1998a; Holvoet et al., 1998b), and has proatherogenic properties (Berliner et al., 1990; Watson et al., 1997; Witztum and Steinberg, 1991). Both stabilin-1 and stabilin-2 are involved in the endocytic uptake of oxLDL by LSECs. Stabilin-1, however, appears to be more important for the uptake of mildly oxidized LDL, which represents physiological blood-borne oxLDL, while stabilin-2 is important for uptake when there is greater LDL modification (Li et al., 2011).

The morphological changes in the LSEC in old age might also affect its role in endocytosis. Recently, in vivo microscopy was used to examine the real time uptake of scavenger receptor ligands by LSECs (Ito et al., 2007). Endocytosis was clearly diminished in old mice, particularly in the pericentral zone which may indicate hypoxic liver damage. The effect of old age on clearance of oxLDL by LSEC has not been examined yet. However, involvement of stabilin 1 and 2, the two major LSEC scavenger receptors, in the process of oxLDL uptake (Li et al., 2011) makes it likely that oxLDL clearance would be diminished in old age. This change would increase the level of oxLDL in the circulation, thereby promoting its extrahepatic concentration and increasing the risk of the development of atherosclerosis.

6. Conclusions

Age-related changes in morphology and function of LSECs apparently contribute to dyslipidemia and, as a consequence, to the development of cardiovascular disease. Old age is associated with reduced fenestrae in the LSEC which impedes the hepatic uptake of chylomicron remnants and possibly other lipoproteins. In addition, aging is associated with reduced LSEC endocytic capacity which will impact on circulating levels of oxLDL. Thus the LSEC is a novel therapeutic target for the treatment of age-related dyslipidemia and has great potential for the prevention of atherosclerosis and cardiovascular events.

7. References

Akinc, A., M. Goldberg, J. Qin, J. R. Dorkin, C. Gamba-Vitalo, M. Maier, K. N. Jayaprakash, M. Jayaraman, K. G. Rajeev, M. Manoharan, V. Koteliansky, I. Rohl, E. S. Leshchiner, R. Langer, and D. G. Anderson, 2009, Development of lipidoid-siRNA formulations for systemic delivery to the liver: Mol Ther, v. 17, p. 872-9.

Arias, I. M., 1990, The biology of hepatic endothelial cell fenestrae: Prog Liver Dis, v. 9, p. 11-26.

Arii, S., and M. Imamura, 2000, Physiological role of sinusoidal endothelial cells and Kupffer cells and their implication in the pathogenesis of liver injury: J Hepatobiliary Pancreat Surg, v. 7, p. 40-8.

Aschoff, L., 1924, Das reticulo-endotheliale System: Ergebnisse inn. Med Kinderheilk, v. 26, p. 1-118.

Avogaro, P., G. B. Bon, and G. Cazzolato, 1988, Presence of a modified low density lipoprotein in humans: Arteriosclerosis, v. 8, p. 79-87.

Baker, R. W., 2004, Membrane Technology and Applications: Hokoben NJ, John Wiley & Sons Ltd.

Baynes, J. W., and S. R. Thorpe, 1999, Role of oxidative stress in diabetic complications: a new perspective on an old paradigm: Diabetes, v. 48, p. 1-9.

Berliner, J. A., and J. W. Heinecke, 1996, The role of oxidized lipoproteins in atherogenesis: Free Radic Biol Med, v. 20, p. 707-27.

Berliner, J. A., M. C. Territo, A. Sevanian, S. Ramin, J. A. Kim, B. Bamshad, M. Esterson, and A. M. Fogelman, 1990, Minimally modified low density lipoprotein stimulates monocyte endothelial interactions: J Clin Invest, v. 85, p. 1260-6.

Blouin, A., R. P. Bolender, and E. R. Weibel, 1977, Distribution of organelles and membranes between hepatocytes and nonhepatocytes in the rat liver parenchyma. A stereological study: J Cell Biol, v. 72, p. 441-55.

Borel, P., N. Mekki, Y. Boirie, A. Partier, M. C. Alexandre-Gouabau, P. Grolier, and B. Beaufrere, 1998, Comparison of postprandial plasma vitamin A response in young and older adults: J Gerontol, v. 53, p. B133-140.

Brinkley, T. E., B. J. Nicklas, A. M. Kanaya, S. Satterfield, E. G. Lakatta, E. M. Simonsick, K. Sutton-Tyrrell, and S. B. Kritchevsky, 2009, Plasma oxidized low-density lipoprotein levels and arterial stiffness in older adults: the health, aging, and body composition study: Hypertension, v. 53, p. 846-52.

Chang, Y. H., D. S. Abdalla, and A. Sevanian, 1997, Characterization of cholesterol oxidation products formed by oxidative modification of low density lipoprotein: Free Radic Biol Med, v. 23, p. 202-14.

Cogger, V. C., and D. G. Le Couteur, 2009, Fenestrations in the liver sinusoidal endothelial cell, in I. Arias, A. Wolkoff, J. Boyer, D. Shafritz, N. Fausto, H. Alter, and A. Cohen, eds., The Liver: Biology and Pathobiology: Hokoben NJ, John Wiley & Sons, Ltd, p. 387-404.

Cogger, V. C., A. Warren, R. Fraser, M. Ngu, A. J. McLean, and D. G. Le Couteur, 2003, Hepatic sinusoidal pseudocapillarization with aging in the non-human primate: Exp Gerontol, v. 38, p. 1101-1107.

Cooper, A. D., 1997, Hepatic uptake of chylomicron remnants: J Lipid Res, v. 38, p. 2173-92.

Dietschy, J. M., S. D. Turley, and D. K. Spady, 1993, Role of liver in the maintenance of cholesterol and low density lipoprotein homeostasis in different animal species, including humans: J Lipid Res, v. 34, p. 1637-59.

Dobbs, B. R., G. W. Rogers, H. Y. Xing, and R. Fraser, 1994, Endotoxin-induced defenestration of the hepatic sinusoidal endothelium: a factor in the pathogenesis of cirrhosis?: Liver, v. 14, p. 230-3.

Ehara, S., M. Ueda, T. Naruko, K. Haze, A. Itoh, M. Otsuka, R. Komatsu, T. Matsuo, H. Itabe, T. Takano, Y. Tsukamoto, M. Yoshiyama, K. Takeuchi, J. Yoshikawa, and A. E. Becker, 2001, Elevated levels of oxidized low density lipoprotein show a positive relationship with the severity of acute coronary syndromes: Circulation, v. 103, p. 1955-60.

Elvevold, K., J. Simon-Santamaria, H. Hasvold, P. McCourt, B. Smedsrod, and K. K. Sorensen, 2008, Liver sinusoidal endothelial cells depend on mannose receptor-mediated recruitment of lysosomal enzymes for normal degradation capacity: Hepatology, v. 48, p. 2007-15.

Enzan, H., H. Himeno, M. Hiroi, H. Kiyoku, T. Saibara, and S. Onishi, 1997, Development of hepatic sinusoidal structure with special reference to the Ito cells: Microsc Res Tech, v. 39, p. 336-49.

Everitt, A., G. S. Roth, D. G. Le Couteur, and S. N. Hilmer, 2005, Calorie restriction versus drug therapy to delay the onset of aging diseases and extend life: Age, v. 27, p. 1-10.

Fischer-Dzoga, K., R. Fraser, and R. W. Wissler, 1976, Stimulation of proliferation in stationary primary cultures of monkey and rabbit aortic smooth muscle cells. I. Effects of lipoprotein fractions of hyperlipemic serum and lymph: Exp Mol Pathol, v. 24, p. 346-59.

Fraser, R., A. G. Bosanquet, and W. A. Day, 1978, Filtration of chylomicrons by the liver may influence cholesterol metabolism and atherosclerosis: Atherosclerosis, v. 29, p. 113-23.

Fraser, R., L. M. Bowler, W. A. Day, B. Dobbs, H. D. Johnson, and D. Lee, 1980, High perfusion pressure damages the sieving ability of sinusoidal endothelium in rat livers: Br J Exp Pathol, v. 61, p. 222-8.

Fraser, R., W. J. Cliff, and F. C. Courtice, 1968, The effect of dietary fat load on the size and composition of chylomicrons in thoracic duct lymph: Q J Exp Physiol Cogn Med Sci, v. 53, p. 390-8.

Fraser, R., B. R. Dobbs, and G. W. Rogers, 1995, Lipoproteins and the liver sieve: the role of fenestrated sinusoidal endothelium in lipoprotein metabolism, atherosclerosis, and cirrhosis: Hepatology, v. 21, p. 863-874.

Fu, M. X., J. R. Requena, A. J. Jenkins, T. J. Lyons, J. W. Baynes, and S. R. Thorpe, 1996, The advanced glycation end product, Nepsilon-(carboxymethyl)lysine, is a product of both lipid peroxidation and glycoxidation reactions: J Biol Chem, v. 271, p. 9982-6.

Fujioka, Y., and Y. Ishikawa, 2009, Remnant lipoproteins as strong key particles to atherogenesis: J Atheroscler Thromb, v. 16, p. 145-54.

Furrer, K., A. Rickenbacher, Y. Tian, W. Jochum, A. G. Bittermann, A. Kach, B. Humar, R. Graf, W. Moritz, and P. A. Clavien, Serotonin reverts age-related capillarization and failure of regeneration in the liver through a VEGF-dependent pathway: Proc Natl Acad Sci U S A, v. 108, p. 2945-50.

Hansen, B., P. Longati, K. Elvevold, G. I. Nedredal, K. Schledzewski, R. Olsen, M. Falkowski, J. Kzhyshkowska, F. Carlsson, S. Johansson, B. Smedsrod, S. Goerdt, and P. McCourt, 2005, Stabilin-1 and stabilin-2 are both directed into the early endocytic pathway in hepatic sinusoidal endothelium via interactions with clathrin/AP-2, independent of ligand binding: Exp Cell Res, v. 303, p. 160-73.

Hansen, B., D. Svistounov, R. Olsen, R. Nagai, S. Horiuchi, and B. Smedsrod, 2002, Advanced glycation end products impair the scavenger function of rat hepatic sinusoidal endothelial cells: Diabetologia, v. 45, p. 1379-88.

Henriksen, T., E. M. Mahoney, and D. Steinberg, 1981, Enhanced macrophage degradation of low density lipoprotein previously incubated with cultured endothelial cells: recognition by receptors for acetylated low density lipoproteins: Proc Natl Acad Sci U S A, v. 78, p. 6499-503.

Henriksen, T., E. M. Mahoney, and D. Steinberg, 1983, Enhanced macrophage degradation of biologically modified low density lipoprotein: Arteriosclerosis, v. 3, p. 149-59.

Hilmer, S. N., V. C. Cogger, R. Fraser, A. J. McLean, D. Sullivan, and D. G. Le Couteur, 2005a, Age-related changes in the hepatic sinusoidal endothelium impede lipoprotein transfer in the rat: Hepatology, v. 42, p. 1349-54.

Hilmer, S. N., V. C. Cogger, R. Fraser, A. J. McLean, D. Sullivan, and D. G. Le Couteur, 2005b, Age-related changes in the hepatic sinusoidal endothelium impede lipoprotein transfer in the rat: Hepatology, v. 42, p. 1349-1354.

Holvoet, P., J. M. Stassen, J. Van Cleemput, D. Collen, and J. Vanhaecke, 1998a, Oxidized low density lipoproteins in patients with transplant-associated coronary artery disease: Arterioscler Thromb Vasc Biol, v. 18, p. 100-7.

Holvoet, P., J. Vanhaecke, S. Janssens, F. Van de Werf, and D. Collen, 1998b, Oxidized LDL and malondialdehyde-modified LDL in patients with acute coronary syndromes and stable coronary artery disease: Circulation, v. 98, p. 1487-94.

Hughes, D. A., I. P. Fraser, and S. Gordon, 1995, Murine macrophage scavenger receptor: in vivo expression and function as receptor for macrophage adhesion in lymphoid and non-lymphoid organs: Eur J Immunol, v. 25, p. 466-73.

Itabe, H., 2003, Oxidized low-density lipoproteins: what is understood and what remains to be clarified: Biol Pharm Bull, v. 26, p. 1-9.

Itabe, H., and T. Takano, 2000, Oxidized low density lipoprotein: the occurrence and metabolism in circulation and in foam cells: J Atheroscler Thromb, v. 7, p. 123-31.

Ito, Y., K. K. Sorensen, N. W. Bethea, D. Svistounov, M. K. McCuskey, B. H. Smedsrod, and R. S. McCuskey, 2007, Age-related changes in the hepatic microcirculation of mice: Exp Gerontol, v. 48, p. 789-797.

Jamieson, H., S. N. Hilmer, V. C. Cogger, A. Warren, R. Cheluvappa, D. R. Abernethy, A. Everitt, R. Fraser, R. de Cabo, and D. G. Le Couteur, 2007, Caloric restriction reduces age-related pseudocapillarization of the hepatic sinusoid: Experimental Gerontology, v. 42, p. 374-8.

Jialal, I., and S. Devaraj, 1996, Low-density lipoprotein oxidation, antioxidants, and atherosclerosis: a clinical biochemistry perspective: Clin Chem, v. 42, p. 498-506.

Kankaanpaa, J., S. P. Turunen, V. Moilanen, S. Horkko, and A. M. Remes, 2009, Cerebrospinal fluid antibodies to oxidized LDL are increased in Alzheimer's disease: Neurobiol Dis, v. 33, p. 467-72.

Karpe, F., G. Steiner, K. Uffelman, T. Olivecrona, and A. Hamsten, 1994, Postprandial lipoproteins and progression of coronary atherosclerosis: Atherosclerosis, v. 106, p. 83-97.

Kawai, Y., B. Smedsrod, K. Elvevold, and K. Wake, 1998, Uptake of lithium carmine by sinusoidal endothelial and Kupffer cells of the rat liver: new insights into the classical vital staining and the reticulo-endothelial system: Cell Tissue Res, v. 292, p. 395-410.

Knook, D. L., and E. C. Sleyster, 1976, Separation of Kupffer and endothelial cells of the rat liver by centrifugal elutriation: Exp Cell Res, v. 99, p. 444-9.

Knook, D. L., and E. C. Sleyster, 1980, Isolated parenchymal, Kupffer and endothelial rat liver cells characterized by their lysosomal enzyme content: Biochem Biophys Res Commun, v. 96, p. 250-7.

Krasinski, S. D., J. S. Cohn, E. J. Schaefer, and R. M. Russell, 1990, Postprandial plasma retinyl ester response is greater in older subjects compared with younger subjects. Evidence for delayed plasma clearance of intestinal lipoproteins: J Clin Invest, v. 85, p. 883-892.

Lakatta, E. G., and D. Levy, 2003, Arterial and cardiac aging: major shareholders in cardiovascular disease enterprises: Part I: aging arteries: a "set up" for vascular disease: Circulation, v. 107, p. 139-146.

Le Couteur, D. G., V. C. Cogger, S. N. Hilmer, M. Muller, M. Harris, D. Sullivan, A. J. McLean, and R. Fraser, 2006, Aging, atherosclerosis and the liver sieve, in L. V. Clark, ed., New Research on Atherosclerosis: NY, Nova Science, p. 19-44.

Le Couteur, D. G., V. C. Cogger, A. M. A. Markus, P. J. Harvey, Z. L. Yin, A. D. Ansselin, and A. J. McLean, 2001, Pseudocapillarization and associated energy limitation in the aged rat liver: Hepatology, v. 33, p. 537-543.

Le Couteur, D. G., R. Fraser, V. C. Cogger, and A. J. McLean, 2002, Hepatic pseudocapillarisation and atherosclerosis in ageing: Lancet, v. 359, p. 1612-1615.

Le Couteur, D. G., R. Fraser, S. Hilmer, L. P. Rivory, and A. J. McLean, 2005, The hepatic sinusoid in aging and cirrhosis - Effects on hepatic substrate disposition and drug clearance: Clin Pharmacokinet, v. 44, p. 187-200.

Le Couteur, D. G., and A. J. McLean, 1998, The aging liver - Drug clearance and an oxygen diffusion barrier hypothesis: Clin Pharmacokinet, v. 34, p. 359-373.

Le Couteur, D. G., A. Warren, V. C. Cogger, B. Smedsrod, K. K. Sorensen, R. De Cabo, R. Fraser, and R. S. McCuskey, 2008, Old age and the hepatic sinusoid: Anat Rec (Hoboken), v. 291, p. 672-83.

Lee, H. S., 1999, Oxidized LDL, glomerular mesangial cells and collagen: Diabetes Res Clin Pract, v. 45, p. 117-22.

Li, R., A. Oteiza, K. K. Sorensen, P. McCourt, R. Olsen, B. Smedsrod, and D. Svistounov, 2011, Role of liver sinusoidal endothelial cells and stabilins in elimination of oxidized low-density lipoproteins: Am J Physiol Gastrointest Liver Physiol, v. 300, p. G71-81.

Lin, Y., S. S. Mousa, N. Elshourbagy, and S. A. Mousa, Current status and future directions in lipid management: emphasizing low-density lipoproteins, high-density lipoproteins, and triglycerides as targets for therapy: Vasc Health Risk Manag, v. 6, p. 73-85.

Ling, W., M. Lougheed, H. Suzuki, A. Buchan, T. Kodama, and U. P. Steinbrecher, 1997, Oxidized or acetylated low density lipoproteins are rapidly cleared by the liver in mice with disruption of the scavenger receptor class A type I/II gene: J Clin Invest, v. 100, p. 244-52.

Lopes-Virella, M. F., G. Virella, T. J. Orchard, S. Koskinen, R. W. Evans, D. J. Becker, and K. Y. Forrest, 1999, Antibodies to oxidized LDL and LDL-containing immune complexes as risk factors for coronary artery disease in diabetes mellitus: Clin Immunol, v. 90, p. 165-72.

Malerod, L., K. Juvet, T. Gjoen, and T. Berg, 2002, The expression of scavenger receptor class B, type I (SR-BI) and caveolin-1 in parenchymal and nonparenchymal liver cells: Cell Tissue Res, v. 307, p. 173-80.

Malovic, I., K. K. Sorensen, K. H. Elvevold, G. I. Nedredal, S. Paulsen, A. V. Erofeev, B. H. Smedsrod, and P. A. McCourt, 2007, The mannose receptor on murine liver sinusoidal endothelial cells is the main denatured collagen clearance receptor: Hepatology, v. 45, p. 1454-61.

Martin-Armas, M., J. Simon-Santamaria, I. Pettersen, U. Moens, B. Smedsrod, and B. Sveinbjornsson, 2006, Toll-like receptor 9 (TLR9) is present in murine liver sinusoidal endothelial cells (LSECs) and mediates the effect of CpG-oligonucleotides: J Hepatol, v. 44, p. 939-46.

Martinez-Hernandez, A., and P. S. Amenta, 1993, The hepatic extracellular matrix. I. Components and distribution in normal liver: Virchows Arch A Pathol Anat Histopathol, v. 423, p. 1-11.

McCourt, P. A., B. H. Smedsrod, J. Melkko, and S. Johansson, 1999, Characterization of a hyaluronan receptor on rat sinusoidal liver endothelial cells and its functional relationship to scavenger receptors: Hepatology, v. 30, p. 1276-86.

McLean, A. J., V. C. Cogger, G. C. Chong, A. Warren, A. M. Markus, J. E. Dahlstrom, and D. G. Le Couteur, 2003, Age-related pseudocapillarization of the human liver: J Pathol, v. 200, p. 112-117.

McLean, A. J., and D. G. Le Couteur, 2004, Aging biology and geriatric clinical pharmacology: Pharmacol Rev, v. 56, p. 163-184.

Naito, M., and E. Wisse, 1978, Filtration effect of endothelial fenestrations on chylomicron transport in neonatal rat liver sinusoids: Cell Tissue Res, v. 190, p. 371-82.

Nonaka, H., M. Tanaka, K. Suzuki, and A. Miyajima, 2007, Development of murine hepatic sinusoidal endothelial cells characterized by the expression of hyaluronan receptors: Dev Dyn, v. 236, p. 2258-67.

O'Reilly, J. N., V. C. Cogger, R. Fraser, and D. G. Le Couteur, 2010, The effect of feeding and fasting on fenestrations in the liver sinusoidal endothelial cell: Pathology, v. 42, p. 255-8.

O'Reilly, J. N., V. C. Cogger, and D. G. Le Couteur, 2009, Old age is associated with ultrastructural changes in isolated rat liver sinusoidal endothelial cells: J Electron Microsc (Tokyo).

Oorni, K., M. O. Pentikainen, M. Ala-Korpela, and P. T. Kovanen, 2000, Aggregation, fusion, and vesicle formation of modified low density lipoprotein particles: molecular mechanisms and effects on matrix interactions: J Lipid Res, v. 41, p. 1703-14.

Palinski, W., M. E. Rosenfeld, S. Yla-Herttuala, G. C. Gurtner, S. S. Socher, S. W. Butler, S. Parthasarathy, T. E. Carew, D. Steinberg, and J. L. Witztum, 1989, Low density lipoprotein undergoes oxidative modification in vivo: Proc Natl Acad Sci U S A, v. 86, p. 1372-6.

Politz, O., A. Gratchev, P. A. McCourt, K. Schledzewski, P. Guillot, S. Johansson, G. Svineng, P. Franke, C. Kannicht, J. Kzhyshkowska, P. Longati, F. W. Velten, and S. Goerdt, 2002, Stabilin-1 and -2 constitute a novel family of fasciclin-like hyaluronan receptor homologues: Biochem J, v. 362, p. 155-64.

Popper, H., 1986, Aging and the liver: Prog Liver Dis, v. VIII, p. 659-683.

Schmucker, D. L., 1998, Aging and the liver: an update: J Gerontol, v. 53A, p. B315-B320.

Seternes, T., K. Sorensen, and B. Smedsrod, 2002, Scavenger endothelial cells of vertebrates: a nonperipheral leukocyte system for high-capacity elimination of waste macromolecules: Proc Natl Acad Sci U S A, v. 99, p. 7594-7.

Simons, L. A., J. Simons, Y. Friedlander, and J. McCallum, 2001, Cholesterol and other lipids predict coronary heart disease and ischemic stroke in the elderly, but only in those below 70 years: Atherosclerosis, v. 159, p. 201-208.

Skogh, T., R. Blomhoff, W. Eskild, and T. Berg, 1985, Hepatic uptake of circulating IgG immune complexes: Immunology, v. 55, p. 585-94.

Smedsrod, B., 2004, Clearance function of scavenger endothelial cells: Comp Hepatol, v. 3 Suppl 1, p. S22.

Smedsrod, B., P. J. De Bleser, F. Braet, P. Lovisetti, K. Vanderkerken, E. Wisse, and A. Geerts, 1994, Cell biology of liver endothelial and Kupffer cells: Gut, v. 35, p. 1509-16.

Smedsrod, B., K. Elvevold, and I. Martinez, 2006, The liver sinusoidal endothelial cell: a cell type of controversial and confusing identity: 13th International Symposium on Cells of the Hepatic Sinusoid, v. 13th, p. 61-62.

Smedsrod, B., D. Le Couteur, K. Ikejima, H. Jaeschke, N. Kawada, M. Naito, P. Knolle, L. Nagy, H. Senoo, F. Vidal-Vanaclocha, and N. Yamaguchi, 2009, Hepatic sinusoidal cells in health and disease: Liver Int, v. 29, p. 490-501.

Smedsrod, B., J. Melkko, N. Araki, H. Sano, and S. Horiuchi, 1997, Advanced glycation end products are eliminated by scavenger-receptor-mediated endocytosis in hepatic sinusoidal Kupffer and endothelial cells: Biochem J, v. 322 (Pt 2), p. 567-73.

Smedsrod, B., H. Pertoft, S. Gustafson, and T. C. Laurent, 1990, Scavenger functions of the liver endothelial cell: Biochem J, v. 266, p. 313-27.

Stacchiotti, A., A. Lavazza, M. Ferroni, G. Sberveglieri, R. Bianchi, R. Rezzani, and L. F. Rodella, 2008, Effects of aluminium sulphate in the mouse liver: similarities to the aging process: Exp Gerontol, v. 43, p. 330-8.

Steinberg, D., 1997, Low density lipoprotein oxidation and its pathobiological significance: J Biol Chem, v. 272, p. 20963-6.

Steinberg, D., 2009, The LDL modification hypothesis of atherogenesis: an update: J Lipid Res, v. 50 Suppl, p. S376-81.

Steinbrecher, U. P., S. Parthasarathy, D. S. Leake, J. L. Witztum, and D. Steinberg, 1984, Modification of low density lipoprotein by endothelial cells involves lipid peroxidation and degradation of low density lipoprotein phospholipids: Proc Natl Acad Sci U S A, v. 81, p. 3883-7.

Van Berkel, T. J., Y. B. De Rijke, and J. K. Kruijt, 1991, Different fate in vivo of oxidatively modified low density lipoprotein and acetylated low density lipoprotein in rats. Recognition by various scavenger receptors on Kupffer and endothelial liver cells: J Biol Chem, v. 266, p. 2282-9.

Vidal-Vanaclocha, F., and E. Barbera-Guillem, 1985, Fenestration patterns in endothelial cells of rat liver sinusoids: J Ultrastruct Res, v. 90, p. 115-23.

Warren, A., P. Bertolino, V. C. Cogger, A. J. McLean, R. Fraser, and D. G. Le Couteur, 2005, Hepatic pseudocapillarization in aged mice: Exp Gerontol, v. 40, p. 807-12.

Watson, A. D., N. Leitinger, M. Navab, K. F. Faull, S. Horkko, J. L. Witztum, W. Palinski, D. Schwenke, R. G. Salomon, W. Sha, G. Subbanagounder, A. M. Fogelman, and J. A. Berliner, 1997, Structural identification by mass spectrometry of oxidized phospholipids in minimally oxidized low density lipoprotein that induce monocyte/endothelial interactions and evidence for their presence in vivo: J Biol Chem, v. 272, p. 13597-607.

Watson, K. E., B. N. Horowitz, and G. Matson, 2003, Lipid abnormalities in insulin resistant states: Rev Cardiovasc Med, v. 4, p. 228-36.

Williams, K. J., 2008, Molecular processes that handle -- and mishandle -- dietary lipids: J Clin Invest, v. 118, p. 3247-59.

Wisse, E., 1970, An electron microscopic study of the fenestrated endothelial lining of rat liver sinusoids: J Ultrastruct Res, v. 31, p. 125-50.

Wisse, E., F. Braet, D. Luo, R. De Zanger, D. Jans, E. Crabbe, and A. Vermoesen, 1996, Structure and function of sinusoidal lining cells in the liver: Toxicol Pathol, v. 24, p. 100-11.

Witztum, J. L., and D. Steinberg, 1991, Role of oxidized low density lipoprotein in atherogenesis: J Clin Invest, v. 88, p. 1785-92.

Yla-Herttuala, S., W. Palinski, M. E. Rosenfeld, S. Parthasarathy, T. E. Carew, S. Butler, J. L. Witztum, and D. Steinberg, 1989, Evidence for the presence of oxidatively modified low density lipoprotein in atherosclerotic lesions of rabbit and man: J Clin Invest, v. 84, p. 1086-95.

Young, I. S., and J. McEneny, 2001, Lipoprotein oxidation and atherosclerosis: Biochem Soc
      Trans, v. 29, p. 358-62.
Zhou, B., J. A. Weigel, L. Fauss, and P. H. Weigel, 2000, Identification of the hyaluronan
      receptor for endocytosis (HARE): J Biol Chem, v. 275, p. 37733-41.

2

Dyslipidemia and Cardiovascular Disease

Hossein Fakhrzadeh and Ozra Tabatabaei-Malazy
Endocrinology & Metabolism Research Center,
Tehran University of Medical Sciences,Tehran,
Islamic Republic of Iran

1. Introduction

Four non-communicable diseases (NCDs) including cardiovascular disease (CVD), cancer, chronic respiratory disease, and diabetes were announced by World Health Organization (WHO) as the major causes of mortality in the world in 2008(Alwan, 2008). According to WHO prediction, in the next 10 years, mortality rate caused by NCDs will increase by 17 percent with the highest mortality rate in the regions of Africa (27 percent) and Eastern Mediterranean (EMRO, 25 percent) (Alwan, 2008). Fortunately more than 80 percent of heart disease, stroke, and type 2 diabetes mellitus incidence and almost one third of cancers could be prevented with appropriate interventions to reduce the effect of risk factors (Alwan, 2008).

Dyslipidemia, as a risk factor of CVD, is manifested by elevation or attenuation of plasma concentration of lipoproteins. Several methods have been used to classify the lipoproteins in respect to their density, physical, and chemical properties. Based on these classifications, different types of lipoproteins, including chylomicrones, IDL[1], VLDL[2], LDL[3,] and HDL[4], and apolipoproteins (Apo), including Apo A, Apo B, Apo C, and Apo E, have been introduced. Generally, dyslipidemia is defined as the total cholesterol, LDL, triglycerides, apo B or Lp (a) levels above the 90th percentile or HDL and apo A levels below the 10th percentile of the general population (Dobsn et al., 1996).

CVD is the most common health problem worldwide. This disease is often manifested as coronary heart disease (CHD). According to the international reports, mortality of CHD in the developed countries is expected to reach almost 29 percent in women and 48 percent in men in years 1990-2020. These figures have been estimated to increase by 120 percent in women and 137 percent in men (Thom et al., 1998) in the developing countries.

Atherosclerosis is the most common cause of CHD. According to recent epidemiological studies, hypercholesterolemia and possibly coronary atherosclerosis are suggested as the sole risk factors of ischemic stroke. The results of a meta-analysis of 10 large cohort studies (Law et al., 1994) showed that for each 0.6 mmol/l reduction in serum cholesterol levels in

---

[1] Intermediate Density Lipoprotein
[2] Very Low Density Lipoprotein
[3] Low Density Lipoprotein
[4] High Density lipoprotein

those aged 60 years, the risk of CHD decreased by 27 percent, which manifested a calculated relative risk of 0.73. With three times reduction in serum cholesterol (1.80 mmol/l or 70mg/dl), the relative risk of CHD was 0.39 $(0.73)^3$ and risk reduction reached to 61 percent. The expected benefits of total cholesterol and LDL reduction seem to be in both primary and secondary prevention of CHD. Protective effects of HDL against initial coronary events in secondary prevention (Barter et al., 2007; Rosenson, 2007) was even observed in levels of higher than 75 mg/dl with long lifetime protection (Longevity Syndrome) and emancipation of the relative risk of coronary disease. Based on these observations, current attempt for stroke prevention is mostly focused on intensive treatment with lipid-lowering drugs (Gorelick et al., 1997).

In spite of a decline in cardiac events and coronary mortality rates, many people who are under appropriate treatment are still exposed to these events. In a population-based study regarding hypercholesterolemia awareness (Nieto et al., 1995), only 42% of population were informed of their hypercholesterolemia and only 4% were under lipid-lowering drug treatment. Need assessment to better understand the role of lipids and its subgroups including; VLDL, Small dense LDL, lipoprotein (a), and subgroups of HDL in pathogenesis of CVD calls for a general awareness regarding these topics. In this context, the major challenges would be: 1 – to identify those who need treatment (with or without past history of coronary artery disease), 2 – to develop more effective treatment strategies for patients with coronary artery disease (whether individuals were treated with lipid-lowering drugs or people who have not received adequate treatment), 3 – to adequately treat other high risk individuals such as diabetic, hypertensive, and old subjects.

1.1 Objective

Main objective of this chapter is to express the relationship between lipid disorders and CVD according to the top epidemiological studies in the world. Other minor objectives include; evaluation of role of dyslipidaemia in the incidence of CVD, and also assessment of the role of different types of lipoproteins in this area.

1.2 Expected outcomes

- To increase general awareness regarding the relationship between lipid disorders and CVD
- To reduce the morbidity and mortality of CVD (by primary or secondary prevention)

2. World epidemiological evidences of association between dyslipidemia and CVD

CVD is widespread among general population. Reports received from late 1990s indicate that the ultimate cause of death in adults is CVD (Murray & Lopez, 1997). It has been predicted that CVD will become the ultimate cause of disability in the world between years 2000-2025 (Murray & Lopez, 1997). Common lifestyle determinants such as western diet, physical inactivity, tobacco consumption and also increase in life expectancy are linked to elevation of CVD prevalence (Critchley et al., 1999).

According to data published from the autopsy studies in 1960s, the origin of early lesions of atherosclerosis in adults is mostly caused by consumption of Western diet. The prevalence and severity of fibroid plaques and calcified lesions as signs of CVD were significantly lower in Asia, underdeveloped countries and consumers of Mediterranean diet (Eggen et al., 1964).

2.1 Total and LDL cholesterol

Two decades after World War II, large population studies had been performed in different countries in order to determine risk factors of heart disease. The most famous studies include the Framingham Study, Chicago and Tecumseh in USA (Butler et al., 1985; Dawber et al., 1951; Dyer et al., 1981; Keys, 1970) and Seven Country Studies including studies in England, Sweden and Norway (Fager et al., 1981; Keys et al., 1984; Miller et al., 1977) in European countries. The major finding of these cohort studies was that in addition to serum cholesterol levels, other factors also are involved in development of coronary heart disease. Among the main risk factors, dyslipidemia, especially increase in LDL levels and decrease in HDL concentrations were considered as the important factors. Table-1 demonstrates the Population Attributable Factors (PARs) with its 99 percent confidence interval (CI) associated with lipids by sex and geographic region (Labarthe, 2011; Yusuf et al., 2004). In some countries, PAR estimation in women is based on small numbers which makes them less reliable.

Region	Lipids in men % (CI 99%)	Lipids in women % (CI 99%)	Lipids in both sexes % (CI 99%)
West Europe	36.7 (10.7-73.8)	47.9 (20.3-76.8)	44.6 (23.5-67.8)
Central & eastern Europe	38.7 (20.0-61.4)	26.8 (5.9-68.2)	35.0 (19.2-54.9)
Middle East	72.7 (58.8-83.2)	63.3 (32.0-86.3)	70.5 (57.8-80.7)
Africa	73.7 (55.2-86.4)	74.6 (49.1-90.0)	74.1 (59.7-84.6)
South Asia	60.2 (42.5-75.6)	52.1 (19.0-83.5)	58.7 (42.7-73.1)
China	41.3 (32.4-50.7)	48.3 (36.9-59.9)	43.8 (36.7-51.2)
Southeast Asia and Japan	68.7 (51.2-82.1)	64.5 (29.5-88.7)	67.7 (52.0-80.2)
Australia & New Zealand	48.7 (17.5-80.9)	14.9 (0.0-99.6)	43.4 (16.0-75.6)
South America	41.6 (20.2-66.6)	59.3 (30.5-82.9)	47.6 (29.6-66.2)
North America	60.0 (22.2-88.8)	32.2 (1.1-95.1)	50.5 (18.2-82.4)
Overall adjusted for age, sex & smoking	53.8 (48.3-59.2)	52.1 (44.0-60.2)	54.1 (49.6-58.6)
Overall adjusted for risk factors	49.5 (43.0-55.9)	47.1 (37.4-57.0)	49.2 (43.8-54.5)

Legend: CI: Confidence Interval.

Table 1. Population Attributable Factors (PARs) associated with lipids in men & women by geographic region.

In parallel to these large population studies, a series of case studies were also performed. In one study, serum lipid levels were evaluated in 500 men with a prior history of myocardial infarction. Overall 30 percent of study population had abnormal blood lipid levels (Goldstein et al., 1973). High levels of cholesterol in 8 percent, triglycerides in7 percent and concomitant high cholesterol and triglycerides in15 percent were reported by this study.

In normal individuals from different communities, plasma levels of lipids vary due to differences in genetic background and diet. For example, the average cholesterol levels, according to age, in western and Chinese men are 202 mg/dl and165 mg/dl, respectively (Caroll et al., 2005; Wu et al., 2004). Based on results of the National Health and Nutrition Examination Surveys (NHANES) from 1999 to 2004, the percentage of adults with triglyceride levels above 150 and 200 mg/dl in the United States, were 33 and 18 percent, respectively (Ford et al., 2009). In the United States, the NHANES from 2005 to 2008 found that 98.8 million adults have total cholesterol levels ≥ 200 mg/dl, 33.6% of them having a total cholesterol level ≥ 240 mg/dl (American Heart Association [AHA], 2011).

Table-2 shows the prevalence of high levels of total cholesterol (cholesterol ≥ 200 mg/dl), LDL (LDL cholesterol ≥130 mg/dl), and HDL (HDL cholesterol≤ 40 mg/dl) in adults aged ≥20 years, according to NHANES (American Heart Association [AHA], 2011).

	Non-Hispanic White		Non-Hispanic Black		Mexican-American	
	M	F	M	F	M	F
Total cholesterol						
200-239 mg/dl	41.2	47.0	37.0	41.2	50.1	46.5
≥ 240 mg/dl	13.7	16.9	9.7	13.3	16.9	14.0
LDL cholesterol						
≥130 mg/dl	30.5	32.0	34.4	27.7	41.9	31.6
HDL cholesterol						
≤ 40 mg/dl	29.5	10.1	16.6	6.6	31.7	12.2

Legend: M: Male; F: Female; LDL: Low Density Lipoprotein; HDL: High Density Lipoprotein.

Table 2. Proportion of USA adults aged ≥ 20 years with dyslipidemia by ethnicity and gender

In MONICA[5] project designed for more than 30 countries in different regions of WHO coverage except the US, the percentage of hypercholesterolemia for individuals aged between 35-64 years and total cholesterol levels between 5.2-7.8 mmol/1 (approximately 200-300 mg/dl) was found to be lowest (20%) among the men in China-Beijing and highest (76%) in France-Strasbourg. The lowest percent of women with hypercholesterolemia (5%) was in Australia-Perth population and the highest percent (76%) was observed in Germany-Bremen (WHO MONICA project, 2008). However, these figures were different when the total cholesterol level >7.8 mmol/1 was considered as hypercholesterolemia. None of the China-Beijing's men had the serum cholesterol levels >7.8 mmol/1 (0%) while 15% of Switzerland-Ticino men had hypercholesterolemia (highest percent). for women these figures were 0% in China-Beijing and 14% in Lithuania-Kaunas (WHO MONICA project, 2008).

---

[5] Multinational MONItoring of trends and determinants in CArdiovascular disease

The WHO MONICA project showed (WHO MONICA project, 1989) that the average of total cholesterol in 30 studied areas varied from 158 mg/dl (in the Beijing, China) to 246 mg/dl (Loczamburk, Germany) for men and from 162 mg/dl (Beijing, China) to 246 mg/dl (Glasgow, UK) in women. In addition, there was a difference in prevalence of hypercholesterolemia in different regions, from 2 percent in Beijing, China to nearly 50 percent in Lille, France (WHO MONICA project, 1989). An intermediate reduction in cholesterol level of MONICA project study populations during 5-6 year follow-up was observed. The mean annual decrease in total serum cholesterol was 0.4-3 mg/dl (Dobsn et al., 1996).

The highest incidence of hyperlipidemia is shown in patients with premature coronary artery disease, which occurs before age 55 years in men and 65 years in women. Prevalence of dyslipidemia in these patients is equal to 80-88 percent, compared to 40-48 percent in age-matched controls without CHD (Genest et al., 1992; Roncaglioni et al., 1992). In these conditions, 12.5 percent of patients with a prior history of premature coronary disease and 58.5 percent of age-matched controls without prior history of coronary disease have normal lipid profiles.

MRFIT[6] study performed in more than 350,000 middle-aged men demonstrated (Stamler et al., 1986) that a sigmoid relationship (curvilinear) between total serum cholesterol level and prevalence of coronary artery disease especially in total cholesterol more than 240 mg/dl is presented (Figure-1).

The strongest association was found in population from United States and Finland, the intermediate association was observed in European population, and the least correlation was related to Japanese men and rural area of Greece. The relationship between serum cholesterol and incidence of CVD become stronger when the number of risk factors was increased (Kannel, 1983).

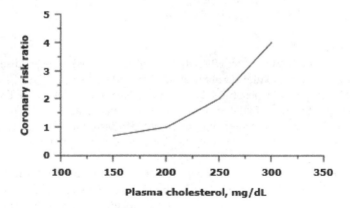

Fig. 1. Association between plasma cholesterol and coronary risk among MRFIT study

---

[6] Multiple Risk Factor Intervention Trial

Similar results were obtained from Framingham and Migration studies (Kannel et al., 1971, 1979). The Migration study is one of the strong studies evaluating the relationship between increased serum cholesterol and risk of CVD. This study was done in 1960 and compared Japanese men residing in Japan with immigrated Japanese to Honolulu and San Francisco. In Japanese men living in their native country, the mean total cholesterol levels and CHD rate were lower compared to immigrated population. In immigrated Japanese, those who live in Hawaii had lower lipid levels than those in San Francisco. Considering race similarity in this study, the reason for observed differences in rate of CHD and cholesterol levels can be related to differences in dietary cholesterol and fat consumption (Kagen et al., 1974).

However the results of other studies on immigrants were not always similar to the Migration study. In one study (Kushi et al., 1985), diet produced no effect on cholesterol levels or heart disease mortality. In General, the importance of age, sex and race on levels of cholesterol has been shown in population-based studies.

Invention of ultracentrifuge has facilitated measurement of the various lipid parameters. LRCP (Lipid Research Clinics Program) was one of the first surveys during 1970 that was conducted to determine the total cholesterol, HDL cholesterol, LDL cholesterol and triglyceride levels in American adults (Heiss et al., 1980). In another study, difference in distribution of cholesterol and its components in the blood in accordance to age were described (Glueek & Stein, 1979). In both sexes, the slope of total cholesterol curve is increased by increase in age until the end of middle-age. After that, by increasing the age, slope of the curve is downward until reaching the old age. Mean total cholesterol in men and women aged between 20 -50 years is similar, however, the levels of HDL cholesterol in women after puberty is higher than men (Rifkind & Segal, 1983).

Among patients with a prior history of myocardial infarction, an elevated total cholesterol following recovery was a major independent risk factor for reinfarction, death from heart disease and total mortality. Cardiovascular mortality is varied in different populations. The highest and lowest mortality rate was found in Finland and Japan, respectively, with a direct relationship to serum cholesterol levels (Rosenson, 2011).

2.2 HDL cholesterol

The negative relationship between low HDL cholesterol and the risk of heart disease is well stablished in the general population (Abbott et al., 1988; Abbott et al., 1998; Castelli, 1983; Gordon et al, 1989; Harper & Jacobson, 1999; Rosenson, 2005) (figure-2). In the Framingham Heart study, the protective role of HDL has been well described (Kannel et al., 1971).

Based on results of this study, by each 5 mg /dl decrease in serum levels of HDL (compared to mean normal values for men and women), the risk of myocardial infarction was increased by 25 percent.

Predictive role of HDL against coronary events was also well documented in patients with known heart disease. The results of Lipid and Care clinical trial showed that low levels of HDL cholesterol is a stronger predictor of heart disease incidence in presence of serum LDL cholesterol < 125 mg/dl than LDL cholesterol ≥ 125 mg/dl (Sacks et al., 2002). They also found that in serum LDL<125 mg/dl, each 10 mg /dl increase in HDL level, will cause 29 percent reduction in the incidence of cardiovascular events , while with the serum LDL cholesterol ≥ 125 mg/dl, this attenuation will be lowered to 10 percent. This association was also seen in post hoc analysis of TNT[7] study, in which 10000 known cases of CVD were under-treatment with different doses of statins (Barter et al., 2007).

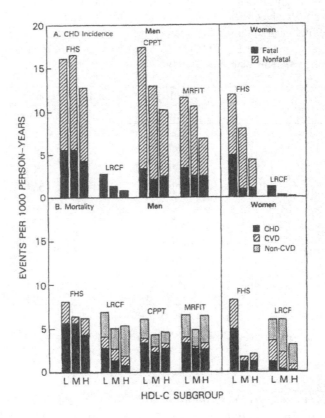

Legend: CHD: Coronary heart disease; L M H HDL: Low, middle, high, high density lipoprotein; CVD: Cardiovascular disease; FHS: Framingham Heart Study; LRCF: Lipid Research Clinics Prevalence Mortality Follow-up Study; CPPT: Lipid Research Clinics Coronary Primary Prevention Trial; MRFIT: Multiple Risk Factor Intervention Trial.

Fig. 2. Inverse association between HDL and CVD events.

As mentioned previously, the cardioprotective effect of HDL was shown to be present at serum levels higher than 60 mg/dl (Castelli et al., 1983). These effects are more prominent when the serum levels of HDL cholesterol reach 75 mg/dl and higher (Table-3).

In assessment of 18 relatives with familial hyperalfa–lipoproteinemia, the life long of these men and women were found to be 5 and 7 years, respectively, more than general population (Glueck et al., 1976).

---

[7] Treating to New Targets trial

In the Lipid Research Clinics study, the Framingham heart Study and the HHS[8] the ratio of LDL to HDL was shown to be the best predictor of cardiovascular events (Manninen et al., 1992; Kinosian et al., 1994). In HHS study, the risk of new coronary events such as myocardial infarction and sudden cardiac death in patients with LDL/HDL ≥ 5 and a concomitant serum triglycerides ≥ 200 mg /dl, was fourfold more than patients with lower LDL/HDL ratio and triglycerides levels. Overall, among men, an LDL/HDL ratio of ≥ 6.4 had 2–14 percent higher predictive value than serum total cholesterol or LDL levels. Among women the predictive value of LDL/HDL ≥ 5.6 was 25–45 percent greater than serum total cholesterol or LDL level (Kinosian et al., 1994).

HDL (mg/dl)	Multiplier for cardiovascular risk	
	men	women
30	1.82	----
35	1.49	----
40	1.22	1.94
45	1.00	1.55
50	0.82	1.25
55	0.67	1.00
60	0.55	0.80
65	0.45	0.64
70	----	0.52
75	Longevity syndrome	Longevity syndrome

Legend: HDL: High Density Lipoprotein.

Table 3. Inverse relation between plasma HDL-cholesterol levels and cardiovascular risk in men and women.

2.3 Triglycerides
The relationship between hypertriglyceridemia and CVD was determined in the population-based Stockholm prospective study (Carlson et al., 1979). In this study, 3,486 subjects were followed for 14.5 years. An independent relation between hypertriglyceridemia and CVD was observed in this study, which was stronger than the relationship between hypercholesterolemia and CVD. Meta-analysis of several large population–based prospective studies showed similar results (Hokanson & Austin, 1996). Based on this study, the univariate risk ratio (RR) of triglyceride, independent of HDL and other CVD risk factors, among men was 1.32 (95 percent CI, 1.26 to 1.39) and among women was 1.76 (95 percent CI, 1.50 to 2.07).

As mentioned previously in the HHS study, not only there is an interaction between triglycerides and total cholesterol/HDL ratio, but also an inverse association between triglycerides and HDL levels exists (Rosenson, 2011). Additionally, hypertriglyceridemia is associated with increased mortality in patients with known CHD and also reduces the

---

[8] Helsinki Heart Study

event–free survival after coronary artery bypass graft surgery (CABG) (Haim et al., 1999; Sprecher et al., 2000).

Nevertheless, because hypertriglyceridemia is an independent risk factor for CVD, measurement of triglycerides as a part of routine cholesterol screening is recommended by NECP ATPIII guidelines (Haim et al., 1999). Fasting triglyceride measurement is important for evaluating the risk of heart disease especially in cases who are suffering from diabetes, glucose intolerance, insulin resistance syndrome, obesity and low HDL. Although, triglyceride measurement is commonly done after 8–12 hours fasting, an association between nonfasting triglyceride levels and CVD is also present (Nordestgaard et al., 2007; Bansal et al., 2007).

2.4 Non-HDL cholesterol

Non–HDL cholesterol is defined as the difference between total and HDL cholesterols. Thus it includes LDL, Lp (a), IDL and VLDL (Ballantyne et al., 2000). In both LRCP study and the Women's Health Study non-HDL cholesterol has been suggested as a better tool for risk assessment of CVD than LDL levels (Cobbaert et al., 1997; Ridker et al., 2005). In the LRCP study in which the patients were followed for an average of 19 years, a 30 mg/dl difference in non–HDL and LDL concentrations, produced 19 and 15 percent, increase in mortality risk of CVD among men, respectively, and 11 and 8 percent, among women, respectively, (Cobbaert et al., 1997).

2.5 Lipoprotein (a)

Lipoprotein (a), also called Lp (a), is established as an independent risk factor for CVD. Lp (a) is a modified form of LDL with a structure similar to plasminogen (Steyrer et al., 1994) that could interfere with fibrinolysis by competing with plasminogen for binding to cells (Loscalzo et al., 1990; Palabrica et al., 1995). Lp (a) also binds to macrophages to promote foam cell formation and deposition of cholesterol in atherosclerotic plaques (Zioncheck et al., 1991). Thus, Lp (a) accelerates atherosclerosis process by impairing fibrinolysis and increasing LDL oxidation (Stein & Rosenson, 1997). Evidences of association between Lp (a) excess [Lp (a) levels above the 95th percentile] and CVD mostly come from 2 large meta-analyses that found positive continuous correlation between Lp (a) and risk of CVD events (Bennet et al., 2008; Emerging et al., 2009). The 24 cohort studies in the meta-analysis (Bennet et al., 2008) found a risk ratio of 1.13 (95 percent CI, 1.09 to 1.18) between the top and third bottom baseline Lp (a) levels after adjustment for multiple traditional cardiovascular risk factors. Lp (a) excess concentration is usually detected in patients with premature CHD. In one study 18.6 percent of patients with premature CHD had excess levels of Lp (a), while 12.7 percent of them had no dyslipidemia (Genest et al., 1992).

LP (a) increases the risk of cerebrovascular disease, peripheral vascular disease, myocardial infarction (MI), re–stenosis after angioplasty, and failure after CABG (Rosengren et al., 1990; Schaefer et al., 1994). 12 years and more follow–up of patients in the Framingham Heart study showed that Lp (a) can increase the risk of premature coronary heart disease by two-times (Bostom et al., 1996), and augment the risk of MI, intermittent claudication, cerebrovascular disease, and coronary artery stenosis. In the 4S[9] study an association between increased Lp (a) levels and overall mortality rate was also observed (Bostom et al., 1994).

---

[9] Scandinavian Simvastatin Survival Study

2.6 Apolipoproteins & atherogenic lipoprotein phenotype

There are limited prospective studies about the relationship between apolipoproteins (apo A-I and apo B) and the CVD risk. The QCS[10] was studied 2155 men aged between 45-76 years and reported a direct correlation between apo B levels and prevalence of ischemic heart disease over the future 5 years, [relative risk (RR) 1.4; 95 percent CI, 1.2 to 1.7] (Lamarche et al., 1996), independent of other risk factors of CVD. For apo A-I, a negative correlation (RR = 0.85; 95 percent CI, 0.7 to 1.0) was reported.

Since the measurement of apo B and apo A-I is an indicator of total atherogenic (lDL, VLDL, and LDL) and antiatherogenic particles (HDL), some studies (Lamarche et al., 1996; Meisinger et al., 2005; Yusuf et al., 2004; Walldius et al., 2001, 2005) proposed that measurements of apo B and apo A are more important predictors of the CVD than above measurements. The AMORIS[11] study evaluated this relationship in 175,553 subjects with 65 months follow up (Walldius et al., 2001). In the multivariate analysis the apo B concentration was significantly higher than LDL levels and served as a better predictor of CVD than LDL.

The results regarding the role of apolipoproteins in prediction of CVD risk are conflicting. Two studies; Women's Health Study and the Framingham Study obtained a similar predictive value for apo B/A-I ratio versus total cholesterol/ HDL ratio (Ridker et al., 2005; Ingelsson & Schaefer, 2007). However, in contrast to Health Professionals Follow-up Study (Pischon et al., 2005; Sniderman, 2005) and AMORIS study, apo A-I and apo B did not have any predictive value for CHD risk in ARIC[12] study (Sharrett et al., 2001). The explanation for these disparate results is not clear. However, it seems apolipoproteins have a potential role in CHD risk stratification. Standardization of laboratory methods and measurements to the same reference system, and establishing threshold and target values for diagnosis could help recognize the full potential of apolipoproteins (Srinivasan & Berenson, 2001; Denke, 2005).

Apo E is important in plasma lipid metabolism and Apo E gene affects plasma levels of LDL. Three major apo E isoforms are E2, E3, and E4, which are encoded by three common alleles at the APO E locus. The less common and the most common isoforms in society are E2 and E3, respectively. E4 allele is associated with higher plasma total cholesterol and LDL cholesterol levels and with risk of heart attack. In contrast, subjects with E2 allele have lower risk of heart attack compared to people with E4 isoform (Song et al., 2004).

Some clinical researches have focused on the relationship between small dense LDL particles and risk of CVD. This status, also called atherogenic lipoprotein phenotype, is usually associated with increased triglyceride, VLDL and LDL levels (Krauss, 1994). The Physician's Health Study showed that small dense LDL particles can increase three times the risk of CVD more than LDL cholesterol (Zambon et al., 1996). In QCS study, during 5 year follow up, 114 cases from a total of 2103 were diagnosed with heart disease. In this study, in multivariate analysis small dense LDL was more important predictor of CVD [odds ratio (OR) = 3.7; 95 percent CI, 1.4 to 9.7) than LDL (OR = 1.8; 95 percent CI, 1.2 to 2.9) (Lamarche et al., 1997). The Familial atherosclerosis Treatment Study (FATS) found that LDL subclasses were the most important predictor of coronary progression (Zambon et al., 1999). In the Pravastatin Limitation of Atherosclerosis in the Coronaries (PLAC–I) study showed that

---

[10] Quebec Cardiovascular Study
[11] Apolipoprotein-related MOrtality RISk
[12] Atherosclerosis risk in Communities

small LDL particle size (≤ 20.5 nm) could increase rate of coronary progression with OR= 5.0 and 95 percent CI, 1 to 9. High numbers of small LDL particles (>30 mg/dl) was the most important lipoprotein predictor in multivariate analysis (OR = 9.1; 95 percent CI, 2.1 to 39) (Otvos et al., 2002).

In the FATS[13] study 95 percent variance in regression of atherosclerosis in coronary arteries were related to changes in lipid profile. Adding the LDL density to the equation showed that almost 45 percent of the variance was related to changes in LDL density (Lamarche et al., 1997). In contrast, the CHS[14] reported that LDL particle concentration and not LDL size acted as a significant predictor of MI and angina in women, in which by every 100 nmol/l increase in LDL particle number, the OR of MI and angina increased by 11 percent (Kuller et al., 2002).

In Women's Health Study which assessed LDL particle size and concentration by NMR[15] , the LDL particle concentration was a strong predictor of CVD after adjustment for traditional risk factors (Blake et al., 2002).

EPIC[16]- Norfolk prospective Population Study examined NMR-measured LDL particle size and concentration (El Harchaoui et al., 2007) and found that LDL particle concentration did not increase the prediction of CHD. After LDL particle concentration adjustment, LDL size was no longer associated with CHD.

Recently, some scientists from the University of Warwick in UK discovered a modified form of LDL, MGmin-LDL, also called super-sticky LDL, or very-bad LDL, that promotes CVD (Rabbani et al., 2011). High levels of this lipid are more common in diabetics and elderly patients. Diabetic subjects present almost four times more serum levels of MGmin-LDL than normal subjects. This may explain the high frequency of CVD in diabetics and elderly patients. Rabbani et al (Rabbani et al., 2011) found that secondary to hyperglycemia, LDL is glycated with methylglyoxal (MG) and makes a type of LDL with smaller, stickier and more atherogenic LDL than normal LDL. The MGmin-LDL can help to build fatty plaques. When these plaques grow, the wall of arteries become narrower and the blood flow reduces. Plaque rapture, an event that would eventually happen, triggers the blood clot cascades that could cause a heart attack or stroke. In elderly, the activity of the enzyme for detoxification of MGmin-LDL is reduced. They (Rabbani et al., 2011) also showed that metformin can block the glycation processes which might explain the cardioprotective effects of this drug. This discovery could lead to invention of new treatments for CVD prevention especially in type 2 diabetics and the elderly subjects.

3. Summary

The relationships described above can be summarized in the figure-3 (Ridker et al., 2005). This figure shows the adjusted Hazard ratios of future cardiovascular events among patients who are in the extreme quintiles of each measured marker. Black bars present 95 percent CI.

---

[13] Familial Atherosclerosis Regression Study
[14] Cardiovascular health Study
[15] Nuclear Magnetic Resonance
[16] European Prospective Investigation into Cancer and Nutrition

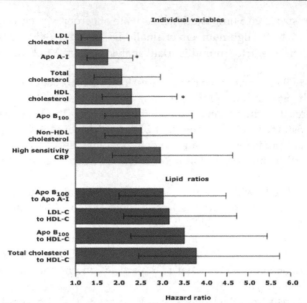

Legend: LDL: Low Density Lipoprotein; Apo A-I: Apolipoprotein A-I; HDL: High Density Lipoprotein; Apo B100: Apolipoprotein B100; CRP: C - reactive protein.

Fig. 3. Adjusted Hazard ratios for future cardiovascular events.

Today, interventional studies have investigated the effects of augmentation of HDL levels. The clinical trials which deal with this matter will be discussed in a separate part. In assessment of dyslipidemia two points should be stipulated:

1. Decline of coronary events could be possible by modifying the serum lipid levels in order to prevent or delay the reduction of vessel diameter, and also to stabilize atheroma plaques. Small plaques are mostly filled with lipid and are prone to disposable rupture, thrombosis, acute, serious and ultimately fatal atherosclerosis. Reduction of LDL leads to removal of fatty deposits from the inside of the atheroma plaque and makes them more stable. In addition, lowering the lipids levels can return the normal activity of vessel wall endothelium and its ability to produce nitric oxide, the main mediator of coronary vasodilation (Krauss, 1994).

2. During lipid-lowering drug therapy the cost-effectiveness of the treatment should be considered. This depends on the price of drugs as well as patient's risk. For example, at least cost-effectiveness includes patients with intermediate elevation of serum cholesterol, who, without any other risk factors, are under- lipid lowering agent therapy. In 4S study which was performed in patients with high risk of CVD, cost per year of life gain, was depended on age, sex and baseline levels of lipid. The range of this cost was varied from 3,800 $ U.S. for men aged 70 years and the mean serum cholesterol 309 mg/dl, to 27,400 $ U.S. for women aged 35 years and the average serum cholesterol 213 mg/dl (Johannessonet al., 1997). In other studies these figures were different from 19,000 $ U.S. to 56,000 $ U.S. which depends on drug dose and formulation used. Also, these costs were three folds, two folds and 1.3 folds more in women at age 40, 60 and 70 years, respectively, when compared with the men at age 40 years (Martens & Guibert, 1994; Thorvik et al., 1996).

4. References

Abbott RD, Wilson PWF, Kannel WB, Castelli WP (1988). High density lipoprotein cholesterol, total cholesterol screening, and myocardial infarction: the Framingham Study. *Arteriosclerosis*; 8: 207–11.

Abbott RD, Yano K, Hakim AA (1998). Changes in total and high - density lipoprotein holesterol over 10- and 20–year periods (the Honolulu Heart program). *Am J Cardiol*; 82: 172–8.

Alwan A (2008). 2008–2013 action plan for the global strategy for the prevention and control of noncommunicable diseases. *Report World Health Organization*.

Ballantyne CM, Grundy SM, Oberman A, et al (2000). Hyperlipidemia: diagnostic and therapeutic perspectives. *J Clin Endocrinol Metab*; 85:2089–112.

Bansal S, Buring JE, Rifai N, et al (2007). Fasting compared with nonfasting triglycerides and risk of cardiovascular events in women. *JAMA*; 298:309–16.

Barter P, Gotto AM, LaRosa JC, Maroni J, Szarek M, Grundy SM, et al (2007). HDL cholesterol, very low levels of LDL cholesterol, and cardiovascular events. *N Engl J Med*; 357: 1301–10.

Bennet A, Di Angelantonio E, Erqou S, et al (2008). Lipoprotein (a) levels and risk of future coronary heart disease: large-scale prospective data. *Arch Intern Med*; 168:598– 608.

Blake GJ, Otvos JD, Rifai N, Ridker PM (2002). Low–density lipoprotein particle concentration and size as determined by nuclear magnetic resonancespectroscopy as predictors of cardiovascular disease in women. *Circulation*; 106: 1930–7.

Blood cholesterol levels by sex, adults aged 35–64, latest available data MONICA project population, 4th August 2008, Available from:
http://www.ktl.fi/publications/monica.

Bostom AG, Gagnon DR, Cupples LA, et al (1994). A prospective investigation of elevated LP (a) detected by electrophoresis and cardiovascular disease in women: the Framingham Heart Study. *Circulation*; 90: 1688–95.

Bostom AG, Cupples LA, Jenner JL, et al (1996). Elevated plasma lipoprotein (a) and coronary heart disease in men aged 55 years and younger: a prospective study. *JAMA*; 276: 544–48.

Butler WJ, Ostrander LDJ, Carman WJ (1985). Mortality from coronary heart disease in the Tecumseh Study: long–term effect of diabetes mellitus, glucose tolerance and other risk factors. *Am J Epidemiol*; 121: 541–7.

Carlson LA, Böttiger LE, Ahfeldt PE (1979). Risk factors for myocardial infarction in the Stockholm prospective study. A 14–year follow-up focussing on the role of plasma triglycerides and cholesterol. *Acta Med Scand*;206(5):351–60.

Caroll MD, Lacher DA, Sorlie PD, Cleeman JI, Gordon DJ, Wolz M, et al. (2005).Trends in serum lipids and lipoproteins of adults, 1960–2002. *JAMA*; 294:1773– 81.

Castelli WP (1983). Cardiovascular disease and multifactorial risk: Challenge of the 1980s. *Am Heart J*; 106: 1191–200.

Cobbaert C, Jukema JW, Zwinderman AH, et al (1997). Modulation of lipoprotein(a) atherogenicity by high density lipoprotein cholesterol levels in middle-aged men with symptomatic coronary artery disease and normal to moderately elevated serum cholesterol. Regression Growth Evaluation Statin Study (REGRESS) Study Group. *J Am Coll Cardiol*; 30:1491–9.

Critchley J, Liu J, Zhao D (2004). Explaining the increase in coronary heart disease mortality in Beijing between 1984 and 1999. *Circulation*; 110: 1236–44.

Dawber TR, Meadors GF, Moore FE Jr (1951). Epidemiological approaches to heart disease: the Framingham Study. *Am J Public Health*; 41: 279–86.

Denke MA (2005). Weighing in before the fight: low–density lipoprotein cholesterol and non–high–density lipoprotein cholesterol versus apolipoprotein B as the best predictor for coronary heart disease and the best measure of therapy. *Circulation*; 112: 3368–70.

Dobsn A, Filipiak B, Kuulasmaa K (1996). Relations of changes in coronary disease rates and changes in risk factor levels: methodological issues and a practical example. *Am J Epidemiol*; 143: 1025–34.

Dyer AR, Stamler J, Paul O (1981). Serum cholesterol and risk of death from cancer and other causes in three Chicago epidemiological studies. *J Chronic Dis*; 39: 249–60.

E'g'gen DA, Strong JP, McGill HCJ (1964). Calcification in the abdominal aorta: relationship to race, sex, and coronary atherosclerosis. *Arch Pathol*; 78: 575– 83.

El Harchaoui K, van der Steeg WA, Stroes ES, et al (2007). Value of low–density lipoprotein particle number and size as predictors of coronary artery disease in apparently healthy men and women: the EPIC–Norfolk Prospective Population Study. *J Am Coll Cardiol*; 49:547–53.

Emerging Risk Factors Collaboration, Erqou S, Kaptoge S, et al (2009). Lipoprotein(a) concentration and the risk of coronary heart disease, stroke, and nonvascular mortality. JAMA; 302:412– 23.

Fager G, Wiklund O, Olofsson SO, Wilhelmsen L, Bondjers G (1981). Multivariate analysis of apolipoproteins and risk factors in relation to acute myocardial infarction. *Arteriosclerosis*; 1: 273–7.

Ford ES, Li C, Zhao G, Pearson WS, Mokdad AH (2009). Hypertriglyceridemia and its pharmacologic treatment among US adults. *Arch Intern Med*; 169: 572–8.

Genest JJ Jr, Martin-Munley SS, McNamara JR, Ordovas JM, Jenner J, Myers RH, et al. (1992). Familial lipoprotein disorders in patients with premature coronary artery disease. *Circulation*; 85: 2025–33.

Glueck CJ, Gartside P, Fallat RW, et al (1976). Longevity syndromes: familial hypobeta and familial hyperalphalipoproteinemia. *J Lab Clin Med*; 88: 941–75.

Glueck CJ, Stein EA (1979). Treatment and management of hyperlipoproteinemia in childhood. In: Levy R, Rifkind B, Dennis B, Ernst N. Nutrition, Lipids, and Coronary Heart Disease, New York: Raven Press; pp. 285–307.

Goldstein JL, Hazzard WR, Schrott HG, Bierman EL, Motulsky AG (1973). Hyperlipidemia in coronary heart disease I. Lipid levels in 500 survivors of myocardial infarction. *J Clin Invest*; 52:1533–43.

Gordon DJ, Probstfield JL, Garrison RJ, Neaton JD, Castelli WP, Knoke JD, et al. (1989). High-density lipoprotein cholesterol and cardiovascular disease. Four prospective American studies. *Circulation*; 79: 8–15.

Gorelick PB, Schneck M, Berglund LF, Feinberg W, Goldstone J (1997). Status of lipids as a risk factor for stroke. *Neuroepidemiology*; 16: 107–15.

Haim M, Benderly M, Brunner D, et al (1999). Elevated serum triglyceride levels and long-term mortality in patients with coronary heart disease: the Bezafibrate Infarction Prevention (BIP) Registry. *Circulation*; 100: 475–82.

Harper CR, Jacobson TA (1999). New perspectives on the management of low levels of high–density lipoprotein cholesterol. *Arch Intern Med*; 159(10):1049–57.

Heiss G, Tamir I, Davis CEo (1980). Lipoprotein –Cholesterol distributions in selected North American populations: the Lipid Research Clinics Program Prevalence Study. *Circulation*; 61: 302–15.

High blood cholesterol and other lipids–statistics, 8 June 2011, Available from: www.americanheart.org

Hokanson IE, Austin MA (1996). Plasma triglyceride level is a risk factor in cardiovascular disease independent of high density lipoprotein cholesterol level: a meta – analysis of population - based prospective studies. *J Cardiovasc Risk*; 3: 213–9.

Ingelsson E, Schaefer EJ, Contois JH, et al (2007). Clinical utility of different lipid measures for prediction of coronary heart disease in men and women. *JAMA*; 298: 776–85.

Johannesson M, Jonsson B, Kjekshns J (1997). Cost–effectiveness of Simvastatin treatment to lower cholesterol levels in patients with coronary heart disease. *N Engl J Med*; 336: 332–6.

Kagan A, Harris BR, Winkelstein W Jr (1974). Epidemiologic studies of coronary disease and stroke in Japanese men living in Japan, Hawaii and California: demographic, physical, dietary and biochemical characteristics. *J Chronic Dis*; 27: 345–64.

Kannel WB, Castelli WP, Gordon T, McNamara PM (1971). Serum cholesterol, lipoproteins, and the risk of coronary heart disease: the Framingham Study. *Ann Intern Med*; 74: 1–12.

Kannel WB, Castelli WP, Gordon T (1979). Cholesterol in the prediction of atherosclerotic disease: new perspective based on the Framingham Heart Study. *Ann Intern Med*; 90: 85–91.

Kannel WB (1983). High–density lipoproteins: epidemiologic profile and risks of coronary artery disease. *Am J Cardiol*; 52:9B–l2B.

Keys A (1970). Coronary heart disease in seven countries. *Circulation*; 41 (suppl 1): 1–199.

Keys A, Menotti A, Aravanis C, Blackburn H, Djordevic BS, Buzina R, et al. (1984). The seven countries study: 2289 deaths in 15 years. *Prev Med*; 13: 141–54.

Kinosian B, Glick H, Garland G (1994). Cholesterol and coronary heart disease: predicting risk s by levels and ratios. *Ann Intern Med*; 121: 641–7.

Krauss RM (1994). Heterogeneity of plasma low–density lipoproteins and atherosclerosis risk. *Curr Opin Lipidol*; 5: 339–49.

Kuller L, Arnold A, Tracy R, et al (2002). Nuclear magnetic resonance spectroscopy of lipoproteins and risk of coronary heart disease in the cardiovascular health study. *Arterioscler Thromb Vasc Biol*; 22:1175–80.

Kushi LH, Lew RA, Stare FJ (1985). Diet and 20–year mortality from coronary heart disease. The Ireland –Boston Diet–Heart Study. *N Engl J Med*; 312: 811–8.

Labarthe DR (2011). Coronary heart disease, In: *Epidemiology and prevention of cardiovascular disease: a global challenge*, Labarthe DR, pp. 59-87, Jones and Bartlett, ISBN-13: 978-0-7637-4689-6, Canada.

Lamarche B, Moorjani S, Lupien PJ, et al (1996). Apolipoprotein AI and B levels and the risk of ischemic heart disease during a five year follow up of men in the Quebec Cardiovascular Study. *Circulation*; 94: 273-278.

Lamarche B, Tchernof A, Mooljani S, et al (1997). Small, dense low–density lipoprotein particles as a predictor of the risk of ischemic heart disease in men: prospective results from the Quebec Study. *Circulation*; 95: 69–75.

Law MR, Wald NJ, Thompson SG (1994). By how much and how quickly does reduction in serum cholesterol concentration lower risk of ischemic heart disease? *BMJ*; 308: 367–72.

Loscalzo J, Weinfeld M, Fless GM, Scanu AM (1990). Lipoprotein(a), fibrin binding, and plasminogen activation. *Arteriosclerosis*; 10:240– 5.

Manninen V, Tenkanen L, Koskinen P, Huttunen JK, Manttar M, Heinonen OP, et al (1992). Joint effects of serum triglyceride and LDL–cholesterol and HDL– cholesterol concentrations on coronary heart disease risk in the Helsinki Heart Study: implications for treatment. *Circulation*: 85: 37–45.

Martens LL, Guibert R (1994). Cost–effectiveness analysis of Lipid – modifying therapy in Canada: comparison of HMG–COA reductase inhibitors in the primary prevention of coronary heart disease. *Clin Therapeut*; 16: 1052–62.

Meisinger C, Loewel H, Mraz W, Koenig W (2005). Prognostic value of apolipoprotein B and A–I in the prediction of myocardial infarction in middle-aged men and women: results from the MONICA/KORA Augsburg cohort study. *Eur Heart J*; 26:271–8.

Miller NE, Thelle DS, Forde OH, Mjos OD (1977). The TromsØ heart study. High–density Lipoprotein and coronary heart disease: a Prospective case–control study. *Lancet*; 1: 965–70.

Murray CJ, Lopez AD (1997). Mortality by cause for eight regions of the world: Global Burden of Disease Study. *Lancet*; 349: 1269–76.

Murray CJ, Lopez AD (1997). Alternative projections of mortality and disability by cause 1990–2020: Global Burden of Disease Study. *Lancet*; 349: 1498–504.

Nieto FJ, Alonso J, Chambliss LE (1995). Population awareness and control of hypertension and hypercholesterolemia: the atherosclerosis in communities study. *Arch Intern Med*; 155: 677–84.

Nordestgaard BG, Benn M, Schnohr P, Tybjaerg-Hansen A (2007). Nonfasting triglycerides and risk of myocardial infarction, ischemic heart disease, and death in men and women. *JAMA*; 298:299–308.

Otvos JD, Shalaurova I, Freedman DS, Rosenson RS (2002). Effects of pravastatin treatment on lipoprotein subclass profiles and particle size in the PLAC–I trial. *Atherosclerosis*; 160:41–8.

Palabrica TM, Liu AC, Aronovitz MJ, Furie B, Lawn RM, Furie BC (1995). Antifibrinolytic activity of apolipoprotein(a) in vivo: human apolipoprotein(a) transgenic mice are resistant to tissue plasminogen activator-mediated thrombolysis. *Nat Med*; 1:256– 9.

Pischon T, Girman CJ, Sacks FM, et al (2005). Non–high–density lipoprotein cholesterol and apolipoprotein B in the prediction of coronary heart disease in men. *Circulation*; 112: 3375–83.

Rabbani N, Godfrey L, Xue M, Shaheen F, Geoffrion M, Milne R, et al (2011). Glycation of LDL by methylglyoxal increases arterial atherogenicity. A possible contributor to increased risk of cardiovascular disease in diabetes. *Diabetes*; 60 (7): 1973–80.

Ridker PM, Rifai N, Cook NR, Bradwin G, Buring JE (2005). Non–HDL cholesterol, apolipoproteins A–I and B100, standard lipid measures, lipid ratios, and CRP as risk factors for cardiovascular disease in women. *JAMA*; 294:326– 33.

Rifkind BM, Segal P (1983). Lipid Research Clinics Program reference values for Hyperlipidemia and hypolipidemia. *JAMA*; 250: 1869–72.

Roncaglioni MC, Santoro L, D'Avanzo B, Negri E, Nobili A, Ledda A, et al. (1992). Role of family history in patients with myocardial infarction. An Italian case- control study. GISSI–EFRIM investigators. *Circulation*; 85: 2065–72.

Rosengren A, Wilhelmsen L, Eriksson E (1990). Lipoprotein (a) and coronary heart disease risk: a prospective case - control study in a general population sample of middle – aged men. *BMJ*; 301: 1248–51.

Rosenson RS (2005). Low HDL–C: a secondary target of dyslipidaemia therapy. *Am J Med*; 118: 1067–77.

Rosenson RS. Screening guidelines for dyslipidemia, May 2011, Available from: www.uptodate.com

Sacks FM, Tonkin AM, Craven T, Pfeffer MA, Shepherd J, Keech A, et al (2002). Coronary Heart disease in patients with low LDL–cholesterol: benefit of pravastatin in diabetics and enhanced role for HDL– cholesterol and triglycerides as risk factors. *Circulation*; 105: 1424–8.

Schaefer EI, Lamon - Fava S, Ianner I (1994). Lipoprotein (a) levels and risk of coronary heart disease in men: the Lipid Research Clinics Primary Prevention Trial. *JAMA*; 271: 999–1003.

Sharrett AR, Ballantyne CM, Coady SA, et al (2001). Coronary heart disease prediction from lipoprotein cholesterol levels, triglycerides, lipoprotein(a), apolipoproteins A–I and B, and HDL density subfractions: The Atherosclerosis Risk in Communities (ARIC) Study. *Circulation*; 104: 1108–13.

Sniderman AD (2005). Apolipoprotein B versus non–high–density lipoprotein cholesterol: and the winner is... *Circulation*; 112: 3366–7.

Song Y, Stampfer MJ, Liu S (2004). Meta–analysis: apolipoprotein E genotypes and the risk for coronary heart disease. *Ann Intern Med*; 141 (2): 137–47.

Sprecher DL, Pearce GL, Cosgrove DM, et al (2000). Relation of serum triglyceride levels to Relation of serum triglyceride levels to survival after coronary artery bypass grafting. *Am J Cardiol*; 86:285–8.

Srinivasan SR, Berenson GS (2001). Apolipoproteins B and A–I as predictors of risk of Coronary artery disease. *Lancet*; 358:2012–3.

Stamler, J, Wentworth, D, Neaton, JD (1986). Is relationship between serum cholesterol and risk of premature death from coronary heart disease continuous and graded? Findings in 356,222 primary screenees of the Multiple Risk Factor Intervention Trial (MRFIT). *JAMA*; 256:2823–8.

Stein IH, Rosenson RS (1997). Lipoprotein LP (a) excess and coronary heart disease. *Arch Intern Med*: 157: 1170–6.

Steyrer E, Durovic S, Frank S, et al (1994). The role of lecithin: cholesterol acyltransferase for lipoprotein (a) assembly. Structural integrity of low density lipoproteins is a prerequisite for Lp(a) formation in human plasma. *J Clin Invest*; 94: 2330- 40.

The WHO MONICA Project: Risk factors (1989). *Int J Epidemiol*; 339: 861–7.

Thom TJ, Kannel WB, Silbershats S (1998). Incidence, prevalence and mortality of cardiovascular diseases in the United States. In: Hurst's the Heart, 9th ed, Alexander R W, Schlant RC, Fuster V, Roberts R (Eds), McGraw Hill, New York, P.3.

Thorvik E, Aursnes I, Kristiansen IS, Waller HT (1996). Cost–effectiveness of cholesterol – lowering drugs :a review of the evidence. *Wiener Klin Wochensch*; 108: 234–43.

Walldius G, Jungner I, Holme I, et al (2001). High apolipoprotein B, low apolipoprotein A- I, and improvement in the prediction of fatal myocardial infarction (AMORIS study): a prospective study. *Lancet*; 358: 2026–33.

Walldius G, Jungner I (2005). Rationale for using apolipoprotein B and apolipoprotein A-I as indicators of cardiac risk and as targets for lipid–lowering therapy. *Eur Heart J*; 26: 210-2.

Wu Z, Yao C, Zhao D, Wu G, Wang W, Liu J, et al. (2004). Cardiovascular disease risk factor levels and their relations to CVD rates in China- results of Sino- MONICA project. *Eur J Cardiovasc Prev Rehabil*; 11: 275–83.

Yusuf S, Hawken S, Ôunpuu S, Dans T, Avezum A, Lanas F, et al. (2004). Effect of potentially modifiable risk factors associated with myocardial infarction in 52 countries (the INTERHEART study): case–control study. *Lancet*; 364: 937–52.

Zambon A, Brown BG, Hokansen LE, Brunzeel IL (1996). Hepatic lipase changes predict coronary artery disease regression in the Familial Atherosclerosis Treatment Study (Abstract). Circulation; 94: 1–539.

Zambon A, Hokanson JE, Brown BG, Brunzell JD (1999). Evidence for a new pathophysiological mechanism for coronary artery disease regression: hepatic lipase–mediated changes in LDL density. Circulation; 99: 1959– 64.

Zioncheck TF, Powell LM, Rice GC, et al (1991). Interaction of recombinant apolipoprotein(a) and lipoprotein(a) with macrophages. J Clin Invest; 87:767–71.

3

Dyslipidemia and Cardiovascular Risk: Lipid Ratios as Risk Factors for Cardiovascular Disease

Telmo Pereira

College of Health Technologies, Polytechnic Institute of Coimbra
Portugal

1. Introduction

There are extensive epidemiological data demonstrating that high blood cholesterol levels increase cardiovascular risk, and that this risk is dependent on the levels of the different blood cholesterol fractions. Moreover, the reduction of total blood cholesterol has been clearly related to a reduction in the risk of stroke, coronary disease and overall cardiovascular death. However, the traditional cholesterol measurements tend to be most accurate at predicting risk for those at the lower and higher ends of the risk spectrum. Recent data has shown LDL-Cholesterol/HDL-Cholesterol ratio and even Total-Cholesterol/HDL-Cholesterol ratio, to be accurate predictors of cardiovascular risk. In fact, changes in ratios have been shown to be better indicators of successful CHD risk reduction than changes in absolute levels of lipids or lipoproteins. In the Helsinki Study, the LDL-C/HDL-C ratio had more prognostic value than LDL-C or HDL-C alone (Manninen, Tenkanen, Koskinen *et al*, 1992). The ratio was especially accurate at predicting risk among those who also had elevated triglyceride levels. The PROSPER trial, a retrospective analysis of 6,000 patients, found that the ratio of LDL-C/HDL-C was the most powerful measure of cardiovascular disease risk in elderly people (Packard, Ford, Robertson *et al*, 2005). The PROCAM Study, which included almost 11,000 men aged 36 to 65 who were studied for 4 to 14 years, found a continuous and graded relationship between the LDL-C/HDL-C ratio and CVD mortality (Cullen, Schulte, Assmann *et al*, 1997). In addition, comparison of individual LDL-C/HDL-C ratios from subjects in the Framingham Study clearly indicates that these ratios are significantly more robust predictors of CVD than the individual levels of LDL-C or HDL-C (Kannel, 2005).

2. Theoretical framework

2.1 Cardiovascular risk – Generalities

Cardiovascular diseases are an unavoidable topic when discussing health related issues, particularly in developed societies. Cardiovascular disease is the leading cause of mortality in these countries (World Health Organization, 2002), assuming a progressively more important role in developing countries and even in less developed countries. In the latter, we may consider the presence of a *double-frontier* of health risk. These countries show coexistence of important mortality indexes related to diseases whose prevalence is a demonstration to their stage of development (perinatal, nutritional and infectious health problems), with a more consistent presence of coronary disease, with increased percentage reaching 137% for males and 120% for females by the year 2010 (Yusuf, Reddy, Ounpuu *et al*, 2001).

In epidemiological terms, coronary heart disease and cerebrovascular disease represent the most significant expressions of cardiovascular disease, and were the main causes of mortality and morbidity worldwide, accounting for one third of total mortality in the year 2001 (American Heart Association, 2003). According to the World Health Organization, every year 16 million deaths occur from cardiovascular disease, and this number is expected to rise to 20 million in the first decade of the XXI century (World Health Organization, 2002). The singular importance of coronary heart disease is extraordinarily important and it is estimated that mortality by this disease had risen to 7.2 million individuals by the year 2001 (World Health Organization, 2002). However, in recent years, there has been a trend towards a decline in this disease in Western countries, with a concomitant increase in other lands, notably in Russia and Eastern European countries. In fact, in Western countries, the number of deaths from coronary per 100,000 inhabitants was 151 in 1972, dropping to 44 in 2004, in men aged 64 or less. Similar reductions were also observed in females (36 to 11 women per 100,000). Paradoxically, in Russia, there was a marked increase of this rate, from 169/100.000, in the year 1980, to 242/100.000 deaths, in the year 2005 (Allender, Scarborough, Black *et al*, 2008).

The onset of cardiovascular disease is consistently related to the presence of a group of cardiovascular risk factors, whose manipulation can be crucial to its prevention (see Table 1).

| **Reversible** |
| Smoking |
| Arterial hypertension |
| Hyperlipidemia |
| Obesity |
| Sedentarism |
| Alcohol |
| Stress |
| **Irreversible** |
| Family history |
| Male gender |
| Age |
| **Partially Reversible** |
| Diabetes |
| Menopause |

Table 1. Conventional cardiovascular risk factors.

Concerning reversible risk factors in which intervention could be decisive, we should highlight the relative importance of smoking, arterial hypertension and hypercholesterolaemia. Although the global fight against all reversible risk factors constitute a therapeutic imperative, the elimination of hypercholesterolemia would result in the single most important benefit against the incidence of coronary heart disease as well as other atherosclerotic vascular problems (Wilson, D'Augustine, Levy *et al*, 1998).

Regarding arterial hypertension, it always presents itself as a major risk factor, given its very high incidence and prevalence. Despite all the research carried out and considering all the remarkable therapeutic advances, the control of blood pressure levels only provides a reduction of about 40% in mortality from cerebrovascular disease and a more modest 20% reduction in mortality from coronary heart disease (Kaplan, 2002).

Diabetes is another important risk factor, with the particularity of becaming the major epidemy of this century given its substantial and consistent epidemiological growth. The high cardiovascular risk that diabetes provides is well illustrated by the prognostic similarity between a diabetic patient without clinical manifestations of coronary heart disease and a patient with a history of acute coronary events (Hafnner, Lethe, Ronnema et al, 1988).

Obesity is undoubtedly a major risk factor for cardiovascular disease (Higgins, Kannel, Garrison et al, 1988), now becoming a public health problem, given the alarming increase of its prevalence in industrialized countries. The pathogenic mechanisms involved in this situation are complex and not just related to the metabolic overload involved, but also determined by its close associations with arterial hypertension, type 2 diabetes, dyslipidemia, and inflammation (Higgins, Kannel, Garrison et al, 1988).

Smoking is consensually assumed as a relevant contributer to cardiovascular disease, both in the active as well as the passive form. Some studies indicate that smokers have a reduced life expectancy of about ten years (although this number is dose-dependent) and that this habit cancells the natural cardioprotection in women (Silva, 2000). In fact, the differences in cardiovascular risk amongst men and women are well known, largely documented by the classic time lag between genders, with a higher risk in males until the fifth decade of life, with a progressive increase in women of cardiovascular risk until the eighth decade of life, when the risk is similar in men and women. The explanation for this is closely linked to the production and subsequent estrogen deficiency (as a consequence of menopause) seen in different phases of a woman's life. But other factors must not be overlooked. For instance, If we consider only the lipid profile changes induced by menopause, on average a 10% increase in LDL-cholesterol, an 8% reduction in HDL-cholesterol and an elevation in triglycerides are expected. Nonetheless, these changes can be normalized by hormonal replacement therapy (Stampfer, Colditz, Willet et al, 1991). Oral contraception, by contrast, tends to cause an adverse impact on lipid profile. At present, the worrying rate of young women with acute coronary events, a situation rarely seen before, has directed special attention to factors that could be blamed for this surprising finding. The association of hormonal contraception with smoking has emerged as very common in this population, likely to concur not only for atherogenic metabolic features but also for potentially thrombotic coagulation disorders (Mosca, Grundy, Judelson et al, 1999).

The cardiovascular impact of alcohollic intake must also be considered. The cardiovascular impact of this behaviour is closely related to the amount of alcohol consumed. A moderate intake may confer some cardiovascular protection, particularly by raising HDL-cholesterol and reducing platelet aggregation, yet it may lead to a higher incidence of arterial hypertension and cerebrovascular disease. Patterns of high alcoholic consumption are an unusually hazardous behaviour, particularly for the heart, greatly increasing the risk of sudden death (Silva, 2000).

2.2 Cardiovascular risk – Dislipidemia

Lipids are a very heterogeneous group of compounds, and their influence on metabolism goes far beyond the misdeeds attributed to him. Lipids constitute an important source of energy storage, represented by triglycerides, and assume a great importance in the constitution of the brain (17% of its dry weight), the formation of hormones, lipoproteins, bile acids, vitamins, and in the structure of cell membranes. Cholesterol and Triglycerides are transported between various components of the organism by specific proteins called apoproteins. These constitute the protein fraction of lipoproteins whose lipid component includes phospholipids, cholesterol and Triglycerides. Lipoproteins are usually divided into six classes according to their composition, size, density and function: Quilomicra, VLDL (very low density lipoproteins), IDL (intermediate density lipoprotein), LDL (low density lipoprotein), HDL (high density lipoprotein) and Lipoprotein (a). The interaction of lipoproteins with a high number of enzymes, transport proteins and receptors, constitutes a complex metabolism where equilibrium is determined by intrinsic and extrinsic factors, and its unbalance leads to the pathophysiological cascade of atherosclerosis, with its well known clinical consequences (Silva, 2000). In very one-dimensional terms, fat from the diet is transported to the intestinal wall and integrated into large lipoprotein particles rich in triglycerides - the Quilomicra - which, when secreted by the lymphatic system eventually reach the bloodstream. The liver, in its turn, synthesizes other lipoproteins with high content of triglycerides, the VLDL. The extracellular lipoprotein-lipase degrades triglycerides of Quilomicra and VLDL into free fatty acids, which are deposited in tissues. Lipoproteins, by reducing their concentration in triglycerides, are converted into IDL, which are usually hydrolyzed by the hepatic lipase, and are than converted into LDL, which bind to specific liver or peripheral receptors. Meanwhile, in another cycle - the reverse transport of cholesterol - HDL particles pick up cholesterol deposited in the arterial wall and provide transportation to the liver, where it is subsequently excreted in the bile (Eckardstein, Hersberger & Roher, 2005).

The disorder of lipid metabolism is a key player for the occurrence of cardiovascular disease and particularly heart disease. For many years, cholesterol has been directly related to cardiovascular prognosis. This relationship is very consistent, as an increase of 2 to 3% in the incidence of coronary heart disease is expected for every 1% increase in total cholesterol (Carlson, Bottiger & Ahfeldt, 1979). A review of internationally published studies showed, however, that this association may be even stronger. Thus, a 10% increase in total cholesterol relates to a 38% increase in the risk of coronary-related mortality (Law, Wald & Thompson, 1994). More recently, several clinical studies on the primary and secondary prevention of coronary heart disease emphasized the importance of the LDL fraction (ILIB International Lipid Information Bureau, 2003) allowing the potential for the discrimination of cardiovascular risk. In fact, the risk of each patient may best be defined by the magnitude of the LDL-cholesterol rather than its total cholesterol, which is why international standards for the treatment of dyslipidemia have been oriented to listing the risk thresholds and treatment goals depending on the plasma levels of this lipoprotein. In practical terms, the determination of LDL-cholesterol may be derived by the Friedewald formula, where LDL Cholesterol = Total Cholesterol - HDL Cholesterol - VLDL cholesterol, VLDL cholesterol are derived from triglycerides/5.

For many years it was difficult to classify unequivocally Triglycerides as an independent risk factor for the occurrence of coronary heart disease, a situation presumably related to the wide fluctuations observed in their concentrations throughout the day, with the heterogeneity of triglyceride-rich lipoproteins (Quilomicra and VLDL) and its inseparable association with other risk factors. However, several studies have demonstrated a clear correlation between their levels and the occurrence of coronary heart disease, indicating that the presence of high levels of Triglycerides leads to a 13% increase in the risk of cardiovascular disease in men and 37% in women (Castelli, 1986; Criqui, Heiss, Cohn et al, 1993; Hokanson & Austin, 1996; Assman, Schulte & von Eckardstein, 1996). With regard to HDL-cholesterol, its inverse relationship with the risk of coronary heart disease is well accepted. In fact, this risk is 2 to 3% lower for each 1mg/dl elevation of HDL-Cholesterol (Gordon, Probstfiel, Garrison et al, 1989). The protective properties of this fraction derive not only from its involvement in reverse cholesterol transport, but are also a consequence of its anti-inflammatory capacity and protection against LDL-cholesterol oxidation (Ansell, Navab, Watson et al, 2004). On the other hand, it is recognized that individuals with very low levels of HDL-cholesterol have a higher cardiovascular risk. This population is often characterized for having concomitant hypertriglyceridemia, obesity, a sedentary lifestyle, active tobacco intoxication and decreased glucose tolerance (World Health Organization, 1999). In fact, an increased occurrence of cardiovascular events is expected for levels of HDL-cholesterol below 40 mg/dl (1.0 mmol/L) in men and less than 46 mg/dl (1.2 mmol/L) in women (UK HDL-C Consensus Group, 2004).

Recent evidence further stresses the importance of determining the non-HDL-cholesterol, defined by the concentration of LDL-cholesterol + VLDL-cholesterol. This parameter can better translate the risk of cardiovascular mortality than LDL-cholesterol, as it expresses more accurately the lipoprotein atherogenicity (Cui, Blumenthal, Flaws et al, 2001).

In recent years, a large number of risk factors for vascular disease have emerged from the international literature (see Table 2), demonstrating the relevance of more complex lipid disorders for the pathophysiology of atherosclerosis. Other emerging risk factors are related to inflammatory markers, as well as by the presence of metabolic changes, subtle changes in coagulation, hormonal disturbances and psychological or behavioral disorders (ILIB International Lipid Information Bureau, 2003).

Lipidic	Coagulation
Lipoproteic remnants	Fibrinogen
Lipoprotein (a)	Von Willebrand Factor
Small and dense LDL	Factor VII
HDL subspecies	Plasminogen activator inhibitor (PAI-1)
apolipoprotein B	
Apolipoprotein A-1	**Psychological / Behavioral**
Inflammatory	Alcoholism
High-sensitivity CRP	Depression
Homocysteine	Social Isolation
Interleukin-6	Loss and social support
Cell adhesion molecule-1	Low socioeconomic status
Selectin-CD40	**Hormonal**
Metabolic	Loss of estrogen production (menopause)
Postprandial hyperinsulinemia (insulin resistance)	

Table 2. Emerging cardiovascular risk factors.

As we have seen, each stated factor conveys a certain risk to the affected population. However, in everyday clinical practice a large majority of patients have associations of these factors and, as such, have cardiovascular risks that express the magnitude of individual risk factors present in an exponential, rather than additive, trend (Yusuf, Giles, Croft et al, 1998; American Heart Association, 2002).

An alternative option, with very promising results in the context of cardiovascular risk stratification and assessment of the effectiveness of lipid-lowering interventions, is the use of lipid ratios, just as the LDL-Cholesterol/HDL-Cholesterol ratio and the Total-Cholesterol/HDL-Cholesterol ratio, which have the added advantage of being easy to use in clinical practice (Gotto, Whitney & Stein, 2000). Changes in these relations have in fact been shown to better indicate the reduction in cardiovascular risk compared with the absolute levels of conventionally used lipid measures (Natarajan, Glick, Criqui et al, 2003; Kannel, 2005). On the other hand, the estimated LDL-Cholesterol/HDL-Cholesterol ratio translates, albeit imperfectly, an approach to the relationship of plasma apolipoproteins (apo) A-1 and apo B (Walldius & Jungner, 2005), thus enriching the lipid characterization of each patient, with the possibility of a better discrimination of cardiovascular risk, particularly among groups at intermediate cardiovascular risk (Gotto, Whitney, Stein et al, 2000).

Several large studies have demonstrated that the LDL-Cholesterol/HDL-Cholesterol ratio is an excellent predictor of risk of coronary disease and an excellent way to monitor the impact of lipid-lowering therapies (Manninen, Tenkanen, Koskinen et al, 1992; Kannel, 2005; Cullen, Schulte, Assmann et al, 1997; Stampfer, Sacks, Salvini et al, 1991; Gaziano, Hennekens, O'Donnell et al, 1997). In the Helsinki Study, a clinical trial with a 5-year follow-up, involving more than 4000 middle-aged men with hyperlipidemia, the LDL-Cholesterol/HDL-Cholesterol ratio had a superior prognostic value compared with isolated values of LDL-Cholesterol and HDL-Cholesterol. The predictive ability of this ratio was particularly strong in patients with concomitant elevation of triglycerides. It was further shown that the LDL-Cholesterol/HDL-Cholesterol ratio together with the fasting triglyceride concentration, allowed the identification of a particular subgroup of patients that had a remarkable 70% reduction in the risk of coronary heart disease with gemfibrozil (lipid-lowering agent) therapy. In the PROSPER trial, a retrospective analysis of 6,000 patients, the LDL-Cholesterol/HDL-Cholesterol ratio was the stronger predictor of cardiovascular events in elderly patients (Packard, Ford, Robertson et al, 2005). From this study has emerged the recommendation of pharmacological intervention whenever the LDL-Cholesterol/HDL-Cholesterol ratio values exceed 3.3 units. Another study (PROCAM study) involving about 11,000 men aged between 36 and 65, followed over 4 to 14 years, has documented an extremely important and linear relationship between the LDL-Cholesterol/HDL-Cholesterol ratio and cardiovascular mortality (Cullen, Schulte, Assmann et al, 1997). In this study, cardiovascular mortality peaked for LDL-Cholesterol/HDL-Cholesterol values between 3.7 and 4.3 units. In line with these results is the Physician's Health Study, involving 15,000 men (40 to 84 years), where there was a 53% increase in the risk of an acute coronary event for each one-unit increase in the LDL-Cholesterol/HDL-Cholesterol ratio (Stampfer, Sacks, Salvini et al, 1991). In another mixed study, involving men and women under the age of 76, the LDL-Cholesterol/HDL-Cholesterol ratio showed a strong relationship with the risk of coronary events (Gaziano, Hennekens, O'Donnell et al, 1997), aspect reinforced in an analysis of patients from the Framingham Heart Study, where a clear superiority of LDL-Cholesterol/HDL-Cholesterol ratio in predicting cardiovascular events compared to the levels of isolated LDL-cholesterol and HDL-cholesterol was depicted (Kannel, 2005).

Another point that reinforces the superiority of the lipid ratios in the stratification of cardiovascular risk arises from the effect of dietary cholesterol on plasma lipid levels. Several studies have demonstrated that these ratios are not affected by dietary cholesterol (Greene, Zerner, Wood et al, 2005; Herron, Vega-Lopez, Earl et al, 2002). On the contrary, some studies have shown that dietary cholesterol interferes with LDL-cholesterol and HDL-cholesterol, with little variation in the ratio (McNamara, 2000). On average, the predicted change in the LDL-Cholesterol/HDL-Cholesterol ratio per 100 milligrams/day increase in dietary cholesterol is quite small, around 0.01 (McNamara, 2000).

2.3 Cardiovascular risk – Atherogenesis

To understand the sequence of events that occur at the vascular level, resulting in devastating clinical manifestations that are all too familiar, we must look a little closer at the physiology of this system.

One of the most important organs we have without doubt is the vascular endothelium. The endothelium is the inner portion of our vessels, which can be compared to a thin membrane that carpets the blood vessels, and its integrity is fundamental for the maintenance of several potentially unstable equilibria. In this sense, a huge amount of vascular wall or circulating factors are present in close relation to the endothelium, endlessly alternating between defense and aggression, aggression, with Nitric Oxide as the key protector. As the most egregious examples of interaction near the endothelium vicinity, we have the following associations: vasodilation/vasoconstriction; anti-trombotic/pro-trombotic; anti-inflamatory/pro-inflamatory, among others. The relative hegemony of each of these interacting factors will determine the final maintenance of endothelial integrity or, conversely, its dysfunction and destruction (Houston, 2002). Endothelial dysfunction is thus the initial phase of a cascade of events that flow until the onset of clinically overt disease. In a very simplified overview, once the endothelial barrier is compromised, an association of events takes place, mainly with a lipid flooding process of the vascular wall, with the mobilization of inflammatory cells, the expression of chemotactic factors, growth and proliferation of smooth muscle and connective tissue, among others. The histologic consequence of these processes ranges from an initial lipid streak that evolves for an atherosclerotic plaque that may progress to calcification, progressively reducing the vascular lumen (Silva, 2000).

Curiously, most clinical cases are not determined directly by the extreme portion of the atherosclerotic continuum. In other words, cardiovascular events do not usually stem from progressive and insidious arterial occlusion, with consequent ischemia of downstream areas. Of course, cardiovascular events tend to be characterized by their acute nature, that is, by their sudden and unpredictable occurrence. As such, the implicit pathophysiology should express facts that support real-life events. In fact, one of the most important factors in the emergence of cardiovascular events is related to the so-called "atherosclerotic plaque stability". Thus, plaques with a small lipid core, with small inflammation infiltrate, and fitted with a thick, tough outer layer will be less susceptible to disruption by various harmful factors, such as blood pressure, sympathetic activity and other vasoconstrictor stimuli. In contrast, plaques with a rich lipid core, inflammatory activity and a significant weak fibrous cap will present a higher risk of fracture and exposure of their internal contents (Ridolfi & Hutchins, 1977). This in turn will lead to the activation of several factors that promote clotting and platelet aggregation in-sito (Falk, 1991), which may also lead to a sudden reduction of the vascular lumen, or even its complete occlusion by thrombosis.

Thus, the atherosclerotic process brings with it a wide array of metabolic, inflammatory and coagulation phenomena, decisively contributing to its clinical expression. Herein lies the justification of the diverse therapeutic targets that aimed for in these patients.

The importance of hypercholesterolemia as a key-player in this cascade of events is unquestioned and widely demonstrated in the published literature. A perfect expression of the interaction between research and practice is surely the publication of recommendations and guidelines that assist clinicians in the rationalization of therapeutic means available. These emerge as regular updates of successive collections of published scientific data, outlined in an admirably succinct way so they can be strategically combined and applied to the most varied health systems worldwide. Regarding the core topic of this paper, we have to address the most relevant recommendations published by the European Society of Cardiology and the National Cholesterol Education Program (NCEP). These recommendations were prepared according to an individual-risk perspective, and the therapeutic goals are defined according to the expected individual risk at long-term. Table 3 sumarizes the NCEP guidelines, revealing a clear therapeutic aggressiveness increase based on individual risk, as well as the adoption of progressively reduced target LDL-cholesterol values.

	Target	Therapeutic options	
High risk 10-year risk> 20% Established cardiovascular disease Equivalents of Cardiovascular Disease	LDL<100 mg/dl	LDL<100 mg/dl-129 mg/dl Dietary intervention Drug treatment?	LDL≥130 mg/dl Dietary intervention Drug treatment
Intermediate risk ≥ 2 Risk Factors 10-year risk ≤ 20%	LDL<130 mg/dl	LDL≥130 mg/dl Dietary intervention Drug treatment	
10-year risk ≤ 10%	LDL<130 mg/dl	LDL 130-160 mg/dl Dietary intervention	LDL≥160 mg/dl Dietary intervention Drug treatment
Low risk 10-year risk ≤ 10% ≤ 1 risk factor	LDL<160 mg/dl	LDL 160-190 mg/dl Dietary intervention Drug treatment?	LDL≥190 mg/dl Dietary intervention Drug treatment

Table 3. Hypercholesterolemia treatment algorithm of the second Report of the Third National Cholesterol Education Program – NCEP (2001).

These recommendations also included some secondary therapeutic goals, including the attempt to reduce non-HDL cholesterol in patients with triglycerides above 200 mg/dl for values 30 mg/dL higher than the individual target for LDL-cholesterol. Another objective lies in promoting an increase in HDL-cholesterol. Although these objectives are based on a very interventionist philosophy, recent studies may impose additional requirements on these recommendations. In fact, the Heart Protection Study (Heart Protection Study

Collaborative Group, 2002) showed that a reduction of 30% compared to the more restrictive goal (LDL cholesterol <100 mg/dl) was related to an additional 30% reduction in the relative risk of coronary heart disease. The PROVE IT study (Cannon, Braunwald, McCabe *et al*, 2004), enrolled patients who had had acute coronary events and showed that larger reductions of LDL-cholesterol, to levels lower than 100 mg/dl, could significantly provide aditional benefit in terms of future cardiovascular mortality and morbidity.

According to these results one has to consider more challenging treatment goals. The aim is to reach values of LDL-cholesterol <70mg/dl in patients with very high cardiovascular risk, such as those combining several primary risk factors (with primary relevance for diabetics), in patients with primary risk factors that are poorly controlled (with special care to the ones that maintain smoking habits), in patients with multiple risk factors of the so-called metabolic syndrome (triglycerides ≥ 200 mg/dl, non-HDL-cholesterol> 130 mg/dl, HDL-cholesterol<40 mg/dl) and in patients with history of acute coronary events.

The establishment of a therapeutic basis grounded in the control of cardiovascular risk factors has demonstrated its strong validity, and is further reinforced for its effectiveness in terms of cost-benefit. Improved control of risk factors almost certainly contributed to the 50% reduction in cardiovascular mortality observed in the United States of America between 1980 and 1990, with 43% attributable to the verified pharmacological advances (Hunink, Glodman, Tosteson *et al*, 1997). In the Netherlands, similar results were observed, and primary prevention was responsible for a 40% decline in mortality from coronary heart disease between 1978 and 1985 (Grobee & Bots, 1996). The adoption of dietary measures in Finland, relying on an increase in the consumption of fruits and vegetables and a reduction of saturated fats intake, has resulted in a 65% reduction in mortality from coronary heart disease in a time horizon of 20 years (Pekka, Pirjo & Ulla, 2002).

Despite the promising results indicated by these data, only 35% of Americans with a formal indication for dietary or pharmacological therapy, according to the recommendations of the NCEP (2001), are complying with it (Hoerger, Bala, Bray *et al*, 1988). In Canada, a study carried out between 1988 and 1993, including patients at high cardiovascular risk admitted to hospitals, showed very low percentages in relation to lipid dosing prescription (28%) and early dietary (22%) or pharmacological (8%) therapy (The Clinical Quality Improvement Network (CQIN) Investigators, 1995).

In Europe, results have fallen below expectations. An important follow-up study - EUROASPIRE - between 1995 and 1996, envolving nine European countries, showed that 86% of the enrolled patients had hypercholesterolaemia. Nevertheless, only 32% were on medication, and among those treated only 21% had achieved the target lipid levels (EUROASPIRE Study Group, 1997; EUROASPIRE I and II Group, 2001).

In Asia and the Pacific, the outlook is not encouraging either. In patients hospitalized for acute coronary events, quite small rates of lipid profile dosing (1 to 58%) were observed, as well as for the prescription of diet (1 to 32%) or pharmacological (6 to 60%) therapy to patients with high Cholesterol levels (Asian-Pacific CHD Risk Factor Collaborative Group, 1998).

The control of risk factors in clinical practice is thus a vaguely realized desideratum. The EUROASPIRE study has clarified some trends from 1995 to 2000. If the positive results have raised expectations, with an improvement seen in the control of hypercholesterolemia and hypertension, they are still accompanied by other rather disappointing indicators, such as those of smoking habits, obesity and diabetes, whose prevalence has been steadily increasing (EUROASPIRE Study Group, 1997; EUROASPIRE I and Group II, 2001). In the

United States of America the results are also somewhat disappointing. In survivors of acute myocardial infarction or stroke, the control percentages for some primary risk factors are below expectations, particularly for smoking habits (18%), control of hypercholesterolemia (46%), diabetes (48%) and hypertension (53%) (Qureshi et al, 2001).

As in almost all chronic conditions, the real picture lags far behind the expectations and available resources. Regarding hypercholesterolemia, the current situation is even less understandable, given its clear and strong association with the prevailing causes of death and incapacity, and the public awareness of the problem and in consideration of the demonstrated effectiveness of the available lipid-lowering drugs, that may have a quite favorable impact upon the prognosis of patients.

3. Original research data

3.1 Aim

Given the demonstrated role-playing of blood cholesterol in the atherosclerotic continuum, we designed two studies to ascertain the usefulness of the LDL-cholesterol/HDL-cholesterol, Triglycerides/HDL-cholesterol and Total-cholesterol/HDL-cholesterol ratios in predicting cardiovascular risk, through its relation to cardiovascular events and peripheral arterial disease (PAD) in two different clinical and experimental settings.

3.2 Study 1 – Usefulness of the lipidic ratios predicting peripheral artery disease in hypertensive patients: A retrospective analysis

The importance of the lipidic profile is well established in atherosclerotic processes related to coronary artery disease. Its relation with atherosclerosis in other vascular territories, particularly the inferior limbs has also received strong support from several experimental settings and in different clinical contexts. In order to address wether the lipid ratios can predict the occurrence of obstructive peripheral artery disease (PAD) we conducted a cross-sectional study in a sample of hypertensive patients. The study population consisted of 920 Portuguese nationals, aged between 20 and 91 years (mean 64.23 + 12.30 years).

3.2.1 Methods

A total of 920 hypertensive patients (51.3% female, age 64.22 ± 12.01 years) were consecutively included in the study. None of the patients were taking drugs or were in situations known to affect lipoprotein metabolism. Total cholesterol, triglycerides and HDL cholesterol were measured. LDL cholesterol was obtained by Friedewald's formula (if triglycerides <3.39 mmol/l) or by ultracentrifugation. The LDL-Cholesterol/HDL-Cholesterol, Total Cholesterol/HDL-Cholesterol and Triglycerides/HDL-Cholesterol ratios were calculated in all patients. Blood pressure and heart rate were measured in standard conditions. Ankle-Brachial index (ABI) was estimated bilaterally as the ratio of ankle (left and right) systolic blood pressure and brachial (highest upper limb) systolic blood pressure. The normal range for ABI was 0.9-1.3 mmHg, and individuals with ABI<0.9 were classified as having peripheral arterial disease.

All data was processed using STATA for Windows, version 11.1. The distribution of the variables was tested for normality using the Kolmogorov-Smirnov test, and for homogeneity of variance by Levene's test. Simple descriptive statistics were used to characterize the sample and the distribution of variables. Logistic regression analysis was used to determine the influence of the lipidic parameters on the occurrence of PAD.

Groups were compared using the $\chi 2$ test for categorical variables and the Student's t test (2 groups) or ANOVA with the post-hoc Tukey test (3 groups) for quantitative variables. A value of P≤0.05 was taken as the criterion of statistical significance for a 95% confidence interval.

3.2.2 Results
The general characteristics of the studied population are summarized in Table 4. Mean age was 64.23±12.30, with a similar proportion of men versus women (49% and 51%, respectively).

	Total (n=920)	No PAD Patients (n=803)	PAD Patients (n=117)	p-value (PAD versus No PAD)
Age, years	64.23±12.30	63.23±12.30	69.88±8.15	<0.01
Sex, men:women	49:51	48:52	52:48	0.462
Body Mass Index, Kg/m²	28.79±11.85	28.92±12.53	27.94±5.31	0.416
CV events history, no:yes	88:12	90:10	75:25	<0.01
Tobacco Consumption, no:yes	89:11	89:11	88:12	0.856
Dyslipidemia, no:yes	40:60	42:58	26:74	<0.01
Diabetes, no:yes	66:34	68:32	54:46	<0.01
SBP, mmHg	150.14±20.69	148.97±19.60	157.81±25.59	<0.01
DBP, mmHg	86.28±10.91	86.59±10.63	84.20±12.43	0.025
Heart Rate, bpm	70.52±10.48	69.12±9.42	71.22±9.21	0.791
Plasma Glucose, mg/dl	112.42±39.65	111.35±39.10	119.61±42.60	0.035
Plasma Creatinine, mg/dl	0.88±0.22	0.87±0.21	0.96±0.26	<0.01
eGFR, ml/min/1.73m²	84.73±23.28	85.86±23.40	76.94±20.88	<0.01
ABI	1.09±0.14	1.12±0.12	0.8±0.10	<0.01

PAD – peripheral artery disease; CV – cardiovascular events; SBP – systolic blood pressure; DBP – diastolic blood pressure; eGFR – estimated Glomerular Filtration Rate; ABI – Ankle-Brachial Index

Table 4. Characteristics of the study population, in general and stratified for the presence or absence of peripheral artery disease.

Mean body mass index was 28.79±11.85, indicating an overwheighted population. With regard to cardiovascular risk factors, all patients were hypertensive, 60% had dyslipidemia and 34% were diabetic; 11% were smokers and 12% had a personal history of cardiovascular events (mainly Stroke). About 37% were medicated for cardiovascular pathologies, with 13.6% of the patients undertaking statins. This factor was controlled in all the multivariable analysis. Peripheral artery disease (PAD) was encountered in 117 patients (12.7%). Patients with PAD were older, and had a worst metabolic and hemodynamic profile. The proportion of patients with a personal history of cardiovascular events was also greater in patients with PAD (25% versus 10%, p<0.01). The Ankle-Brachial Index (ABI) was also significantly lower in patients with PAD, as expected. Interestingly, patients with PAD also had a significantly lower estimated glomerular filtration rate (76.94 ± 20.88 ml/min/1.73m² versus 85.86 ± 23.40 ml/min/1.73m² in patients without PAD).

Regarding the overall and the comparative lipidic profile (depicted in table 5), significant differences amongst patients with and without PAD were only observed for the three considered lipidic ratios, expressing higher values when PAD was present, and for the HDL-cholesterol, with the PAD patients reaching lower HDL levels (although tendencially, p-value=0.073).

	Total (n=920)	No PAD Patients (n=803)	PAD Patients (n=117)	*p-value* (PAD versus No PAD)
Plasma Total Cholesterol, mg/dl	196.61±41.15	197.06±41.18	193.68±40.98	0.400
Plasma LDL-Cholesterol, mg/dl	116.31±37.62	116.17±41.18	193.68±40.98	0.763
Plasma HDL-Cholesterol, mg/dl	54.46±21.47	54.96±21.56	51.14±20.65	0.073
Plasma Triglicerides, mg/dl	134.84±67.88	134.20±41.18	139.09±66.02	0.460
LDL-Colesterol/HDL-Colesterol Racio	2.55±2.45	2.48±2.11	3.04±2.03	<0.01
Total Cholesterol/HDL-Colesterol Racio	4.15±2.95	4.06±2.48	4.80±2.05	<0.01
Triglicerídeos/HDL-Colesterol Racio	2.97±2.98	2.88±2.44	3.59±2.33	<0.01

Table 5. Lipid profile of the study population.

Figure 1 further ilustrates the differences in the lipidic ratios among patients with and without PAD, with all three considered ratios presenting significant differences between the considered groups.

A multivariable logistic regression analysis was also performed considering PAD as the dependent variable (dichotomized in normal/abnormal), and forcing each lipidic parameter (either individual lipis or lipid ratios) in a model adjusted for the conventional Framingham cardiovascular risk factors (age, sex, diabetes, blood pressure, smoking status and body mass index). The observed Odds Ratios (OR) with 95% confidence intervals is depicted in figure 2. Although there's an appreciable tendency of association with PAD in all lipid variables, it reaches statistical significancy only for the lipidic ratios. In fact, the OR for LDL-cholesterol, Total-cholesterol, HDL-cholesterol and Triglycerides were respectively 1.004 (IC: 0.999-1.010, p=0.1), 1.001 (IC: 0.996-1.007, p=0.4), 0.993 (IC: 0.980-1.004, p=0.2) and 1.001 (IC: 0.998-1.004, p=0.2). For the LDL-cholesterol/HDL-cholesterol ratio, the multiadjusted OR was 1.06 (IC: 0.999-1.120, p=0.052), with a marginally significant association with PAD. For the Total-cholesterol/HDL-cholesterol and the Triglycerides/HDL-cholesterol ratios, the adjusted OR were respectively 1.051 (IC: 1.011-1.200, p=0.01) and 1.050 (IC: 1.002-1.110, p=0.04). A further analysis showed that the association of the lipid ratios with PAD was tendencially linear, particularly for the Total-cholesterol/HDL-cholesterol ratio.

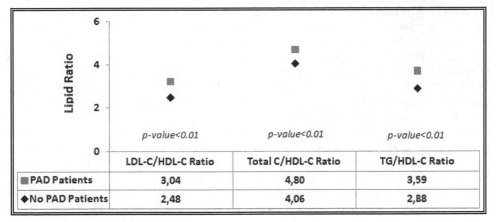

PAD – peripheral artery disease

Fig. 1. Representation of the comparative lipid ratios in patients with and without peripheral arterial disease.

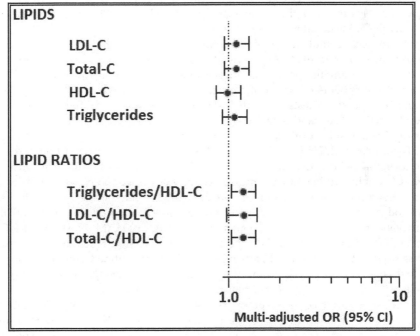

OR – Odds Ratio

Fig. 2. Adjusted Odds Ratios for Peripheral Artery Disease for the individual lipidic variables and for the lipidic ratios. The Odds Ratios are multi-adjusted to conventional Framingham cardiovascular risk factors.

3.3 Study 2 – Usefulness of the lipidic ratios in a low-to-moderate cardiovascular risk population: A sub-analysis of the EDIVA (Estudo de Distensibilidade Vascular) project

The EDIVA project was an epidemiological study assessing cardiovascular risk through sequential Pulse Wave Velocity measurement (Maldonado, Pereira, Polónia *et al*, 2011), but since serum lipids were available for all the included patients, we re-analyzed the EDIVA database aiming to address the delineated objective: to ascertain the usefulness of The LDL-Cholesterol/HDL-Cholesterol, Total Cholesterol/HDL-Cholesterol and Triglycerides/HDL-Cholesterol ratios in the general population. The study population consisted of 2200 Portuguese nationals (1290 men and 910 women), aged between 18 and 91 years (mean 46.33±13.76 years). Of these, 668 had low cardiovascular risk, and 1532 were patients with hypertension, diabetes and/or dyslipidemia. Individuals defined as having low cardiovascular risk were those who had had no chronic disease, had never been prescribed chronic pharmacological therapy, and had a normal physical exam, electrocardiogram, blood and urine tests, these characteristics having remained unchanged for at least two annual assessments. The patient group was under pharmacological therapy for at least one of the above pathologies.

3.3.1 Methods

The study's aims were explained to all participants and their informed consent was obtained. The methodology used to collect the data was approved by the Portuguese Data Protection Commission and the study was approved by the Ethics Committees of the hospitals involved. Mean follow-up was 2 years.

This was a prospective, multicenter, observational study monitoring the occurrence of major adverse cardiovascular events (MACE) – death, stroke, transient ischemic attack, myocardial infarction, unstable angina, peripheral arterial disease, revascularization or renal failure. Follow-up of the patients consisted of annual assessments including, blood pressure (BP) measurement, laboratory tests, including serum lipids, and clinical observation. Total cholesterol, triglycerides and HDL cholesterol were measured. LDL cholesterol was obtained by Friedewald's formula (if triglycerides <3.39 mmol/l) or by ultracentrifugation. The LDL-Cholesterol/HDL-Cholesterol, Total Cholesterol/HDL-Cholesterol and Triglycerides/HDL-Cholesterol ratios were calculated in all patients. At each consultation, the subjects' weight and height were measured and body mass index (BMI) was calculated in kg/m2. Blood pressure and heart rate were measured in standard conditions, in a supine position and after a 10-minute resting period, by an experienced operator and using a clinically validated (class A) sphygmomanometer (Colson MAM BP 3AA1-2®; Colson, Paris) (Pereira & Maldonado, 2005).Three measurements were taken and the arithmetic mean was used in the analysis. All participants underwent routine fasting laboratory tests. At the first consultation they filled out a questionnaire concerning relevant personal and family history, smoking habits, alcohol consumption and medication.

Data from the sample subjects were processed using STATA for Windows, version 11.1. The distribution of the variables was tested for normality using the Kolmogorov-Smirnov test, and for homogeneity of variance by Levene's test. Simple descriptive statistics were used to characterize the sample and the distribution of variables. Cox proportional hazards analysis was used to determine the influence of the lipidic parameters on the occurrence of the specified cardiovascular events. C-Statistics was calculated to address the reliability of the lipidic parameters as prognostic variables.

Groups were compared using the $\chi 2$ test for categorical variables and the Student's t test (2 groups) or ANOVA with the post-hoc Tukey test (3 groups) for quantitative variables. A value of $P \le 0.05$ was taken as the criterion of statistical significance for a 95% confidence interval.

3.3.2 Results

The general characteristics of the study population are summarized in Table 6. Mean age was 46.33±13.77, indicating a relatively young sample, with similar proportions of men and women (59% and 41%, respectively). With regard to cardiovascular risk factors, 52% of the patients were hypertensive, 33% had dyslipidemia and 11% were diabetic; 17% were smokers and 15% had a family history of cardiovascular events. About 37% were medicated for cardiovascular pathologies, with 13.6% of the patients undertaking statins. This factor was controlled in all the multivariable analysis. Mean follow-up is currently 21.42±10.76 months. A total of 50 non-fatal MACE (2.2% of the sample) were recorded, including 27 cases of stroke, 19 of coronary events, 2 of renal failure and 2 of occlusive peripheral arterial disease.

	Total	No MACE Low Risk Patients	Patients	MACE Patients	p-value (MACE vs No MACE)
N,%	2200	32%	66%	2%	
Age, years	46.33±13.77	40.00±13.42	49.03±13,14	50.00±10,21	0.360
Sex, men:women*	59:41	60:40	58:42	46:54	0.104
Body Mass Index, Kg/m²	27.18±5.50	25.90±4.21	27.71±4.45	28.59±5.75	0.348
Waist, cm	89.82±11,05	86.83±10,30	90.63±11,00	90.00±13,06	0.917
Family History, no:yes*	85:15	92:8	83:17	60:40	0.020
Tobacco Consumption, no:yes*	83:17	78:22	85:15	78:22	0.243
Hypertension, no:yes*	48:52	100:0	26:74	14:86	0.109
Dyslipidemia, no:yes*	67:33	100:0	53:47	60:40	0.311
Diabetes, no:yes*	89:11	100:0	85:15	86:14	0.941
SBP, mmHg	142.51±21.05	129.17±14.33	147.83±14.33	161.08±17.34	<0.001
DBP, mmHg	84.52±12.29	77.43±10.11	87.32±11.87	92.08±10.07	<0.001
PP, mmHg	57.99±15.29	51.74±11.90	60.05±15.86	66.20±12.93	<0.001
MAP, mmHg	103.85±14.02	94.68±1.26	107.48±13.52	117.14±11.43	<0.001
Heart Rate, bpm	70.56±12.24	68.21±12.58	71.49±11.87	78.20±13.01	0.001
Plasma Glucose, mg/dl	100.44±31.54	90.86±9.16	103.70±3.75	110.32±39.64	0.406
Plasma Creatinine, mg/dl	1.31±5.08	0.90±1.77	1.43±5.99	1.53±2.92	0.996

MACE – major acute cardiovascular events; SBP – systolic blood pressure; DBP – diastolic blood pressure; PP – pulse pressure; MAP – mean blood pressure

Table 6. General characteristics of the study cohort, depending on the presence of MACE and conventional cardiovascular risk factors.

Regarding the lipidic profile, patients with MACE presented higher levels of the different lipidic parameters, as illustrated in table 7, in particular the lipidic ratios were significantly higher in patients with MACE (5.76±1.74 versus 6.75±1.98 for Total Cholesterol/HDL-Cholesterol ratio, 3.24±1.32 versus 4.51±1.49 for LDL-Cholesterol/HDL-Cholesterol ratio, 3.17±1.34 versus 4.35±1.67 for Triglycerides/HDL-Cholesterol ratio, *p-value*<0.01). So, overall, the patients with MACE were characterized by an unfavorable metabolic profile compared to the asymptomatic patients.

	No MACE (n=2150)	MACE (n=50)	*p-value*
Plasma Total Cholesterol, mg/dl	221.37±34.01	238.43±36.12	<0,01
Plasma LDL-Cholesterol, mg/dl	141.37±31.22	163.26±41.12	<0,01
Plasma HDL-Cholesterol, mg/dl	41.22±11.07	36.19±7.28	<0,01
Plasma Triglicerides, mg/dl	156.37±34.01	181.43±36.12	<0,01
LDL-Colesterol/HDL-Colesterol Ratio	2.98±2.32	4.51±1.49	<0,01
Total Cholesterol/HDL-Colesterol Ratio	4.76±2.11	6.75±1.98	<0,01
Triglicerídeos/HDL-Colesterol Ratio	3.17±2.32	4.35±1.67	<0,01

MACE – major acute cardiovascular events; SBP – systolic blood pressure; DBP – diastolic blood pressure; PP – pulse pressure; MAP – mean blood pressure

Table 7. Lipid profile of the study cohort, stratified for the presence or absence of of MACE.

In the multivariable model analysis, adjusting for all conventional Framingham cardiovascular risk factors (age, sex, diabetes, blood pressure, smoking status and body mass index), the lipids ratios were associated with MACE, with stronger associations than the ones observed for the individual lipidic variables. Overall, the Total-Cholesterol/HDL-Cholesterol was found to be the best single predictor of MACE. In figure 3 we plot the hazard ratios for quintiles of the lipid ratios. A linear increase of the hazard ratios across quintiles of the Total-Cholesterol/HDL-Cholesterol is clearly depicted, while for the other ratios only the upper-extreme quintiles showed an important association with cardiovascular events.

Comparative data of risk association for those in the extreme quintiles of each lipidic variable is presented in figure 4. Of note, one can see that the combination of two individual lipidic components into a single variable provides stronger association with cardiovascular risk, as expressed by the depicted hazard ratios for the lipid ratios. On the other hand, the lipid ratio with the strongest association was the Total-Cholesterol/HDL-Cholesterol ratio, in line with the data depicted in figure 3.

The ROC curve analysis provided the Areas-Under-the-Curve (AUC, equivalent to the C-statistics) for the different lipid parameter considered in the analysis. The parameters with the biggest AUC were the Total-cholesterol/HDL-cholesterol ratio (AUC=0.703, IC:0.65-0.77) and the LDL-cholesterol/HDL-cholesterol (AUC=0.701, IC:0.64-0.79).

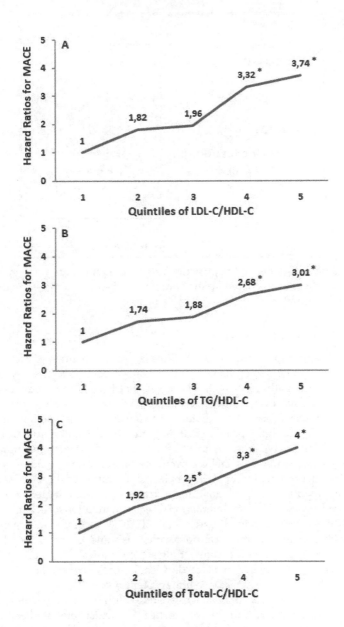

*p-value<0.01.

Fig. 3. Adjusted Hazard Ratios for major acute cardiovascular events distributed according to quintiles of the lipid ratios. A) Hazard ratios for quintiles of the LDL-Cholesterol/HDL-Cholesterol ratio; B) Hazard ratios for quintiles of the Triglycerides/HDL-Cholesterol ratio; C) Hazard ratios for quintiles of the Total-Cholesterol/HDL-Cholesterol ratio. The hazard ratios are multi-adjusted to conventional Framingham cardiovascular risk factors.

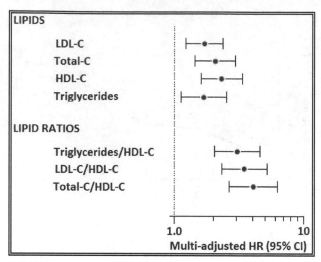

Fig. 4. Adjusted Hazard Ratios for major acute cardiovascular events amongst those in the extreme quintiles of each considered lipidic parameter. The hazard ratios are multi-adjusted to conventional Framingham cardiovascular risk factors.

4. Discussion and conclusions

As previously mentioned, cardiovascular disease, as an expression of atherosclerotic processes, is the leading cause of death in industrialized countries. The key role played by cholesterol in essential pathophysiologic processes that lead to the occurrence of clinically significant cardiovascular events is well recognized. In contemporary clinical practice, this notion is well entrenched, and the individual cardiovascular risk definition incorporates, among other factors, the lipid profile, including the Total Cholesterol, LDL Cholesterol, HDL Cholesterol and triglycerides. A practical evidence of the aforementioned is the fact that the major cardiovascular risk tables currently available (e.g. the Framingham score or the EuroSCORE), incorporate lipid parameters in the definition of thresholds of risk. On the other hand, therapeutic decisions and monitoring have been largely centered on the conventional lipid profile. Even the international recommendations (such as those issued by the National Cholesterol Education Program - NCEP, 2001) recommend target levels of LDL and HDL -cholesterol to determine cardiovascular risk and evaluate the effectiveness of lipid-lowering therapies. However, some studies have indicated important limitations of these parameters in the prediction of cardiovascular risk, particularly in patients with intermediate cardiovascular risk (Gotto, Whitney, Stein *et al*, 2000).

However, more recent evidence has suggested other lipidic components to optimize the definition of cardiovascular risk in clinical practice. In fact, several studies have expressed the superiority of the levels of apolipoprotein (apo) B, apo A-1 and its ratio, both in predicting cardiovascular events and in the evaluation of treatment efficacy (Packard & Marcovina, 2006; Yusuf , Hawken, Ounpuu, *et al*, 2004; Meisinger, Loewel, Mraz *et al*, 2005; Barter, Ballantyne, Carmena *et al*, 2006; Kim, Chang, Choi *et al*, 2005). In fact, considering that each lipidic particle contains one molecule of the atherogenic apo B, then its levels are a direct measure of the number of potentially atherogenic particles in the different conventional lipid components (Walldius & Junger, 2006). In contrast, the concentration of apo A-1 translates the number of anti-atherogenic particles contained in the HDL-cholesterol, thus enclosing the conceptual framework of apoB/apoA-1 ratio as a measure of the ratio of atherogenic particles versus anti-atherogenic particles transported in the blood. Despite the growing enthusiasm about the potential of these emerging parameters for their best performance in the definition of cardiovascular risk, there still remain some questions that limit their dissemination in clinical practice. The central question is very practical, and focuses on the cost-benefit relation associated with a change in the traditional clinical approach. In fact, it is not yet clear whether the superiority of these new lipid parameters over the more conventional ones for risk stratification is enough to justify the additional cost inherent to their laboratory determination (Pischon, Girman, Sacks et al, 2005). Furthermore, despite the current literature supporting apolipoproteins as better predictors of cardiovascular events, its use may not be the most practical operational perspective. Moreover, it is not yet clear whether the replacement of conventional parameters for emerging ones will translate into clear clinical benefit, or if, conversely, it will confuse the various protagonists over the clinical decision frame.

In contrast to this line of argument, several studies have also emerged affirming quite clearly the advantages of using lipid ratios, based on conventional parameters, such as those studied in this work. This is based on the fact that, on the one hand, they add cardiovascular risk discriminative capacity to the individual lipid parameters, and on the other, they are more favorable than the apolipoproteins considering cost and immediate operationalization (Gotto, Whitney & Stein, 2000). As mentioned earlier, several studies have shown fairly consistently that changes in these ratios are favorable indicators of cardiovascular disease risk, above the absolute levels of individual lipids (Natarajan, Glick, Criqui et al, 2003; Kannel, 2005). Accumulating evidence in this regard is quite broad, spreading over several clinical frameworks (Manninen, Tenkanen, Koskinen et al, 1992; Kannel, 2005; Cullen, Schulte, Assmann et al, 1997; Stampfer, Sacks, Salvini et al, 1991; Gaziano, Hennekens, O'Donnell et al, 1997; Packard, Ford, Robertson et al, 2005). The results presented here clearly fall into this line, reinforcing the belief in the superiority of the lipid ratios, particularly the Total-Cholesterol/HDL-Cholesterol and the LDL-Cholesterol/HDL-Cholesterol ratios, over the classic lipid parameters, predicting peripheral arterial disease in hypertensive patients (in a high cardiovascular risk) and predicting future major cardiovascular events (including stroke and myocardial infarction) in a low-to-intermediate cardiovascular risk population. One of the curious aspects extracted from the second presented study was the existence of a linear relationship for the Total-Cholesterol/HDL-Cholesterol ratio with the risk of MACE, something not apparent in the LDL-Cholesterol/HDL-Cholesterol ratio. This same result was reproduced in the Quebec Cardiovascular Study, in which more than 2.000 middle-aged men were followed for 5 years, monitoring the occurrence of major cardiovascular events (Lemieux, Lamarche, Couillard et al, 2001). The lipid parameters with better performance in predicting risk in this study were the Total-Cholesterol/HDL-Cholesterol ratio and the LDL-Cholesterol/HDL-Cholesterol ratio, although only the first stated ratio expressed a linear relationship with risk. One possible explenation for this result is metabolic in nature. In fact, it is well documented that patients with dyslipidemia showing high triglycerides and low HDL-cholesterol (generally patients with abdominal obesity and insulin resistance), often have marginal or even normal levels of LDL-Cholesterol (Lamarche, Després, Moorjani et al, 1996). Moreover, LDL-Cholesterol concentrations are often estimated indirectly from 3 measurements (Total-Cholesterol, Triglycerides and HDL-

Cholesterol), which may include a variation that can reach 25% (Schectman & Sasse, 1993), with a potential and quite significant impact in the LDL-Cholesterol/HDL-Cholesterol ratio, eventually under-estimated. By contrast, the two components included in the Total-Cholesterol/HDL-Cholesterol ratio are measured directly. Supporting the superiority of these ratios over the isolated lipid parameters, is their unique ability to reflect the bidirectional cholesterol traffic (in and outward) through the arterial intima in a way that the individual LDL and HDL-Cholesterol levels cannot reach (Kannel, 2005). Consistent with this assumption, another recent cohort prospective study, involving over 15.000 women followed over a period of 10 years, demonstrated that the Total-Cholesterol/HDL-Cholesterol ratio alongside the non-HDL Cholesterol were predictors of future cardiovascular events, as good or better than apolipoprotein fractions (Ridker, Rifai, Cook *et al*, 2005).

Of course, there are still unresolved issues, such as the definition of a cut-off in these ratios from which lipid-lowering therapy should be considered. The current guidelines of the NCEP (2001) recommend a cut-off of 2.5 for the ratio LDL-cholesterol/HDL-cholesterol. However, recent studies suggest that the risk of cardiovascular events begins to have significant expression for values between 3.3-3.7 (Cullen, Assmann & Schulte, 1997), in line with the results we reported here.

Given all the data currently available, as long as the fundamental reservations to the routine use of apolipoproteins are not exceeded, the use of lipid ratios in clinical practice is strongly advised, both in risk stratification and therapeutic decision and in monitoring its effectiveness.

5. Acknowledgments

The author sincerely thanks Dr Markus Carpenter for the linguistic assistance.

6. References

Allender, S.; Scarborough, P.; Preto, V., et al. (2008). *European cardiovascular disease statistics*. European Heart Network, Belgium.

American Heart Association. (2002). *Heart disease and stroke statistics – 2003 update*. Dallas, Tex: American Heart Association.

American Heart Association. (2003). Statistical facts sheet-populations. *International Disease Statistics*. Dallas, Tex: American Heart Association.

Ansell, B.J.; Navab, M.; Watson, K.E.; *et al.* (2004). Anti-inflamatory properties of HDL. *Rev Endocr Metab Disord*, 5:351-358.

Asian-Pacific CHD Risk Factor Collaborative Group. (1998). Risk factor management in CHD patients in Asia: current status. Atherosclerosis, 136:S31.

Assman, G.; Schulte, H.; von Eckardstein, A. (1996). Hypertriglyceridemia and elevated lipoprotein (a) are risk factors for major coronary events in middle-aged men. Am J Cardiol, 77: 1179-1184.

Barter, P.J.; Ballantyne, C.M.; Carmena, R.; *et al.* (2006). Apo B versus cholesterol in estimating cardiovascular risk and in guiding therapy: report of the thirty-person/ten-country panel. *J Intern Med*, 259:247–258.

Bots, M.L.; Grobee, D.E. (1996). Decline of coronary heart disease mortality in The Netherlands from 1987 to 1985: contributions of medical care and changes over time in presence of major cardiovascular risk factors. *J Cardiovasc Risk*, 3:271-276.

Cannon, C.P.; Braunwald, E.; McCabe, C.H.; *et al.* (2004). Pravastatin or Atorvastatin evaluation and infection therapy: thrombolisis in myocardial infarction 22 investigators. Intensive versus moderate lipi lowering with statins after acute coronary syndromes. *N Eng J Med*, 350:1495-1504.

Carlson, L.A.; Bottiger, L.E.; Ahfeldt, P.E. (1979). Risk factors for myocardial infarction in the Stockholm Prospective Study . A 14-year follow-up focusing on the role of plasma triglycerides and cholesterol. *Acta Med Scand*, 206:351-360.

Castelli, W.P. (1986). The triglyceride issue: a view from the Framingham. *Am Heart J*, 112:432-437.

Criqui, M.H.; Heiss, G.; Cohn, R. *et al.* (1993). Plasma triglyceride level and mortality from coronary heart disease. *N Eng J Med*, 328:1120-1125.

Cui, Y.; Blumenthal, R.S.; Flaws, J.A.; *et al.* (2001). Non-high-density lipoprotein cholesterol level as a predictor of cardiovascular disease mortality. *Arch Intern Med*, 161:1413-1419.

Cullen, P.; Schulte, H.; Assmann, G. (1997). The Munster Heart Study (PROCAM) Total Mortality in Middle-Aged Men is increased at low total and LDL cholesterol concentrations in smokers but not in nonsmokers. *Circulation*, 96:2128 - 2136.

Eckardstein, A.; Hersberger, M.; Roher, L. (2005). Current understanding of the metabolism and biological actions of HDL. Curr Opin Clin Nutr Metab Care, 8:147-152.

EUROASPIRE I and II Group. (2001). Clinical reality of coronary prevention guidelines: a comparison of EUROASPIRE I and II in nine countries. *Lancet*, 357:995-1001.

EUROASPIRE Study Group. (1997). EUROASPIRE: A European Society of Cardiology survey of secondary prevention of coronary heart disease: principal results. *Eur Heart J*, 18:1569-1582.

European guidelins on cardiovascular disease prevention in clinical practice. (2003). Third joint task force of european and other societies on cardiovascular disease prevention in clinical practice. *European J Card Prev and Rehab*, 10:S1-S10.

Falk, E. (1991). Coronary thrombosis: pathogenesis and clinical manifestations. *Am J Cardiol*, 68:28B-35B.

Gaziano, J.M.; Hennekens, C.H.; O'Donnell, C.J.; *et al.* (1997). Fasting triglycerides, high-density lipoprotein, and risk of myocardial infarction. *Circulation*, 96:2520 - 2525.

Gordon, D.J.; Probstfield, J.L.; Garrison, R.J.; *et al.* (1989). High-density lipoprotein cholesterol and cardiovascular disease: four prospective american studies. *Circulation*, 79:8-15.

Gotto, A.M.; Whitney, E.; Stein, E.A.; *et al.* (2000). Relation between baseline and on-treatment lipid parameters and first acute major coronary events in the Air Force/Texas Coronary Atherosclerosis Prevention Study (AFCAPS/Tex CAPS). *Circulation*, 101:477 - 484.

Gotto, A.M.; Whitney, E.; Stein, E.A.; *et al.* (2000). Relation between baseline and on-treatment lipid parameters and first acute major coronary events in the Air Force/Texas Coronary Atherosclerosis Prevention Study (AFCAPS/Tex CAPS). *Circulation*, 101:477–484.

Greene, C.M.; Zern, T.L.; Wood, R.J.; et al. (2005). Maintenance of the LDL cholesterol: HDL cholesterol ratio in an elderly population given a dietary cholesterol challenge. *J Nutr*, 135:2793 – 2798.

Haffner, S.M.; Letho, S.; Ronnema, T.; et al. (1988). Mortality from coronary heart disease in subjects with typo 2 diabetes and in non diabetic subjects with and without prior myocardial infarction. *N Eng J Med*, 339:229-234.

Heart Protection Study collaborative group.(2002). MRC/BHF Heart Protection Study of cholesterol lowering with sinvastatin in 20.536 high-risk individuals: a randomised placebo-controlled trial. Lancet, 360(9326):7-22.

Herron, K.J.; Vega-Lopez, S.; Conde, K.; et al. (2002). Pre-menopausal women classified as hypo-or hyper-responders, do not alter their LDL/HDL ratio following a high dietary cholesterol challenge. *J Am Coll Nutr*, 21:250 – 258.

Higgins, M.; Kannel, W.; Garrison, R.; et al. (1988). Hazards of obesity: the Framingham experience. *Acta Med Scand*, Suppl 723:23-36.

Hoerger, T.J.; Bala, M.V.; Bray, J.W.; et al. (1988). Treatment patterns and distribution of low-density lipoprotein cholesterol levels in treatment-eligible United States adults. *Am J Cardiol*, 82:61-65.

Hokanson, J.E.; Austin, M.A. (1996). Plasma triglyceride level is a risk factor for cardiovascular disease independent of high-density lipoprotein choloesterol level: a meta-analysis of population-based prospective studies. *J Cardiovasc Risk*, 3:213-219.

Houston, M. (2002). *Vascular Biology and Clinical Practice*. Hanley & Belfus Inc. Philadelphia.

Hunink, M.L.; Glodman, L.; Tosteson, A.N.A.; et al. (1997). The recent decline in mortality from coronary heart disease, 1980-1990: the effect of secular trends in risk factors and treatment. *JAMA*, 277:535-542.

ILIB International Lipid Information Bureau. (2003). *Dyslipidemia and coronary heart disease*. 3th Edition. 2003 International Lipid Information Bureau. New York.

Implications of recent clinical trials for the National Cholesterol Education Program Adult Treatment Panel III Guidelines. (2004). *Circulation*, 110:227-239.

Kannel, W.B. (2005). Risk stratification of dyslipidemia: Insights from the Framingham Study. *Curr Med Chem Cardiovasc Hematol Agents*, 3:187 – 193.

Kaplan's Clinical Hypertension. (2002). Lippincot Williams & Wilkins.

Kim, H.K.; Chang, S.A.; Choi, E.K.; et al. (2005). Association between plasma lipids, and apoliproteins and coronary artery disease: a cross-sectional study in a low-risk Korean population. *Int J Cardiol*, 101:435-440.

Lamarche, B.; Després, J.P.; Moorjani, S.; et al. (1996). Triglycerides and HDL.cholesterol as risk factors for ischemic heart disease: results from the Quèbec Cardiovascular Study. *Atherosclerosis*, 119:235-245.

Law, M.R.; Wald, N.J.; Thompson, S.G. (1994). By how much and how quickly does reduction in serum cholesterol concentratio lower risk of ischemic heart disease ? *BMJ*, 308:367-372.

Lemieux, I.; Lamarche, B.; Couillard, C ; et al. (2001). Total cholesterol/HDL cholesterol ratio vs LDL cholesterol/HDL cholesterol ratio as indices of ischemic heart disease risk in men. Arch Intern Med, 161:2685-2692.

Maldonado, J.; Pereira, T.; Polónia, J.; et al. (2011). Arterial stiffness predicts cardiovascular outcome in a low-to-moderate cardiovascular risk population: the EDIVA (Estudo de DIstensibilidade VAscular) project. *J Hypertens*, 29(4):669-75.

Manninen, V.; Tenkanen, L.; Koskinen, P.; *et al.* (1992). Joint effects of serum triglyceride and LDL cholesterol and HDL cholesterol concentrations on coronary heart disease risk in the Helsinki Heart Study. Implications for treatment. *Circulation*, 85:37 - 45.

Marcovina, S.; Packard, C.J. (2006). Measurement and meaning of apolipoprotein AI and apolipoprotein B plasma levels. *J Intern Med*, 259:437–446.

McNamara, D.J. (2000). The impact of egg limitations on coronary heart disease risk: Do the numbers add up? *J Am Coll Nutr*, 19:540S - 548S.

Meisinger, C.; Loewel, H.; Mraz, W.; *et al.* (2005). Prognostic value of apolipoprotein B and A-I in the prediction of myocardial infarction in middle-aged men and women: results from the MONICA/KORA Augsburg cohort study. *Eur Heart J*, 26:271–278.

Mosca, J.; Grundy, S.M.; Judelson, D.; *et al.* (1999). Guide to preventive cardiology in women. AHA/ACC scientific statement: consensus panel statement. *Circulation*, 99:2480-2484.

Natarajan, S.; Glick, H.; Criqui, M.; *et al.* (2003). Cholesterol measures to identify and treat individuals at risk for coronary heart disease. *Am J Prev Med*, 25:50 - 57.

Packard, C.J.; Ford, I.; Robertson, M.; *et al.* (2005). The PROSPER Study Group: Plasma lipoproteins and apolipoproteins as predictors of cardiovascular risk and treatment benefit in the PROspective Study of Pravastatin in the Elderly at Risk (PROSPER). *Circulation*, 112:3058 - 3065.

Pekka, P.; Pirjo, P.; Ulla, U. (2002). Influencing public nutrition for non-communicable disease prevention: from community intervention to national programme – experiences from Finland. *Public Health Nutr*, 5:245-251.

Pereira, T.; Maldonado, J. (2005). Performance of the Colson MAM BP 3AA1-2 automatic blood pressure monitor according to the European Society of Hypertension validation protocol. *Rev Port Cardiol*, 24:1341–1351.

Pischon, T.; Girman, C.J.; Sacks, F.M.; *et al.* (2005). Non-high-density lipoprotein cholesterol and apolipoprotein B in the prediction of coronary heart disease in men. *Circulation*, 112:3375–3383.

Qureshi, A.I.; Suri, M.F.K.; Guterman, L.R.; et al. (2001). Ineffective Secondary Prevention in Survivors of Cardiovascular Events in the US Population: Report From the Third National Health and Nutrition Examination Survey. Arch Intern Med, 161:1621-1628.

Ridker, P.M.; Rifai, N.; Cook, N.R.; *et al.* (2005). Non-HDL cholesterol, apolipoproteins A-1 and B100, standard lipid measures, lipid ratios, and CRP as risk factors for cardiovascular disease in women. JAMA, 294 (3):326-333.

Ridolfi, R.L.; Hutchins, G.M. (1977). Relationship between coronary artery lesions and myocardial infarcts: ulceration of atherosclerotic plaques precipitating coronary thrombosis. *Am Heart J*, 93:468.

Schectman, G.; Sasse, E. (1993). Variability of lipid measurements: relevance for the clinician. *Clin Chem*, 39:1495-1503.

Silva, J. (2000). *Colesterol, lípidos e doença vascular*. Lidel, Edições Técnicas Lda.

Stampfer, M.J.; Colditz, G.A.; Willet, W.C.; *et al.* (1991). Postmenopausal estrogen therapy and cardiovascular disease:ten-year follow-up from the Nurses Health Study. *N Eng J Med*, 325:756-762.

Stampfer, M.J.; Sacks, F.M.; Salvini, S.; *et al.* (1991). A prospective study of cholesterol apolipoproteins and the risk of myocardial infarction. *N Engl J Med*, 325:373 - 381.

The Clinical Quality Improvement Network (CQIN) Investigators. (1995). Low incidence of assessment and modification of risk factors in acue care patients at high risk for cardiovascular events, particularly among females and the elderly. *Am J Cardiol*, 76:570-573.

UK HDL-Consensus Group. (2004). Role of fibrates in reducing coronary risk: a UK consensus. *Curr Med Res Opin*, 20:241-247.

Walldius, G.; Junger, N. (2006). The apo B/apoA-I ratio: a strong, new risk factor for cardiovascular disease and a target for lipid-lowering therapy - a review of evidence. J Int Med, 259:493-519.

Walldius, G.; Jungner, I. (2005). Rationale for using apoliprotein B and apolipoprotein A-1 as indicators of cardiac risk and as targets for lipid-lowering therapy. *Eur Heart J*, 26:210 - 212.

Wilson, p.; D'Agostinho, R.B.; Levy, D.; *et al.* (1998). Prediction of coronary heart disease using risk factor categories. *Circulation*, 97:1837-1847.

World Health Organization. (1999). *Definition, diagnosis and classification of diabetes mellitus and its complications: report of a WHO consultation*. Part 1: Diagnosis and classification of diabetes mellitus. Geneva: World Health Organization.

World Health Organization. (2002). *The world health report 2002: reducing risks, promoting life*. Geneva: Worlf Health Organization.

Yusuf, H.R.; Giles, W.H.; Croft, J.B.; et al. (1998). Impact of multiple risk factor profiles on determining cardiovascular disease risk. Prev Med, 27:1-9.

Yusuf, S.; Hawken, S.; Ounpuu, S ; *et al.* (2004). Effect of potentially modifiable risk factors associated with myocardial infarctin in 52 countries (the INTERHEART study): case-control study. *Lancet*, 364:937–952.

Yusuf, S.; Reddy, S.; Ounpuu, S.; et al. (2001). Global burden of cardiovascular diseases part I: general considerations. *Circulation*, 104:2746-2753.

4

Dyslipidemia Induced by Stress

Fernanda Klein Marcondes[1], Vander José das Neves[1],
Rafaela Costa[1], Andrea Sanches[1], Tatiana Sousa Cunha[1,2],
Maria José Costa Sampaio Moura[3], Ana Paula Tanno[4]
and Dulce Elena Casarini[5*]

1. Introduction

The pioneering work of Hans Selye (1936) led to the use of the word "stress" in a biological context gaining popularity world-wide. Stress is as an organic response to stressors that can be aversive stimuli or unknown situations capable of compromising homeostasis. During the stress reaction, the sympathetic nervous system and hypothalamic–pituitary–adrenal axis are stimulated. Consequently, serum concentrations of classical stress hormones, namely catecholamines and glucocorticoids, are increased and act on cells and tissues inducing adaptive changes in order to protect the organism and allow its survival. In addition, the stress reaction can also modulate immune system activities and the secretion of other hormones (gonadotrophins, estrogen, testosterone, thyroid, angiotensins).

Considering that organic homeostatic systems are subject to frequent environmental and internal variations, Sterling and Eyer (1988) proposed the term alostasis to describe the adaptative processes that actively maintain stability through physiological changes.

The terms eustress and efficient allostasis describe facile adaptation, such as a quick peak stress response to mobilize energy to deal with an acute stressor, and a rapid return to baseline, when the stressor terminates. On the other hand, distress or allostatic load refers to an imbalance in systems that promote adaptation (Epel, 2009; Korte et al., 2005). This imbalance can simply be the result of too much repeated stress, but it can also be the result of adaptive systems that are out of balance and fail to shut-off or, alternatively, systems that fail to return to normal (Epel, 2009). Therefore the shut-off of the stress response is particularly important, because, when systems do not shut off in time, they can cause damage or promote pathology (McEwen, 1998).

The classical stress hormones, glucocorticoids (cortisol) and catecholamines (epinephrine and norepinephrine), are catabolic and modulate the breakdown of glycogen, triglycerides and proteins into molecules that can be rapidly metabolized in order to generate energy (Black, 2002). These responses enable energy substrates to be directed to organs and tissues

*[1]Department of Physiological Sciences, Piracicaba Dental School, University of Campinas, Piracicaba, Brazil
[2]Science and Technology Institute, Federal University of São Paulo, São José dos Campos, Brazil
[3]Life Sciences Center, Pontifical Catholic University of Campinas, Campinas, Brazil
[4]Division of Pharmacy, Faculty of Americana, Americana, Brazil
[5]Department of Medicine, Federal University of São Paulo, São Paulo, Brazil

with the greatest demand during the stress reaction, and support the fight or flight reaction to a stressor.

During acute stress, there is a rapid and transient increase in blood concentrations of total cholesterol, low-density lipoprotein (LDL), apoprotein B, triglycerides, and free fatty acids (Stoney, 2007). This increase persists as along as the stressor is maintained (Black, 2002), and disappears in stress-free periods (Stoney et al., 1999). In chronic stress situations, it has been shown that dyslipidemia is maintained and may persist even after the stressor is no longer present (Neves et al., 2009).

2. Dyslipidemia induced by stress: Physiological mechanisms

Many studies have shown the effect of stress on lipid metabolism. Stress associated with a major disaster, such as an earthquake or loss of job and income is associated with increased total cholesterol, LDL, and triglycerides in the bloodstream (Stoney, 2007). The perception of increased stress during a period of high workload is associated with elevated cholesterol in the bloodstream and ingestion of foods that increase cholesterol (McCann et al., 1990). Acute psychological stress in healthy men and women reduces the clearance rate of exogenous fat (Stoney et al., 2002). Chronic psychological stress increased the plasma cholesterol level in medical students (O'Donnell et al., 1987). In a more recent study, Yoo et al., 2011, showed high prevalence of hypercholesterolemia in stressed female law enforcement officers in comparison with the general female population. Moreover, elevated basal cortisol concentrations and lower circadian cortisol variability can induce dyslipidemia in patients with depressive and anxiety disorders (Venn et al., 2009; Vogelzangs et al., 2007). These patients presented hypercortisolism, increased serum levels of total cholesterol, LDL, and triglycerides and decreased serum levels of HDL (Venn et al., 2009).

In animal studies, it has been shown that electric shock stress increases plasma cholesterol concentrations (Berger et al., 1980), and unpredictable immobilization stress decreases HDL, increases blood LDL, and very-low-density lipoprotein (VLDL) concentrations in rats (Bryant et al., 1988). Chronic mild unpredictable stress increases triglycerides, total cholesterol, VLDL, and LDL concentrations in the bloodstream of stressed rats compared with control rats and this effect was observed 15 days after the stress protocol had ended (Neves et al., 2009).

The stressful modern lifestyle exerts a strong influence on lipid metabolism (Black, 2002) and may transform adaptive responses to pathophysiological changes. Acute increases in blood lipids are necessary for the individual to survive and adapt to the stressor. However prolonged changes in lipid metabolism induced by chronic stress can result in cardiovascular diseases such as atherosclerosis, coronary heart disease, and stroke (Brindley et al., 1993).

The negative effects of sustained stress-induced dyslipidemia are related to a bidirectional relationship between stress hormones and insulin. Catecholamines directly stimulate free fatty acid and glycerol secretion in the bloodstream from fat depots, a process that may result from increased blood flow through adipose tissue or from adipose-β_2 adrenoceptor stimulation (Stoney, 2007). Stress-induced high glucocorticoid concentration exerts a permissive effect on these lipolytic actions of catecholamines (Brindley et al., 1993). Since insulin regulates triglyceride synthesis and hepatic VLDL production, insulin resistance results in unregulated triglyceride synthesis and VLDL production (Stoney, 2007) and triglycerides are secreted by the liver in large quantities within the VLDL particles (Black, 2003). Therefore both catecholamines and glucocorticoids antagonize the actions of insulin, contributing to insulin resistance (Kyrou & Tsigos, 2009; Lafontan & Langin, 2009).

Moreover, hyperinsulinemia acts centrally to stimulate sympathetic nervous system activity, resulting in increased secretion of catecholamines (Black, 2003), and the absence of satisfactory insulin action facilitates the actions of cortisol and glucagon, which in turn stimulate phosphatidate phosphohydrolase activity to synthesize hepatic triglyceride (Brindley et al., 1993).

The cortisol also induces apoprotein B (apo B) secretion from the liver in the proportion of one apo B molecule per VLDL particle (Brindley et al., 1993), consequently increasing the VLDL concentrations in the bloodstream. As each VLDL particle is metabolized to intermediate-density lipoprotein (IDL) or LDL, the action of the cortisol that stimulates apo B secretion also results in increased LDL particles in the blood. Furthermore, in the presence of stress-induced insulin resistance, high levels of glucocorticoids suppress the hepatic LDL receptors, which delay LDL clearance (Stoney, 2007).

Contributing to all these processes, it has been shown that perilipin, which coats the surface of lipid droplets to restrict lipase access to the triglyceride core within the droplet, may suffer phosphorylation and/or down-regulation by glucocorticoid action, thereby facilitating the lipolysis of triglycerides in fatty acids and glycerol (Xu et al., 2001). This sets off a vicious cycle, leading to more and more triglycerides being produced by the liver and secreted in VLDL particles, as a result of the stimulation of glucocorticoids and fatty acids.

In addition, norepinephrine and cortisol inhibit lipoprotein lipase activity, leading to diminished triglyceride clearance, decrease in HDL concentration, and increase in VLDL, IDL, and LDL concentrations in the bloodstream (Stoney, 2007). Norepinephrine also diminishes hepatic triglyceride lipase activity, which in turn promotes high concentrations of lipoproteins rich in triglycerides in the blood (Stoney, 2007).

In the context of stress-induced dyslipidemia, changes in food ingestion must also be considered. During acute stress, transient dyslipidemia and food intake inhibition are mediated by β-adrenergic activation and increased hypothalmic corticotrophin releasing hormone (CRH) levels which act as catabolic signals. On the other hand, chronic activation of the hypothalamic-pituitary-adrenal axis has been associated with overeating and obesity (Dallman et al., 2004; Nishitani & Sakakibara, 2006). Many studies have supported this relationship. Lemieux & Coe, 1995, related that approximately 50% of women with posttraumatic stress disorder as a result of childhood sexual abuse were overweight, and also showed high concentrations of norepinephrine, epinephrine, and dopamine in urine. Changes in sleep-wake cycles associated with stress, resulting in sleep loss, induce decreased leptin levels, increased ghrelin levels, and increased hunger and appetite (Pejovic et al., 2010; Spiegel et al., 2004). In addition, the parent's lifestyle can influence metabolism, and individuals exposed to maternal stress during intrauterine life can exhibit deregulation of body weight control mechanisms and blood lipid profile (De Moura, 2008). The relationship between excessive glucocorticoids and visceral fat accumulation has also been discussed by Björntorp & Rosmond, 1999.

Thus, the typical response to chronic stress is not by way of avoiding food but by increasing the intake of sugar- and fat-rich comfort foods, which make people feel better

(Stoney, 2007; Torres & Nowson, 2007). Dallman et al., 2003, suggested that people or animals eat comfort food in an attempt to reduce activity in the 'chronic stress-response network' with its attendant anxiety. They suggested the following mechanism: first, in the periphery, glucocorticoids stimulate accretion of mesenteric energy stores; second, as the abdominal energy-generated (unidentified) signal increases, the negative input to catecholaminergic cells in the nucleus tractus solitarius reduces the synthesis of enzymes required for norepinephrine synthesis; third, the decreased noradrenergic signal to the hypothalamic paraventricular nucleus (PVN), in turn, decreases CRH synthesis and secretion. Thus, there is a powerful metabolic feedback control of CRH in the PVN, which may indirectly decrease glucocorticoid-action in the central nucleus of the amygdala; and thereby control anxiety (Korte et al., 2005). Consequently, all these mechanisms can lead to obesity and dyslipidemia due to overeating. In addition, it has been proposed that when chronic stress, to which animals and humans cannot easily adapt, is combined with high-fat high-sugar diets, it stimulates the sympathetic nerves to upregulate the expression of neuropeptide Y, an adrenergic cotransmitter and stress mediator. Stress and hypercaloric diets also increase glucocorticoid concentration in visceral fat, which in turn upregulates the expression of neuropeptide Y and its receptor Y2R, resulting in fat growth, hyperinsulinemia and hyperlipidemia (Bartolomucci et al., 2009; Kuo et al., 2008).

Some studies have also shown that glucocorticoid actions in the target tissues depend not only on circulating hormone levels, but also on intracellular glucocorticoid receptors and activities of both 11β-Hydroxysteroid dehydrogenase type 1 (11β-HSD1) and 2 (Bose et al., 2009). The effects of glucocorticoid are enhanced by the enzyme 11β-HSD1 in the stromal cells of visceral fat, since this enzyme catalyzes the conversion of inactive cortisone to active glucocorticoid in local tissue. It has been shown that transgenic knockout mice, which overexpress 11β-HSD1 in adipose tissue, present accumulation of visceral adipose tissue, hypertension, dyslipidemia and glucose intolerance (Masuzaki et al., 2001; Masuzaki & Flier, 2003). Therefore 11β-HSD1 plays an important role in the development of metabolic disease associated with stress (Bose et al., 2009; Walker & Stewart, 2003).

In addition, cytokines such as interleukin 6 (IL-6), tumor necrosis factor (TNF)-α, and leptin released from fatty cells also contribute to dyslipidemia induced by stress. IL-6 increases the activity of 11β-HSD1 with consequent expansion of visceral fat. TNF-α induces lipolysis in adipose tissue. Both IL-6 and TNF-α decrease lipoprotein lipase activity, contributing to the increase in triglyceride levels induced by stress (Black, 2003). Moreover, TNF-α induces insulin resistance because it depresses insulin receptor activity (Yudkin et al., 2000). TNF-α also induces IL-6 synthesis, and stimulates leptin synthesis, which acts centrally to decrease appetite and increase thermogenesis to decrease fat storage (Black, 2003). Leptin increases the activity of sympathetic nervous system centrally (Mohamed-Ali et al., 1998), which in turn stimulates increased release of TNF-α and IL-6 from adipocytes (Black, 2003). This sympathetic nervous system hyperactivity induced by high levels of leptin in the bloodstream would provide an additional effect of catecholamines on the genesis of insulin resistance and dyslipidemia associated with stress in obese individuals.

Therefore, dyslipidemia induced by stress involves complex interactions among stress hormones, insulin, adipose tissue metabolism and cytokines. Figure 1 indicates the physiological mechanisms of dyslipidemia induced by stress.

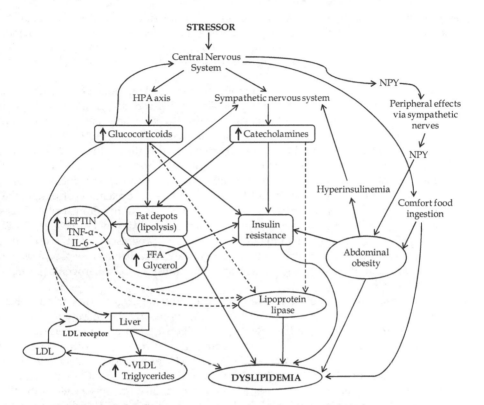

Fig. 1. Schematic representation of physiological mechanisms of dyslipidemia induced by stress. Hypothalamic-pituitary-adrenal axis (HPA), low-density lipoprotein (LDL), very-low-density lipoprotein (VLDL), free fatty acids (FFA), neuropeptide Y (NPY), tumor necrosis factor (TNF-α), interleukin 6 (IL-6). Solid arrows show stimulatory effects; dashed arrows indicate inhibitory effects.

3. Stress, dyslipidemia and atherosclerosis: Putative mechanisms

Atherogenic dyslipidemia is a major underlying cause of the development of atherosclerosis, which is an inflammatory disease (Mullick et al., 2006; Sheril et al., 2009). Since the stress-induced atherogenic lipid profile potentiates the effects of dietary and genetic factors in atherogenesis (Brindley et al., 1993), stress has been recognized as a risk factor for atherosclerosis (Kyrou & Tsigos, 2009; Shively et al., 2009). However, despite the association between dyslipidemia and atherosclerosis, many individuals develop severe atherosclerotic lesions associated with low serum lipid concentration, and others develop far more severe atherosclerosis than would be expected on the basis of a modest elevation of serum lipids (Kaplan et al., 1983). In this context, other effects of stress, not related specifically to dyslipidemia, are also involved in atherogenesis (Bierhaus et al., 2003; Gu et al., 2009) and approximately 40% of cases without known causal factor, have been attributed to stressful situations (Black, 2002).

The atherogenic effects of stress include changes in nitric oxide (NO) and cytokine production, vascular smooth muscle mitogenesis, occurrence of insulin resistance, neuropeptide Y (NPY) actions and modulation of the renin-angiotensin system activity. These effects are directly and indirectly related to stress-induced dyslipidemia, as will be pointed out below.

The healthy endothelium provides a smooth barrier that limits the activation of proinflammatory factors, blocks the transfer of Apo-B 100-containing atherogenic lipid particles into subendothelial space, inhibits the release of chemokines and cytokines, and prevents platelet and monocyte adhesion to the vascular wall (Cersosimo & DeFronzo, 2006). A high amount of NO is produced by endothelial nitric oxide synthase (eNOS). It is a vasodilator, has antithrombogenic properties, is an inhibitor of smooth muscle cell proliferation and of leukocyte- and monocyte-adhesion (Badimón & Martínez-González, 2002; Sudano et al., 2006). Decrease in NO bioavailability is a key feature of endothelial dysfunction resulting in lower responses to vasodilator agents (Codoñer-Franch et al., 2011), and represents an early stage of atherosclerosis (Badimón & Martínez-González, 2002). Endothelial dysfunction contributes to the development and progression of atherosclerosis by favoring coagulation, inflammatory cell adhesion, imbalance between vasoconstriction and vasodilation, and by enhancing transendothelial transport of atherogenic particles (Cersosimo & DeFronzo, 2006).

High stress-induced glucocorticoid levels reduce the expression of guanosine triphosphate cyclohydrolase 1 messenger ribonucleic acid (mRNA), necessary for tetrahydrobiopterin cofactor (BH_4) synthesis, which stabilizes eNOS (Mitchell et al., 2004). If BH_4 levels decrease, endothelial eNOS becomes uncoupled and transfers electrons to molecular oxygen generating superoxide anions (Rizzo et al., 2009), which react avidly with NO to form peroxynitrites (Förstermann & Münzel, 2006), resulting in diminished NO bioavailability, and favoring the traffic of oxidized lipids across the endothelium. Associated with this injurious effect of glucorticoids, the high LDL levels induced by stress also decrease eNOS mRNA expression (Liao et al., 1995).

Considering dyslipidemia induced by stress, it has been reported that before structural changes appear, chronic elevations of cholesterol in the bloodstream are frequently associated with impaired endothelium-dependent NO production due to increased interaction between caveolin and eNOS (Feron et al., 1999). Caveolin proteins are expressed in the majority of the cell types that play a role in atherogenesis, including endothelial cells, macrophages, and smooth muscle cells (Frank & Lisanti, 2004). High levels of LDL-cholesterol increase the caveolin concentration in endothelial cells (Feron et al., 1999), strengthen the calveolin-eNOS complex, and reduce the interaction between Ca^{2+}-calmodulin and eNOS. These effects decrease eNOS translocation from caveolae to the cytoplasm and considerably diminish NO production (Feron et al., 1999; Frank & Lisanti, 2004). In addition, lipid peroxidation induced by stress also impairs nitric oxide production (NO), stimulates inflammatory response, and increases the traffic of inflammatory molecules and oxidized LDL to sub-endothelial space, leading to vascular endothelial dysfunction (Black, 2002; Black, 2003; Black & Garbutt, 2002; Rizzo et al., 2009).

Insulin resistance is also involved in the atherogenic effects of stress. Insulin stimulates NO production by the endothelium (Muniyappa & Quon, 2007). During chronic stress cortisol-induced insulin resistance (Black, 2002; Kyrou & Tsigos, 2009) decreases this effect, and endothelial dysfunction may occur. In addition, insulin resistance is associated with inhibition of the phosphatidylinositol 3-kinase pathway and over-stimulation of the mitogen-activated protein kinase pathway in endothelial cells. Impairment of the phosphatidylinositol 3-kinase pathway reduces eNOS activity, and accentuates free fatty acid-evoked oxidative stress. These effects decrease NO bioavailability and promote an imbalance between vasoconstriction and vasodilation (Cersosim & DeFronzo, 2006; Muniyappa & Quon, 2007) predisposing the individual to atherosclerosis and arterial hypertension. In addition insulin resistance increases the reactive oxygen species, reducing eNOS activity (Muniyappa et al., 2008).

Morphological changes in blood vessels are also associated with atherosclerosis. The increase in intima media thickness (IMT) in the carotid artery has been used as a marker of target organ damage in human hypertension (Sierra & de la Sierra, 2008). In experimental studies, the IMT of the aorta observed in stressed rats (Okruhlicová et al., 2008) was related to the atherogenic effects of stress. In healthy blood vessels, NO produced by the endothelium maintains the mitogenic quiescence of smooth muscle cells. Decreased NO bioavailability induced by stress-related glucocorticoid levels or -insulin resistance results in the loss of this effect and consequently vessel wall hypertrophy may occur (Costa & Assreuy, 2005). In fact, it has been observed that rats submitted to chronic mild unpredictable stress presented higher IMT and lower relaxation response to acetylcholine in the thoracic aorta, in comparison with non stressed animals. These effects were observed 15 days after the end of the stress protocol and were associated with insulin resistance and dyslipidemia. However, in this study, the dyslipidemia induced by the hypercaloric diet alone, did not promote morphological or functional changes in the thoracic aorta, or insulin resistance evidencing the role of stress in pro-atherogenic effects (Neves et al., 2011).

NPY, a hormone known as orexigenic peptide, may also be involved in the atherogenic effects of stress. Some stressors such as cold and aggression, increase the release of NPY from sympathetic nerves (Kuo et al., 2007). The peripheral actions of NPY are stimulatory, synergizing with glucocorticoids and catecholamines to potentiate the stress response. It causes prolonged vasoconstriction, potentiating the effect of norepinephrine, induces hyperlipidemia, and vascular remodeling via smooth muscle cell proliferation, in addition to stimulating monocyte migration and activation (Kuo et al., 2007). NPY upregulates its Y2 receptors in a glucocorticoid-dependent manner in abdominal fat, consequently leading to abdominal obesity, hyperinsulinemia and dyslipidemia (Kuo et al., 2008). In blood vessels, Y1 and Y5 receptor activation promotes pro-atherogenic responses (Zukowska, 2005).

In addition to all the above-mentioned mechanisms, the inflammatory process also forms part of the stress response (Black, 2003), and is pathophysiologically linked to atherosclerosis (van Oostrom et al., 2004). In the atherogenic process, the high level of catecholamines induced by stress stimulates endothelial permeability to the traffic of oxidized LDL. Once trapped in the endothelium of an artery, LDL can undergo progressive oxidation, cross the endothelial barrier, and be internalized by macrophages expressing scavenger receptors, leading to lipid peroxide formation and accumulation of cholesterol esters, culminating in foam cells formation (Ross, 1999; Singh & Mehta, 2003). Oxidized LDL upregulates the expression of adhesion molecules and secretion of chemokines, which contributes to the recruitment of circulating monocytes and leukocytes (Cersosimo & DeFronzo, 2006; Steinberg, 2002). One of the initial steps in the formation of atherosclerosis is the adhesion of monocytes to the endothelium, their entry into sub-endothelial space, followed by their differentiation into macrophages (Lamharzi et al., 2004). These cells are then responsible for taking up LDL and other particles, thereby starting the atherogenesis process (Lamharzi et al., 2004). In foam cell formation, the macrophages in the endothelial space also have VLDL receptors, which bind the apolipoprotein (apo) E-containing lipoproteins, including VLDL, intermediate density lipoprotein, and β-migrating VLDL. The LDL-receptor-related protein in macrophages is also capable of binding apo E-containing lipoproteins, lipoprotein lipase, and lipoprotein lipase-triglyceride-rich lipoprotein complex (Nakazato, 1996), leading to a sequence in the development of atherosclerosis.

In addition, high levels of free fatty acids also may amplify monocyte inflammation via toll-like receptors in the presence of high glucose levels (Dasu & Jialal, 2011). Lamharzi et al., 2004, showed that free fatty acids in concert with glucose stimulate machrophage proliferation involving glucose-dependent oxidation of LDL in atherosclerotic lesions. Toll like receptors are expressed by machrophages in murine and human lipid-rich atherosclerotic plaques and upregulated by oxidized LDL (Xu et al., 2001). Recently Gu et al., 2009, showed the importance of toll-like receptor 4 in atherosclerosis induced by chronic mild stress in aortas from apolipoprotein-E-knockout-mice. Toll-like receptor 4 is present in T cells, monocytes, and macrophages, and is a key signaling receptor of innate immunity. Toll-like receptor 4 plays an important role in atherogenesis because it recognizes pathogen-associated molecular patterns and activates inflammatory cells via the nuclear factor kB (NF-kB) pathway (Bierhaus et al., 2003; Gu et al., 2009). During the stress reaction, glucocorticoids and catecholamines can induce cytokine production by endothelial cells and macrophages (Black, 2003; Chae et al., 2001) and activation of the NF-kB pathway leads to the synthesis of the following proinflammatory chemokines: interleukin 1-β, inteleukin 6, TNF-α, monocyte chemoattractant protein-1, intercellular adhesion molecule-1. Interleukin 1-β and inteleukin 6 influences smooth muscle cell proliferation and/or migration (Gu et al., 2009), and inhibits eNOS activity (Muniyappa et al., 2008). TNF-α increases endothelin-1 secretion, decreases NO production in endothelial cells, inducing vasoconstriction (Muniyappa & Quon, 2007), and can induce interleukin 6 production (Black, 2003). Monocyte chemoattractant protein-1 is correlated with neointimal proliferation and plays a role in the transition from the stable state of lesion to the more complex state of atherosclerosis (Tellez et al., 2011). Intercellular adhesion molecule-1 may contribute to accelerating atherosclerosis in insulin-resistant states (Muniyappa et al., 2008). Hypertriglyceridemia associated with stress may also increase NF-kB, consequently activating proinflammatory molecules (Fitch et al., 2011).

In addition, the accumulation of macrophages may also be associated with increased plasma concentration of C-reactive protein (CRP) (Ross, 1999). CRP is the principal down-stream mediator of inflammatory acute phase response, which is primarily derived via interleukin 6-dependent hepatic biosynthesis (Pradhan et al., 2001). CRP interacts with oxidized LDL to form proatherogenic oxidized LDL/CRP complexes, perpetuating vascular inflammation, triggering an autoimmune response, and accelerating atherogenesis (Matsuura et al., 2009; Sitia et al., 2010).

Activation of the renin-angiotensin system (RAS) by stress also plays a role in the pathogenesis of endothelial dysfunction, hypertension and atherosclerosis. Lipid accumulation in blood vessels enhances the expression of RAS components, which in turn stimulates accumulation of oxidized LDL in blood vessels (Singh & Mehta, 2003). Activation of the angiotensin II-type 1 receptor (AT_1R) leads to vasoconstriction and neurohumoral activation, and is associated with reduced NO bioavailability, vascular cell apoptosis, increased oxidized LDL receptor expression, and proinflammatory cytokine production (Sitia et al., 2010). According Nickening et al., 1999, LDL-cholesterol can accumulate in vascular smooth muscle cells, and this effect is mediated via AT_1R. Angiotensin II increases LDL uptake by arterial wall macrophages (Keidar et al., 1994). Angiotensin II binds LDL and the angiotensin II-modified LDL is taken up by macrophages via scavenger receptors, leading to cellular cholesterol accumulation (Keidar et al., 1996). In atherogenic dyslipidemia, hypercholesterolemia increases AT_1R density and its functional responsiveness to vasoconstrictors, whereas the administration of statins reduces AT_1R expression and deregulates its functions. Moreover, the localization of angiotensin-converting enzyme in atherosclerotic lesions suggests a capacity for local generation of angiotensin II and proinflammatory substances (Sitia et al., 2010). There is also evidence that hypercholesterolemia increases plasma angiotensinogen and angiotensin peptide production (Sitia et al., 2010), and that AT_1R antagonism improves hypercholesterolemia-associated endothelial dysfunction, resulting in an anti-atherosclerotic effect (Taguchi et al., 2011).

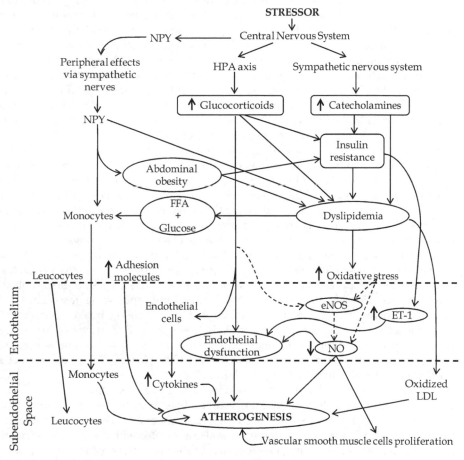

Fig. 2. Schematic representation of putative mechanisms involved in the relations between among stress, dyslipidemia, and atherosclerosis. Hypothalamic-pituitary-adrenal axis (HPA), neuropeptide Y (NPY), low-density lipoprotein (LDL), very-low-density lipoprotein (VLDL), free fatty acids (FFA), endothelial nitric oxide synthase (eNOS), nitric oxide (NO), endothelin 1 (ET-1). Solid arrows show stimulatory effects; dashed arrows indicate inhibitory effects.

Atherosclerosis is an inflammatory disease and stress contributes to its development. Therefore, if we can block or minimize the stress components that directly or indirectly induce atherogenesis, it will be possible to preserve the protective components of vascular function and structure, thereby developing new preventive and therapeutic possibilities. Figure 2 illustrates the putative mechanisms of the relations between stress, dyslipidemia, and atherosclerosis.

4. Reduction of dyslipidemia induced by stress: Physical exercise and nutritional intervention

The role of stress in the etiology of chronic degenerative diseases is increasingly recognized (Gerber & Pühse, 2009; Holmes et al., 2010; Tsatsoulis & Fountoulakis, 2006; Yin et al., 2005). Moreover, it has been reported that obese people have an exaggerated response to stress, which may further increase the risk of weight gain, leading to the development of insulin resistance, hyperlipidemia, diabetes mellitus, hypertension and atherosclerosis in both men and women. This burden of chronic degenerative diseases is strongly influenced by several lifestyle factors, including the way an individual perceives a stressful situation, i.e., "mental fitness" and also his/her general physical condition or "physical fitness" (McEwen, 1998). Tsatsoulis & Fountoulakis, 2006, demonstrated that stress-mediated allostatic load, in the presence of physical inactivity, is associated with an increased risk of mental and physical illness, and direct evidence for this notion has been provided by several studies. A strong inverse association between physical activity and the metabolic syndrome has been demonstrated, and several years ago this association was shown to be much steeper in unfit individuals (Kriska et al., 1993; Lindgärde & Saltin, 1981). Evidence for this view was also provided by the MacArthur studies of successful aging based on a large cohort of elderly men and women (Seeman et al., 1997), showing that subjects with low levels of physical and mental fitness had higher prevalence of cardiometabolic disease when compared with those with high fitness levels. Moreover, a strong association between physical inactivity, excessive food consumption, high-fat diet and increasing incidence of insulin resistance, Type 2 diabetes, (Hawley, 2004; Steanovv et al., 2011), development of obesity (Venables & Jeukendrup, 2009; Vessby, 2000) and depression (Win et al., 2011) has also been described in the literature. Considering that stress, physical inactivity, and aging (associated with declining physical activity and metabolic rate, coupled with an energy intake not matched to the declining need), in addition to a high-fat diet, are the very features of our current lifestyle, the incidence of this "stress-induced/exercise deficient" phenotype is becoming increasingly prevalent in modern society (Davy et al., 1996, Hawley, 2004, Poehlman et al., 1995, Schiut et al., 1998, Tsatsoulis & Fountoulakis, 2006).

Based on the above mentioned findings, it is reasonable to assume that physical inactivity may potentiate the stress-related allostatic load and comorbidities, since the energy substrate that is mobilized during stress is not oxidized but is stored in visceral fat depots. This adaptation creates a vicious cycle, in which perceived stress is also associated with decreased participation in several health behaviors including exercise, social behaviors, stress management/rest, and safety/environmental behaviors, as shown by Padden et al., 2011, in the study on health behavior of military spouses during deployment separation. In this context, physical exercise practiced as a non-pharmacological alternative, either with or without the association of pharmacological therapies, is very important, and a great deal of attention should be given to the barriers imposed, especially by mood disorders, including depression. Individuals in this condition are at disadvantage, since most of the time they lack the energy and motivation to exercise, and this overwhelming feeling of lethargy seems very difficult to shift (Chaput et al., 2011). In this situation, when psychological stress is not accompanied by physical activity (such as the fight or flight reaction) and by effective use and fast clearance of free fatty acids, triggered by stimulation of the sympathetic nervous system, these are converted into triglycerides by the liver and then circulate in the blood within the VLDL (Howard et al., 1993). In fact, this maladaptive situation can lead to the development of dyslipidemia, reflected by elevated plasma triglyceride and reduced HDL concentration, overproduction of VLDL-apolipoprotein (apo) B-100, decreased catabolism of apoB containing particles, and increased catabolism of HDL apoA-I particles (Watts et al., 2008; Watts et al., 2009).

While physical inactivity may potentiate the stress-induced allostatic load, there is accumulating evidence suggesting that the adoption of an active lifestyle, including exercise training, may play a protective role in stress system dysregulation, reducing vulnerability to stress, and possibly delaying or preventing the future development of comorbidities, such as dyslipidemia, hypertension and insulin resistance (Roberts & Barnard, 2005; Tsatsoulis & Fountoulakis, 2006). In addition, physical activity may induce favorable changes in traditional and emerging coronary heart disease biomarkers among individuals with, or at high risk of coronary heart disease (Chainani-Wu et al., 2011). Assuming that the stress response is a neuroendocrine mechanism that occurs in anticipation of physical action, it is reasonable to assume that physical activity should provide the vehicle to prevent or combat the somatic and emotional consequences of stress. Thus, physical activity may promote physical and psychological benefits that are involved in both the indirect action of exercise in reducing stress, and a direct effect on various metabolic functions of the body (McMurray & Hanckney, 2005).

The first rationale for using exercise as a stress reduction strategy was based on the cross-stressor adaptation, a promising hypothesis first presented in the 1990s (Sothmann et al., 1996), which has not received strong support since the publication of recent meta-analyses (Forcier et al., 2006; Hamer et al., 2006; Jackson & Dishman, 2006). According to Chaput et al., 2011, the key question now is whether physical activity, which seems to modulate the level of stress, may interact in the relationship between stress and obesity. Different possible mechanisms have been proposed, suggesting that exercise training might protect against stress induced obesity. Regular exercise has been demonstrated to have positive effects on plasma lipid and lipoprotein profiles (Durstine et al., 2002) and these results may have a significant independent effect on HDL cholesterol (Thompson et al., 1988). During physical activity, exercise increases lipid oxidation and lipolysis to ensure an adequate oxygen supply (McMurray & Hanckney, 2005), increases the ability of muscle tissue to take up and oxidize nonesterified fatty acids, and increases muscle lipoprotein lipase activity (Eriksson et al., 1997). Although studies indicate that exercise training changes gene expression in adipose tissue in different ways, affecting some types of adipose tissue more than others (Company et al., 2010), the lowering of plasma triglycerides proves the effects of exercise on VLDL kinetics. Moreover, it is important to highlight that a single 90-min bout of whole body resistance exercise (Tsekouras et al., 2009) or 2h of cycling (Magkos et al., 2006) was proven to be enough to decrease fasting plasma VLDL-triglyceride concentrations by increasing VLDL-triglyceride removal from plasma. These results may be due to the increase in blood flow and hepatic insulin sensitivity associated with an increase in lipoprotein lipase activity.

In addition to its possible direct effect modulating the stress response, exercise training improves insulin sensitivity, which might counteract the insulin resistance state produced by chronic hypercortisolemia (Tsatsoulis & Fountoulakis, 2006). Insulin secretion could then be reduced, and thereby, its deleterious impact on energy intake may be diminished. Moreover, exercise training improves glucose tolerance among non-diabetic, non-obese subjects with hypertriglyceridemia (Lampman & Schteingart, 1991) and enhances the oxidative capacity of skeletal muscle (Tsatsoulis & Fountoulakis, 2006). Together, these beneficial adaptations could prevent stress-induced fat deposition by routing the energy mobilized in response to the stressor toward oxidation rather than storage.

Apart from the protective effects of exercise on the physical and metabolic aspects related to stress, a number of psychological and cognitive benefits have also been reported in the literature. These include improvements in depression and anxiety scores and general improvement in mood, cognitive functioning (Callaghan, 2004; Tsatsoulis & Fountoulakis, 2006), well-being and self esteem, leading to a decrease in body fat, triglycerides, LDL/HDL cholesterol ratio in stressed patients (De Geus & Stubbe, 2007). Physical activity can improve mental health by reducing depressive symptoms in young men (McGale et al., 2011) and in patients with metabolic syndrome (Rubenfire et al., 2011). Moreover exercise induces the elevation of circulating brain derived neurotrophic factor, which is known to improve the health and survival of nerve cells, suggesting that exercise influences brain health (Yarrow et al., 2010). Using animal models, exercise has also been shown to induce antidepressant responses (Greenwood et al., 2003). In rats, swimming exercise induces a remission of anhedonic symptoms suggesting that exercise training might induce biological alterations similar to those provided by antidepressant drugs. In addition, exercise plays an important role in hippocampal protection from damage caused by exposure to glucocorticoids (Sigwalt et al., 2011). In this context, physical activity was able to stimulate the proliferation of hippocampal cells (Ehninger & Kempermann, 2003), promote alterations in synaptic plasticity, neurogenesis and synaptogenesis (Castrén, 2005), and may also be linked to increased levels of brain testosterone (Mukai et al., 2006).

Another beneficial effect of exercise is related to feeding behavior. Stressful situations have been shown to affect feeding behavior (Wallis & Hetherington, 2009) that result in increased energy intake through the stimulation provided by ingesting palatable foods that may serve as feedback signals that reduce the perception and discomfort of stress, thereby contributing to the development of dyslipidemia and obesity (Dallman et al., 2005). Moreover glucorticoids are associated with high neuropeptide Y secretion, which has an orexigenic activity and increases the intake of sugar- and fat-rich- comfort foods (Kuo et al., 2008) and can lead to a state of leptin resistance and elevated levels of this hormone (Zakrzewska et al., 1997). In this context, it has been demonstrated that physical activity has the potential to modulate appetite control by improving the sensitivity of the physiological satiety signalling system, by adjusting macronutrient preferences or food choices and by altering the hedonic response to food (Blundell et al., 2003). Indeed, dietary modification, associated with physical activity has been shown to exert significantly favorable effects on the treatment and prevention of stress-induced comorbidities, improving glycemia, blood pressure, body weight, fat distribution, and lipid profile, which in turn suggest that chronic degenerative diseases are largely preventable (Dagogo et al., 2010). Although exercise cannot change total cholesterol and LDL-cholesterol unless dietary fat intake is reduced, this result may be dependent on the amount of energy expenditure during exercise (Durstine et al., 2002). Furthermore, depending on the time that the exercise is performed (before or after ingestion of fatty foods), its acute responses related to improvement in lipoprotein metabolism may be different (Hashimoto et al., 2011). In a review of several studies realized by Leon & Sanchez

2001, one of proposals evaluated was the effects of aerobic exercise training on blood lipids and the relationship between these effects and diet. The results showed that majority of physically active individuals had an increase in HDL cholesterol, but this could be changed if there was a concomitant reduction in fat intake. The association between low-fat diet and exercise reduces LDL and HDL-cholesterol levels. Furthermore, reductions in total cholesterol, LDL-cholesterol and triglyceride levels were less frequently observed. As regards body weight loss, there was considerable variability between the groups, ranging from 7.2 Kg in the group that was not exposed to dietary intervention to 17.9 Kg in the group that underwent dietary intervention. In addition, Rubenfire et al., 2011, demonstrated that the association between changes in diet and exercise was effective in reducing cardiovascular risk in patients with metabolic syndrome. In this study, the nutritional component was based on a Mediterranean food pattern, and all the participants were provided with the information needed to optimize their nutritional choices in order to improve blood lipid and glucose levels, decrease body weight and blood pressure, and decrease insulin resistance (Rubenfire et al., 2011). It has also been proposed that high-fiber diets protect against obesity and cardiovascular disease by lowering insulin levels (Ludwig et al., 1999). In obese men, the implementation of a high-fiber and low-fat diet associated with regular physical activity resulted in significant reductions in inflammation and dyslipidemia by reducing serum lipids, insulin, oxidative stress, leukocyte-endothelial interactions (Roberts & Barnard, 2005).

Dietary fat influences glucose and lipid metabolism by altering cell membrane function, enzyme activity, insulin signaling, and gene expression (Risérus et al., 2009; Yamazaki et al., 2011) and dietary fructose consumption appears to induce dyslipidemia, obesity (Stanhope et al., 2009) and hypertension (Cunha et al., 2007; Farah et al., 2006). A combination of social stress and high-fat diet resulted in a significant imbalance in lipid regulation associated with changes in the expression of hepatic genes, responsible for its regulation (Chuang et al., 2010). Therefore, clinical strategies based on low fat and sugar intake associated with increase in physical exercise have been used, and have contributed to reducing the risks of developing coronary and metabolic diseases.

5. Conclusion

Dyslipidemia induced by stress is part of the body's response to cope with stressors. The mobilization of lipids, glucose and proteins, allows the organs and tissues to maintain homeostasis and adapt to the stressor. Any deficiency in the activation of this mobilization of energetic fuels can compromise the survival of the individual. Therefore, the increase in blood lipids induced by stress is adaptive and it should return to normal levels when the stressor ends. However, when the stressor is maintained over a long period, the dyslipidemia induced by stress persists and may have deleterious effects, contributing to the occurrence of insulin resistance, obesity, hypertension and atherosclerosis. Considering that physical inactivity may potentiate these effects, the association of physical exercise and control of hypercaloric food consumption have been used in the treatment of dyslipidemia. Knowledge about the physiological mechanisms involved in the adaptive role of transient dyslipidemia induced by acute stress, and in the deleterious effects of sustained dyslipidemia induced by chronic stress is very important in the improvement and development of preventive and therapeutic approaches because in modern society we are continuously exposed to stressors.

6. Acknowledgment

The authors thank Margery Galbraith for English editing.

7. References

Badimón, L. & Martínez-González J. (2002). Endothelium and vascular protection: an update. *Revista española de cardiología*, Vol.55, No.1 (January 2002), pp. 17-26, ISSN 0300-8932.

Bartolomucci, A.; Cabassi, A.; Govoni, P.; Ceresini, G.; Cero, C.; Berra, D.; Dadomo, H.; Franceschini, P.; Dell'Omo, G.; Parmigiani, S. & Palanza, P. (2009). Metabolic consequences and vulnerability to diet-induced obesity in male mice under chronic social stress. *PloS one [electronic resource]*. Vol.4, No.1, (January 2009), pii. e4331, ISSN 1932-6203 online.

Berger, D.F.; Starzec, J.J.; Mason, E.B. & DeVito, W. (1980). The effects of differential psychological stress on plasma cholesterol levels in rats. *Psychosomatic medicine*, Vol.42, No.5, (September 1980), pp.481-492, ISSN 0033-3174.

Bierhaus, A.; Wolf, J.; Andrassy, M.; Rohleder, N.; Humpert, P.M.; Petrov, D.; Ferstl, R.; von Eynatten, M.; Wendt, T.; Rudofsky, G.; Joswig, M.; Morcos, M.; Schwaninger, M.; McEwen, B.; Kirschbaum, C. & Nawroth, P.P. (2002). A mechanism converting psychosocial stress into mononuclear cell activation. *Proceedings of the National Academy of Sciences of the United States of America*, Vol.100, No.4, (February 2003), pp. 1920-1925, ISSN 0027-8424.

Björntorp, P. & Rosmond, R. (1999). Hypothalamic origin of the metabolic syndrome X. *Annals of the New York Academy of Sciences*, Vol.892, (November 1999), pp. 297-307, ISSN 0077-8923.

Black, P.H. (2002). Stress and the inflammatory response: a review of neurogenic inflammation. *Brain, behavior, and immunity*, Vol.16, No.6, (December 2002), pp. 622-653, ISSN 0889-1591.

Black, P.H. (2003). The inflammatory response is an integral part of the stress response: Implications for atherosclerosis, insulin resistance, type II diabetes and metabolic syndrome X. *Brain, behavior, and immunity*, Vol.17, No.5, (October 2003), pp. 350-364, ISSN 0889-1591.

Black, P.H. & Garbutt, L.D. (2002). Stress, inflammation and cardiovascular disease. *Journal of psychosomatic research*, Vol.52, No.1, (January 2002), pp. 1-23, ISSN 0022-3999.

Blundell, J.E.; Stubbs, R.J.; Hughes, D.A.; Whybrow, S. & King, N.A. (2003). Cross talk between physical activity and appetite control: does physical activity stimulate appetite? *The Proceedings of the Nutrition Society*, Vol.62, No.3, (August 2003), pp. 651-661, ISSN 0029-6651.

Bose, M.; Oliván, B. & Laferrère, B. (2009). Stress and obesity: the role of the hypothalamic-pituitary-adrenal axis in metabolic disease. *Current opinion in endocrinology, diabetes, and obesity*, Vol.16, No.5, (October 2009), pp. 340-346, ISSN 1752-296X.

Brindley, D.N.; McCann, B.S.; Niaura, R.; Stoney, C.M. & Suarez, E.C. (1993). Stress and lipoprotein metabolism: modulators and mechanisms. *Metabolism: clinical and experimental*, Vol.42, No.9 Suppl 1, (September 1993), pp. 3-15, ISSN 0026-0495.

Bryant, H.U; Story, J.A. & Yim G.K. (1988). Assessment of endogenous opioid mediation in stress-induced hypercholesterolemia in the rat. *Psychosomatic medicine*, Vol.50, No.6, (November-December 1988), pp. 576-585, ISSN 0033-3174.

Callaghan, P. (2004). Exercise: a neglected intervention in mental health care? *Journal of psychiatric and mental health nursing*, Vol.11, No.4, (Áugust 2004), pp. 476-483, ISSN 1351-0126.

Castrén, E. (2005). Is mood chemistry? *Nature reviews. Neuroscience*, Vol.6, No.3, (March 2005), pp. 241-246, ISSN 1471-003X.

Cersosimo, E. & DeFronzo, R.A. (2006). Insulin resistance and endothelial dysfunction: the road map to cardiovascular diseases. 2006. Diabetes/metabolism research and reviews, Vol.22, No.6, (November/December 2006), pp. 423-436, ISSN 1520-7552.

Chae, C.U.; Lee, R.T.; Rifai, N. & Ridker, P.M. (2001). Blood pressure and inflammation in apparently healthy men. *Hypertension*, Vol.38, No.3, (September 2001), pp. 399-403, ISSN 0194-911X.

Chainani-Wu, N.; Weidner, G.; Purnell, D.M.; Frenda, S.; Merritt-Worden, T.; Pischke, C.; Campo, R.; Kemp, C.; Kersh E.S. & Ornish, D. (2011). Changes in Emerging Cardiac Biomarkers After an Intensive Lifestyle Intervention. *The American journal of cardiology*, Epub ahead of print, doi:10.1016/j.amjcard.2011.03.077, ISSN 1879-1913.

Chaput, J.P.; Klingenberg, L.; Rosenkilde, M.; Gilbert, J.A.; Tremblay, A. & Sjödin, A. (2010). Physical activity plays an important role in body weight regulation. *Journal of obesity [electronic resource]*, Vol.2011 (2011), pii. 360257, ISSN 2090-0716 on line, ISSN 2090-0708 print.

Chuang, J.C.; Cui, H.; Mason, BL.; Mahgoub, M.; Bookout, A.L.; Yu, H.G.; Perello, M.; Elmquist, J.K.; Repa, J.J.; Zigman, J.M. & Lutter, M. (2010). Chronic social defeat stress disrupts regulation of lipid synthesis. *Journal of lipid research*, Vol.51, No.6, (June 2010), pp. 1344-1353, ISSN 0022-2275.

Codoñer-Franch, P.; Tavárez Alonso, S.; Murria-Estal, R.; Megías-Vericat, J.; Torlajada-Girbés, M. & Alonso-Iglesias, E. (2011). *Nitric oxide production is increased in severely obese children and related to markers of oxidative stress and inflammation*. Atherosclerosis, Vol.215, No.2, (April 2011), pp. 475-480, ISSN 0021-9150.

Company, J.M.; Booth, F.W.; Laughlin, M.H.; Arce-Esquivel, A.A.; Sacks, H.S.; Bahouth, S.W. & Fain, J.N. (2010). Epicardial fat gene expression after aerobic exercise training in pigs with coronary atherosclerosis: relationship to visceral and subcutaneous fat. *Journal of applied physiology*, Vo.109, No.6, (December 2010), pp. 1904-1912, ISSN 8750-7587.

Costa, R.S. & Assreuy J. (2005). Multiple potassium channels mediate nitric oxide-induced inhibition of rat vascular smooth muscle cell proliferation. *Nitric oxide: biology and chemistry/official journal of the Nitric Oxide Society*, Vol.13, No.2, (September 2005), pp. 145-51, ISSN 1089-8603.

Cunha, T.S.; Farah, V.; Paulini, J.; Pazzine, M.; Elased, K.M.; Marcondes, F.K.; Irigoyen, M.C.; De Angelis, K.; Mirkin, L.D. & Morris, M. (2007). Relationship between renal and cardiovascular changes in a murine model of glucose intolerance. *Regulatory peptides*, Vol.139, No.1-3, (March 2007), pp. 1-4, ISSN 0167-0115.

Dagogo-Jack, S.; Egbuonu, N. & Edeoga, C. (2010). Principles and practice of nonpharmacological interventions to reduce cardiometabolic risk. *Medical principles and practice: international journal of the Kuwait University, Health Science Centre*, Vol.19, No.3, (March 2010), pp. 167-175, ISSN 1011-7571.

Dallman, M.F.; La Fleur, S.E.; Pecoraro, N.; Gomez, F.; Houshyar, H. & Akana, S.F. (2004). Minireview: Glucocorticoids - food intake, abdominal obesity, and wealthy nations in 2004. *Endocrinology*, Vol.145, No.6, (June 2004), pp. 2633-2638, ISSN 0013-7227.

Dallman, M.F.; Pecoraro, N.; Akana, S.F.; La Fleur, S.E.; Gomez, F.; Houshyar, H.; Bell, M.E.; Bhatnagar, S.; Laugero, K.D. & Manalo, S. (2003). Chronic stress and obesity: a new view of "comfort food". *Proceedings of the National Academy of Sciences of the United States of America,* Vol.100, No.20, (September 2003), pp. 11696-11701, ISSN 0027-8424.

Dallman, M.F.; Pecoraro, N.C. & la Fleur, S.E. (2005). Chronic stress and comfort foods: self-medication and abdominal obesity. *Brain, behavior, and immunity,* Vo.19, No.4 (July 2005), pp. 275-280. ISSN 0889-1591.

Dasu, M.R. & Jialal, I. (2010). Free fatty acids in the presence of high glucose amplify monocyte inflammation via Toll-like receptors. American *journal of physiology. Endocrinology and metabolism,* Vol. 300, No.1, (January 2011), pp. E145-154, ISSN 1522-1555 online, ISSN 0193-1849 print.

Davy, K.P.; Evans, S.L.; Stevenson, E.T. & Seals, D.R. (1996). Adiposity and regional body fat distribution in physically active young and middle age women. *International journal of obesity and related metabolic disorders: journal of the International Association for the Study of Obesity,* Vol.20, No.8, (August 1996), pp. 777-783, ISSN 0307-0565.

De Geus, E.J.C. & Stubbe, J.H. (2007). Aerobic exercise and stress reduction, In: *Encyclopedia of Stress,* pp. 73-78, George Fink (editor), ELSEVIER, ISBN 978-0-12-088503-9, San Diego, CA – USA.

De Moura, E.G.; Lisboa, P.C. & Passos, M.C. (2008). Neonatal programming of neuroimmunomodulation-role of adipocytokines and neuropeptides. *Neuroimmunomodulation,* Vol.15, No.3, (October 2008), pp.176-188, ISSN 1021-7401.

Durstine, J.L.; Grandjean, P.W.; Cox, C.A. & Thompson, P.D. (2002). Lipids, lipoproteins, and exercise. *Journal of cardiopulmonary rehabilitation,* Vol.22, No.6, (November/December 2002), pp. 385-398, ISSN 0883-9212.

Dzubur Kulenović, A.; Kucukalić, A. & Malec, D. (2008). Changes in plasma lipid concentrations and risk of coronary artery disease in army veterans suffering from chronic posttraumatic stress disorder. *Croatian medical journal,* Vol.49, No.4, (August 2008), pp. 506-514, ISSN 0353-9504.

Ehninger, D. & Kempermann, G. (2003). Regional effects of wheel running and environmental enrichment on cell genesis and microglia proliferation in the adult murine neocortex. *Cerebral Cortex,* Vol.13, No.8, (August 2003), pp. 845-851, ISSN 1047-3211.

Epel E.S. (2009). Psychological and metabolic stress: a recipe for accelerated cellular aging? *Hormones (Athens),* Vol.8, No.1, (January-March 2009), pp. 7-22, ISSN 1109-3099.

Eriksson, J.; Taimela, S. & Koivisto, V.A. (1997). Exercise and the metabolic syndrome. *Diabetologia,* Vol.40, No.2, (February 1997), pp. 125-135, ISSN 0012-186X.

Farah, V.; Elased, K.M.; Chen, Y.; Key, M.P.; Cunha, T.S.; Irigoyen, M.C. & Morris, M. (2006). Nocturnal hypertension in mice consuming a high fructose diet. *Autonomic neuroscience: basic & clinical.* Vol.130, No.1-2, (December 2006), pp. 41-50, ISSN 1566-0702.

Feron, O.; Dessy, C.; Moniotte, S.; Desager, J.P. & Balligand, J.L. (1999). Hypercholesterolemia decreases nitric oxide production by promoting the interaction of caveolin and endothelial nitric oxide synthase. *The Journal of clinical investigation,* Vol.103, No.6, (March 1999), pp. 897-905, ISSN 0021-9738.

Fitch, K.V.; Stavrou, E.; Looby, S.E.; Hemphill, L.; Jaff, M.R. & Grinspoon, S.K. (2011). Associations of cardiovascular risk factors with two surrogate markers of subclinical atherosclerosis: Endothelial function and carotid intima media thickness. *Atherosclerosis,* Epub ahead of print, doi: 10.1016/j.atherosclerosis. 2011.04.009, (April 2011), ISSN 0021-9150.

Forcier, K.; Stroud, L.R.; Papandonatos, G.D.; Hitsman, B.; Reiches, M.; Krishnamoorthy, J. & Niaura, R. (2006). Links between physical fitness and cardiovascular reactivity and recovery to psychological stressors: a meta-analysis. *Health psychology: official journal of the Division of Health Psychology, American Psychological Association*, Vol.25, No.6, (November 2006), pp. 723–739, ISSN 0278-6133.

Förstermann, U. & Münzel, T. (2006). Endothelial nitric oxide synthase in vascular disease: from marvel to menace. *Circulation*, Vol.113, No.13, (April 2006), pp. 1708-1714, ISSN 0009-7322.

Frank, P.G. & Lisanti, M.P. (2004). Caveolin-1 and caveolae in atherosclerosis: differential roles in fatty streak formation and neointimal hyperplasia. *Current opinion in lipidology*, Vol.15, No.5, (October 2004), pp. 523-529, ISSN 0957-9672.

Gerber, M. & Pühse, U. (2009). Review article: do exercise and fitness protect against stress-induced health complaints? A review of the literature. *Scandinavian journal of public health*, Vol.37, No.8, (November 2009), pp. 801-819, ISSN 1403-4948.

Greenwood, B.N.; Foley, T.E.; Day, H.E.; Campisi, J.; Hammack, S.H.; Campeau, S.; Maier, S.F. & Fleshner, M. (2003) Freewheel running prevents learned helplessness/behavioral depression: role of dorsal raphe serotonergic neurons. *The Journal of neuroscience: the official journal of the Society for Neuroscience*, Vol.23, No.7, (April 2003), pp. 2889–2898, ISSN 0270-6474.

Gu, H.; Tang, C.; Peng, K.; Sun, H. & Yang, Y. (2009). Effects of chronic mild stress on the development of atherosclerosis and expression of toll-like receptor 4 signaling pathway in adolescent apolipoprotein E knockout mice. *Journal of biomedicine & biotechnology*, Vol.2009, (August 2009), pp. 1-13, ISSN 1110-7243.

Hamer, M.; Taylor, A. & Steptoe, A. (2005). The effect of acute aerobic exercise on stress related blood pressure responses: a systematic review and meta-analysis. *Biological psychology*, Vol.71, No.2, (2006), pp. 183-190, ISSN 1873-6246 online, ISSN 0301-0511 print.

Hawley, J.A. (2004). Exercise as a therapeutic intervention for the prevention and treatment of insulin resistance. *Diabetes/metabolism research and reviews*, Vol.20, No.5, (Sepember/October 2004), pp. 383–393, ISSN 1520-7552.

Hashimoto, S.; Ootani, K.; Hayashi, S. & Naito, M. (2011). Acute Effects of Shortly Pre-Versus Postprandial Aerobic Exercise on Postprandial Lipoprotein Metabolism in Healthy but Sedentary Young Women. *Journal of atherosclerosis and thrombosis*, Epub ahead of print, doi: 10.5551/jat.8482 (June 2011), ISSN 1880-3873.

Holmes, M.E.; Ekkekakis, P. & Eisenmann, J.C. (2009). The physical activity, stress and metabolic syndrome triangle: a guide to unfamiliar territory for the obesity researcher. *Obesity reviews: an official journal of the International Association for the Study of Obesity*, Vol.11, No.7, (July 2010), pp. 492-507, ISSN 1467-789X online, 1467-7881 print.

Howard, B.V. (1993). Insulin, insulin resistance, and dyslipidemia. *Annals of the New York Academy of Sciences*, Vol.683, (June 1993), pp. 1-8, ISSN 1749-6632.

Jackson, E.M. & Dishman, R.K. (2006). Cardiorespiratory fitness and laboratory stress: a meta-regression analysis. *Psychophysiology*, Vol.43, No.1, (January 2006), pp. 57–72, ISSN 0048-5772.

Kaplan, J.R.; Manuck, S.B.; Clarkson, T.F.; Lusso, F.M.; Taub, D.M. & Miller, E.W. (1983). Social stress and atherosclerosis in normocholesterolemic monkeys. *Science*, Vol.220, No.4598, (May 1983), pp. 733-735, ISSN 0036-8075.

Keidar, S.; Kaplan, M.; Shapira, C.; Brook, J.G. & Aviran, M. (1994). Low density lipoprotein isolated from patients with essential hypertension exhibits increased propensity for oxidation and enhanced uptake by macrophages: a possible role for angiotensin II. *Atherosclerosis*, Vol.107, No.71, (May 1994), pp. 71-84, ISSN 0021-9150.

Keidar, S.; Kaplan, M. & Aviram, M. (1996). Angiotensin II-modified LDL is taken up by macrophages via the scavenger receptor, leading to cellular cholesterol accumulation. *Arteriosclerosis, thrombosis, and vascular biology*, Vol.16, No.1, (January 1996), pp.97-105, ISSN 1079-5642.

Korte, S.M.; Koolhaas, J.M.; Wingfield, J.C. & McEwen, B.S. (2004). The Darwinian concept of stress: benefits of allostasis and costs of allostatic load and the trade-offs in health and disease. *Neuroscience and behavioral reviews*, Vol.29, No.1, (February 2005), pp. 3–38, ISSN 1873-7528 online, ISSN 0149-7634 print.

Kriska, A.M.; LaPorte, R.E.; Pettitt, D.J.; Charles, M.A.; Nelson, R.G.; Kuller, L.H.; Bennett, P.H. & Knowler, W.C. (1993). The association of physical activity with obesity, fat distribution and glucose intolerance in Pima Indians. *Diabetologia*, Vol.36, No.9, (September 1993), pp. 863-869, ISSN 0012-186X.

Kuo, L.E.; Abe, K. & Zukowska, Z. (2007). Stress, NPY and vascular remodeling: Implications for stress-related diseases. *Peptides*, Vo.28, No.2 (February 2007), pp. 435-440, ISSN 0196-9781.

Kuo, L.E.; Czarnecka, M.; Kitlinska, J.B.; Tilan, J.U.; Kvetnanský, R. & Zukowska, Z. (2008). Chronic stress, combined with a high-fat/high-sugar diet, shifts sympathetic signaling toward neuropeptide Y and leads to obesity and the metabolic syndrome. *Annals of the New York Academy of Sciences*, Vol.1148, (December 2008), pp. 232–237. ISSN 0077-8923.

Kyrou, I & Tsigos, C. (2009). Stress hormones: physiological stress and regulation of metabolism. *Current opinion in pharmacology*, Vol.9, No.6, (December 2009), pp. 787-793, ISSN 1471-4892.

Lafontan, M. & Langin, D. (2009). Lipolysis and lipid mobilization in human adipose tissue. Progress in lipid research, Vol.48, No.5, (September 2009), pp. 275-297, ISSN 0163-7827.

Lamharzi, N.; Renard, C.B.; Kramer, F.; Pennathur, S.; Heinecke, J.W.; Chait, A. & Bornfeldt, K.E. (2004). Hyperlipidemia in concert with hyperglycemia stimulates the proliferation of macrophages in atherosclerotic lesions: potential role of glucose-oxidized LDL. *Diabetes*, Vol.53, No.12, (December 2004), pp. 3217-3225, ISSN 0012-1797.

Lampman, R.M. & Schteingart, D.E. (1991). Effects of exercise training on glucose control, lipid metabolism, and insulin sensitivity in hypertriglyceridemia and non-insulin dependent diabetes mellitus. *Medicine and science in sports and sxercise*, Vol.23, No.6, (June 1991), pp. 703-712, ISSN: 0195-9131.

Lemieux, A.M. & Coe, C.L. (1995). Abuse-related posttraumatic stress disorders: evidence for chronic neuroendocrine activation in women. *Psychosomatic medicine*, Vol. 57, No.2, (March/April 1995), pp.105-115, ISSN 0033-3174.

Leon, A.S. & Sanchez, O.A. (2001). Response of blood lipids to exercise training alone or combined with dietary intervention. *Medicine and science in sports and exercise*, Vol.33, No.6, (June 2001), pp. S502-S515, ISSN 0195-9131.

Liao, J.K.; Shin, W.S.; Lee, W.Y. & Clark, S.L. (1995). Oxidized low-density lipoprotein decreases the expression of endothelial nitric oxide synthase. *The Journal of biological chemistry*, Vol.270, No.1, (January 1995), pp. 319-324, ISSN 0021-9258.

Lindgärde, F. & Saltin, B. (1981). Daily physical activity, work capacity and glucose tolerance in lean and obese normoglycaemic middle-aged men. *Diabetologia*, Vol.20, No.2, (February 1981), pp. 134-138, ISSN 0012-186X.

Ludwig, D.S.; Pereira, M.A.; Kroenke, C.H.; Hilner, J.E.; Van Horn, L.; Slattery, M.L. & Jacobs, D.R. Jr. (1999). Dietary fiber, weight gain, and cardiovascular disease risk factors in young adults. *JAMA*, Vol.282, No.16, (October 1999), pp. 1539-1546, ISSN 0098-7484.

Magkos, F.; Wright, D.C.; Patterson, B.W.; Mohammed, B.S. & Mittendorfer, B. (2005). Lipid metabolism response to a single, prolonged bout of endurance exercise in healthy young men. *American journal of physiology. Endocrinology and metabolism*, Vol.290, No.2, (February 2006), pp. E355-E362. ISSN 1522-1555 online, 0193-1849 print.

Masuzaki, H. & Flier JS. (2003). Tissue-specific glucocorticoid reactivating enzyme, 11 beta-hydroxysteroid dehydrogenase type 1 (11 beta-HSD1)--a promising drug target for the treatment of metabolic syndrome. *Current drug targets. Immune, endocrine and metabolic disorders*, Vol.3, No.4, (December 2003), pp. 255-262, ISSN 1568-0088.

Masuzaki, H.; Paterson, J.; Shinyama, H.; Morton, N.M.; Mullins, J.J.; Seckl, J.R. & Flier, J.S. (2001). A transgenic model of visceral obesity and the metabolic syndrome. *Science*, Vol.294, No.5549, (December 2001), pp. 2166-2170, ISSN 0036-8075.

Matsuura, E.; Kobayashi, K.; Matsunami, Y.; Shen, L.; Quan, N.; Makarova, M.; Suchkov, S.V.; Ayada, K.; Oguma, K. & Lopez, L.R. (2009). Autoimmunity, infectious immunity, and atherosclerosis. *Journal of clinical immunology*, Vol.29, No.6, (November 2009), pp. 714-721, ISSN 0271-9142.

McEwen, B.S. (1998). Protective and damaging effects of stress mediators: central role of the brain. *Dialogues in clinical neuroscience*, Vol.8, No.4, (2006), pp. 367-381, ISSN 1294-8322.

McCann, B.S.; Warnick, G.R. & Knopp, R.H. (1990). Changes in plasma lipids and dietary intake accompanying shifts in perceived workload and stress. *Psychosomatic medicine*, Vol.52, No.1, (January/February 1990), pp. 97-108, ISSN 0033-3174.

McGale, N.; McArdle, S. & Gaffney, P. (2011). Exploring the effectiveness of an integrated exercise/CBT intervention for young men's mental health. *British journal of health psychology*, Vol.16, No.3, (September 2011), pp.457-471, ISSN 1359-107X.

McMurray, R.G. & Hackney, A.C. (2005). Interactions of metabolic hormones, adipose tissue and exercise. *Sports medicine*, Vol.35, No.5, (2005), pp. 393-412, ISSN 0112-1642.

Mitchell, B.M.; Dorrance, A.M.; Mack, E.A. & Webb, R.C. (2004). Glucocorticoids decrease GTP cyclohydrolase and tetrahydro-biopterin-dependent vasorelaxation through glucocorticoid receptors. *Journal of cardiovascular pharmacology*, Vol.43, No.1, (January 2004), pp. 8-13, ISSN 0160-2446.

Mohamed-Ali, V.; Pinkney, J.H. & Coppack, S.W. (1998). Adipose tissue as an endocrine and paracrine organ. *International journal of obesity and related metabolic disorders: journal of the International Association for the Study of Obesity*, Vol.22, No.12, (December 1998), pp. 1145-1158, ISSN 0307-0565.

Mukai, H.; Tsurugizawa, T.; Ogiue-Ikeda, M.; Murakami, G.; Hojo, Y.; Ishii, H.; Kimoto, T. & Kawato, S. (2006). Local neurosteroid production in the hippocampus: influence on synaptic plasticity of memory. *Neuroendocrinology*, Vol.84, No.4, (2006), pp. 255-263, ISSN: 0028-3835.

Mullick, A.E.; Tobias, P.S. & Curtiss, L.K. (2006). Toll-like receptors and atherosclerosis: key contributors in disease and health? *Immunologic research*, Vol.34, No.3, (2006), pp. 193-209, ISSN 0257-277X.

Muniyappa, R. & Quon, M.J. (2007).Insulin action and insulin resistance in vascular endothelium. *Current opinion in clinical nutrition and metabolic care*, Vol.10, No.4, (July 2007), pp. 523-530, ISSN 1363-1950.

Muniyappa, R.; Iantorno, M. & Quon, M.J. (2008). An integrated view of insulin resistance and endothelial dysfunction. *Endocrinology and metabolism clinics of North America*, Vol.37, No.3, (September 2008), pp. 685-711, ISSN 0889-8529.

Nakazato, K.; Ishibashi, T.; Shindo, J.; Shiomi, M. & Maruyama, Y. (1996). Expression of very low density lipoprotein receptor mRNA in rabbit atherosclerotic lesions. *The American journal of pathology*, Vol.149, No.6, (December 1996), pp. 1831-1838, ISSN 0002-9440.

Neves, V.J.; Moura, M.J.C.S.; Almeida, B.S.; Costa, R.; Sanches, A.; Ferreira, R.; Tamascia, M.L.; Romani, E.A.O.; Novaes, P.D. & Marcondes, F.K. (2011). Chronic stress, but not hypercaloric diet, impairs vascular function in rats. *Stress: the international journal on the biology of stress*, (2011), Epub ahead of print, doi:10.3109/10253890.2011.601369, ISSN 1025-3890.

Neves, V.J.; Moura, M.J.C.S.; Tamascia, M.L.; Ferreira, R.; Silva, N.S.; Costa, R.; Montemor, P.L.; Narvaes, E.A.O.; Bernardes, C.F.; Novaes, P.D. & Marcondes, F.K. (2009). Proatherosclerotic effects of chronic stress in male rats: Altered phenylephrine sensitivity and nitric oxide synthase activity of aorta and circulating lipids. *Stress: the international journal on the biology of stress*, Vol.12, No.4, (July 2009), pp. 320-327, ISSN 1025-3890.

Nickenig, G.; Bäumer, A.T.; Temur, Y.; Kebben, D.; Jockenhövel, F. & Böhm, M. (1999). Statin-sensitive dysregulated AT1 receptor function and density in hypercholesterolemic men. *Circulation*, Vol.100, No.21, (November 1999), pp. 2131-2134, ISSN 0009-7322.

Nishitani, N. & Sakakibara, H. (2005). Relationship of obesity to job stress and eating behavior in male Japanese workers. International journal of obesity : journal of the International Association for the Study of Obesity, Vol.30, No.3, (March 2006), pp. 528-533, ISSN 1476-5497 online, ISSN 0307-0565 print.

O'Donnell, L.; O'Meara, N.; Owens, D.; Johnson, A.; Collins, P. & Tomkin, G. (1987). Plasma catecholamines and lipoproteins in chronic psychological stress. *Journal of the Royal Society of Medicine*, Vol.80, No.6, (June 1987), pp. 339-342, ISSN 0141-0768.

Okruhlicová, L; Dlugosová, K.; Mitasíková, M. & Bernátová, I. (2008). Ultrastructural characteristics of aortic endothelial cells in borderline hypertensive rats exposed to chronic social stress. *Physiological research /Academia Scientiarum Bohemoslovaca*, Vol.57, Suppl.2, (March 2008), pp. S31-37, ISSN 0862-8408.

Padden, D.L.; Connors, R.A. & Agazio, J.G. (2011). Determinants of health-promoting behaviors in military spouses during deployment separation. *Military medicine*, Vol.176, No.1, (January 2011), pp.26-34, ISSN: 0026-4075.

Pejovic, S.; Vgontzas, A.N.; Basta, M.; Tsaoussoglou, M.; Zoumakis, E.; Vgontzas, A.; Bixler, E.O. & Chrousos, G.P. (2010). Leptin and hunger levels in young healthy adults after one night of sleep loss. Journal of sleep research, Vol.19, No.4, (December 2010), pp. 552-558, ISSN 0962-1105.

Poehlman, E.T.; Toth, M.J.; Bunyard, L.B.; Gardner, A.W.; Donaldson, K.E.; Colman, E.; Fonong, T. & Ades, P.A. (1995). Physiological predictors of increasing total and central adiposity in aging men and women. *Archives of internal medicine*, Vol.155, No.22, (December 1995), pp. 2443-2448, ISSN 0003-9926.

Pradhan, A.D.; Manson, J.E.; Rifai, N.; Buring, J.E.& Ridker, P.M. (2001).C-reactive protein, interleukin 6, and risk of developing type 2 diabetes mellitus. *JAMA*, Vol.286, No.3, (July 2001), pp. 327-334, ISSN 0098-7484.

Risérus, U.; Willett, W.C. & Hu, F.B. (2008). Dietary fats and prevention of type 2 diabetes. *Progress in lipid research*, Vol.48, No.1, (January 2009), pp. 44-51, ISSN 1873-2194 online, 0163-7827 print.

Rizzo, M.; Kotur-Stevuljevic, J.; Berneis, K.; Spinas, G.; Rini, G.B.; Jelic-Ivanovic, Z.; Spasojevic-Kalimanovska, V. & Vekic, J. (2009). Atherogenic dyslipidemia and oxidative stress: a new look. *Translational research: the journal of laboratory and clinical medicine*, Vol.153, No.5, (May 2009), pp. 217-223. ISSN 1931-5244.

Roberts, C.K. & Barnard, R.J. (2005). Effects of exercise and diet on chronic disease. *Journal of applied physiology*, Vol.98, No.1, (January 2005), pp. 3-30, ISSN: 8750-7587.

Ross, R. (1999). Atherosclerosis--an inflammatory disease. *The New England journal of medicine*, Vol.340, No.2, (January 1999), pp. 115-126, ISSN. 0028-4793.

Rubenfire, M.; Mollo, L.; Krishnan, S.; Finkel, S.; Weintraub, M.; Gracik, T.; Kohn, D. & Oral, E.A. (2011). The Metabolic Fitness Program: Lifestyle modification for the metabolic syndrome using the resources of cardiac rehabilitation. *Journal of cardiopulmonary rehabilitation and prevention*, Epub ahead of print doi: 10.1097/HCR. 0b013e318220a7eb, (July 2011), ISSN 1932-751X.

Schuit, A.J.; Schouten, E.G.; Miles, TP.; Evans, W.J.; Saris, W.H.M. & Kok, F.J. (1998). The effect of six months training on weight, body fatness and serum lipids in apparently healthy elderly Dutch men and women International. *International journal of obesity and related metabolic disorders: journal of the International Association for the Study of Obesity*, Vol.22, No.9, (September 1998), pp. 847-853, ISSN 0307-0565.

Seeman, T.E.; Singer, B.H.; Rowe, J.W.; Horwitz, R.I. & McEwen, B.S. (1997). Price of adaptation--allostatic load and its health consequences. MacArthur studies of successful aging. *Archives of internal medicine*, Vol.157, No.19, (October 1997), pp. 2259-2268, ISSN 0003-9926.

Selye, H. (1936). A syndrome produced by diverse nocuous agents. *Nature*, Vol.138, (July 1936), p.32, ISSN 1476-4687.

Sheril, A.; Jeyakumar, S.M.; Jayashree, T.; Giridharan, N.V. & Vajreswari A. (2008). Impact of feeding polyunsaturated fatty acids on cholesterol metabolism of dyslipidemic obese rats of WNIN/GR-Ob strain. *Atherosclerosis*, Vol.204, No.1, (May 2009), pp.136-140, ISSN 1879-1484 online, ISSN 0021-9150 print.

Shively, C.A.; Register, T.C. & Clarkson, T.B. (2009). Social stress, visceral obesity, and coronary artery atherosclerosis: product of a primate adaptation. American journal of primatology, Vol.71, No.9, (September 2009), pp. 742-751, ISSN 0275-2565.

Sierra, C. & de la Sierra, A. (2008). Early detection and management of the high-risk patient with elevated blood pressure. *Vascular health and risk management*, Vol.4, No.2, (April 2008), pp. 289-296, ISSN 1176-6344.

Sigwalt, A.R.; Budde, H.; Helmich, I.; Glaser, V.; Ghisoni, K.; Lanza, S.; Cadore, E.L.; Lhullier, F.L.; F de Bem A.; Hohl, A.; J de Matos, F.; de Oliveira, P.A.; S Prediger, R.D.; A Guglielmo, L.G. & Latini, A. (2011). Molecular aspects involved in swimming exercise training reducing anhedonia in a rat model of depression. *Neuroscience*, Epub ahead of print, doi:10.1016/j.physletb.2003.10.071, (June 2011), ISSN 1873-7544.

Singh, B.M. & Mehta, J.L. (2003). Interactions between the renin-angiotensin system and dyslipidemia: relevance in the therapy of hypertension and coronary heart disease. *Archives of internal medicine*, Vol.163, No.11, (June 2003), pp. 1296-1304, ISSN 0003-992

Sitia, S.; Tomasoni, L.; Atzeni, F.; Ambrosio, G.; Cordiano, C.; Catapano, A.; Tramontana, S.; Perticone, F.; Naccarato, P.; Camici, P.; Picano, E.; Cortigiani, L.; Bevilacqua, M.; Milazzo, L.; Cusi, D.; Barlassina, C.; Sarzi-Puttini, P. & Turiel, M. (2010). From endothelial dysfunction to atherosclerosis. *Autoimmunity reviews*, Vol.9, No.12, (October 2010), pp. 830-834, ISSN 1568-9972.

Sothmann, M.S.; Buckworth, J.; Claytor, R.P.; Cox, R.H.; White-Welkley, J.E. & Dishman, R.K. (1996). Exercise training and the cross-stressor adaptation hypothesis. *Exercise and sport science reviews*, Vol.24, (1996), pp. 267-287, ISSN 0091-6331.

Spiegel, K.; Tasali, E.; Penev, P. & Van Cauter E. (2004). Brief communication: Sleep curtailment in healthy young men is associated with decreased leptin levels, elevated ghrelin levels, and increased hunger and appetite. *Annals of internal medicine*, Vol. 141, No.11, (December 2004), pp. 846-850, ISSN 0003-4819.

Stanhope, K.L.; Schwarz, J.M.; Keim, N.L.; Griffen, S.C.; Bremer, A.A.; Graham, J.L.; Hatcher, B.; Cox, C.L.; Dyachenko, A.; Zhang, W.; McGahan, J.P.; Seibert, A.; Krauss, R.M.; Chiu, S.; Schaefer, E.J.; Ai, M.; Otokozawa, S.; Nakajima, K.; Nakano, T.; Beysen, C.; Hellerstein, M.K.; Berglund, L. & Havel, P.J. (2009). Consuming fructose-sweetened, not glucose-sweetened, beverages increases visceral adiposity and lipids and decreases insulin sensitivity in overweight/obese humans. *The journal of Clinical Investigation*, Vol.119, No.5, (May 2009), pp. 1322-1334, ISSN 0021-9738.

Steanovv, T.S.; Vekova, A.M.; Kurktschiev, D.P. & Temelkova-Kurktschiev, T.S. (2011). Relationship of physical activity and eating behaviour with obesity and type 2 diabetes mellitus: Sofia Lifestyle (SLS) study. *Folia Medica*, Vol.53, No.1, (January/March 2011), pp. 11-18, ISSN 0204-8043.

Steinberg, D. (2002). Atherogenesis in perspective: hypercholesterolemia and inflammation as partners in crime. *Nature medicine*, Vol.8, No.11, (November 2002), pp. 1211-1217, ISSN 1078-8956.

Sterling, P. & Eyer, J. (1988). Allostasis: a new paradigm to explain arousal pathology. In: *Handbook of Life Stress, Cognition and Health*, Fisher, S. & Reason, J (editors), pp. 629-649, JOHN WILEY & SONS, ISBN-10: 0471912697/ISBN-13: 978-0471912699, New York – USA.

Stoney, C.M. (2007). Cholesterol and Lipoproteins, In: *Encyclopedia of Stress*, George Fink (editor), pp. 478-483, ELSEVIER, ISBN 978-0-12-088503-9, San Diego, CA – USA.

Stoney, C.M.; Niaura, R.; Bausserman, L. & Matacin, M. (1999). Lipid reactivity to stress: I. Comparison of chronic and acute stress responses in middle-aged airline pilots. *Health psychology : official journal of the Division of Health Psychology, American Psychological Association*, Vol.18, No.3, (May 1999), pp. 241-250, ISSN 0278-6133.

Stoney, C.M.; West, S.G.; Hughes, J.W.; Lentino, L.M.; Finney, M.L.; Falko, J. & Bausserman, L. (2002). Acute psychological stress reduces plasma triglyceride clearance. *Psychophysiology*, Vol.39, No.1, (January 2002), pp. 80-85, ISSN 0048-5772.

Sudano, I.; Spieker, L.E.; Hermann, F.; Flammer, A.; Corti, R.; Noll, G. & Lüscher, T.F. (2006). Protection of endothelial function: targets for nutritional and pharmacological interventions. *Journal of cardiovascular pharmacology*, Vol.47, No.2, (June 2006), pp. S136-S150, ISSN 0160-2446.

Taguchi, I.; Inoue, T.; Kikuchi, M.; Toyoda, S.; Arikawa, T.; Abe, S. & Node, K. (2011). Pleiotropic effects of ARB on dyslipidemia. *Current vascular pharmacology*, Vol.9, No.2, (March 2011), pp. 129-135, ISSN 1570-1611.

Tellez, A.; Schuster, D.S.; Alviar, C.; López-Berenstein, G.; Sanguino, A.; Ballantyne, C.; Perrard, X.Y.; Schulz, D.G.; Rousselle, S.; Kaluza, G.L. & Granada, J.F. (2011). Intramural coronary lipid injection induces atheromatous lesions expressing proinflammatory chemokines: implications for the development of a porcine model of atherosclerosis. *Cardiovascular revascularization medicine: including molecular interventions*, Epub ahead of print, doi:10.1016/j.carrev.2011.03.007, (May 2011), ISSN 1878-0938.

Thompson, P.D.; Cullinane, E.M.; Sady, S.P.; Flynn, M.M.; Bernier, D.N.; Kantor, M.A.; Saritelli, A.L. & Herbert, P.N. (1988). Modest changes in high-density lipoprotein concentration and metabolism with prolonged exercise training. *Circulation*, Vol.78, No.1, (July 1988), pp. 25-34, ISSN 0009-7322.

Torres, S.J. & Nowson, C.A. (2007). Relationship between stress, eating behavior, and obesity. *Nutrition*, Vol.23, No.11-12, (November/December 2007), pp. 887-894, ISSN 0899-9007.

Tsatsoulis, A. & Fountoulakis, S. (2006). The protective role of exercise on stress system dysregulation and comorbidities. . *Annals of the New York Academy of Sciences*, Vol.1083 (November 2006), pp. 196-213, ISSN 0077-8923.

Tsekouras, Y.E.; Magkos, F.; Prentzas, K.I.; Basioukas, K.N.; Matsama, S.G.; Yanni, A.E.; Kavouras, S.A. & Sidossis, L.S. (2009). A single bout of whole-body resistance exercise augments basal VLDL-triacylglycerol removal from plasma in healthy untrained men. *Clinical science*, Vol.116, No.2, (January 2009), pp. 147-156, ISSN 0143-5221.

van Oostrom, A.J.; van Wijk, J. & Cabezas, M.C. (2004). Lipaemia, inflammation and atherosclerosis: novel opportunities in the understanding and treatment of atherosclerosis. *Drugs*, Vol.64, No.2 (2004), pp. 19-41, 0012-6667.

Veen, G.; Giltay, E.J.; DeRijk, R.H.; van Vliet, I.M.; van Pelt, J. & Zitman, F.G. (2009). Salivary cortisol, serum lipids, and adiposity in patients with depressive and anxiety disorders. *Metabolism: clinical and experimental*, Vol.58, No.6, (June 2009), pp. 821-827, ISSN 0026-0495.

Venables, M.C. & Jeukendrup, A.E. (2009). Physical inactivity and obesity: links with insulin resistance and type 2 diabetes mellitus. *Diabetes/metabolism research and reviews*, Vol.25, No.1, (September 2009), pp. S18-S23, ISSN 1520-7552.

Vessby, B. (2000). Dietary fat and insulin action in humans. *The British journal of nutrition*, Vol.83, No.1, (March 2000), pp. S91-S96, ISSN 0007-1145.

Vogelzangs, N.; Suthers, K.; Ferrucci, L.; Simonsick, E.M.; Ble, A.; Schrager, M.; Bandinelli, S.; Lauretani, F.; Giannelli, S.V. & Penninx, B.W. (2007). Hypercortisolemic depression is associated with the metabolic syndrome in late-life. *Psychoneuroendocrinology*, Vol.32, No.2, (February 2007), pp.151-159, ISSN 0306-4530.

Walker, E.A. & Stewart, P.M. (2003). 11beta-hydroxysteroid dehydrogenase: unexpected connections. *Trends in endocrinology and metabolism: TEM*, Vol.14, No.7, (September 2003), pp.334-339, ISSN 1043-2760.

Wallis, D.J. & Hetherington M.M. (2008). Emotions and eating: Self-reported and experimentally induced changes in food intake under stress. *Appetite*, Vol.52, No.2, (April 2009), pp. 355-362, ISSN 1095-8304 online, 0195-6663 print.

Watts, G.F.; Barrett, P.H.R. & Chan, D.C. (2008). HDL metabolism in context: looking on the bright side. *Current opinion in lipidology,* Vol.19, No.4, (August 2008), pp. 395-404, ISSN 0957-9672.

Watts, G.F.; Ooi, E.M.M. & Chan, D.C. (2009). Therapeutic regulation of apoB100 metabolism in insulin resistance in vivo. *Pharmacology & therapeutics,* Vol.123, No.3, (September 2009), pp. 281–291, ISSN: 0163-7258.

Win, S.; Parakh, K.; Eze-Nliam, C.M.; Gottdiener, J.S.; Kop, W.J. & Ziegelstein, R.C. (2011). Depressive symptoms, physical inactivity and risk of cardiovascular mortality in older adults: the Cardiovascular Health Study. *Heart: official journal of the British Cardiac Society,* Vol.97, No.6, (March 2011), pp. 500-505, ISSN 1355-6037.

Xu, C.; He, J.; Jiang., H.; Zu, L.; Zhai, W.; Pu, S. & Xu, G. (2009). Direct effect of glucocorticoids on lipolysis in adipocytes. *Molecular endocrinology,* Vol.23, No.8, (May 2009), pp. 1161-1170, ISSN 0888-8809.

Xu, X.H.; Shah, P.K.; Faure, E.; Equils, O.; Thomas, L.; Fishbein, M.C.; Luthringer, D.; Xu, X.P.; Rajavashisth, T.B.; Yano, J.; Kaul, S. & Arditi, M. (2001). Toll-like receptor-4 is expressed by macrophages in murine and human lipid-rich atherosclerotic plaques and upregulated by oxidized LDL. *Circulation,* Vol.104, No.25 (December 2001), pp. 3103-3108, ISSN 0009-7322.

Yamazaki, Y.; Hashizume, T.; Morioka, H.; Sadamitsu, S.; Ikari, A.; Miwa, M. & Sugatani, J. (2011). Diet-induced lipid accumulation in liver enhances ATP-binding cassette transporter g5/g8 expression at bile canaliculi. *Drug metabism and pharmacokinetics,* Epub ahead of print, doi:10.2133/dmpk.DMPK-11-RG-025, (May 2011), ISSN 1880-0920.

Yarrow, J.F.; White, L.J.; McCoy, S.C. & Borst, S.E. (2010). Training augments resistance exercise induced elevation of circulating brain derived neurotrophic factor (BDNF). *Neuroscience letters,* Vol.479, No.2, (July 2010), pp. 161-165, ISSN 0304-3940.

Yin, Z.; Davis, C.L.; Moore, J.B. & Treiber, F.A. (2005). Physical activity buffers the effects of chronic stress on adiposity in youth. *Annals of behavioral medicine: a* publication *of the Society of Behavioral Medicine,* Vol.29, No.1, (February 2005), pp. 29-36, ISSN 0883-6612.

Yoo, H. & Franke, W.D. (2010). Stress and cardiovascular disease risk in female law enforcement officers. *International archives of occupational and environmental health,* Vol.84, No.3, (March 2011), pp. 279-286, ISSN 1432-1246 online, ISSN 0340-0131 print.

Yudkin, J.S.; Kumari, M.; Humphries, S.E. & Mohamed-Ali, V. (2000). Inflammation, obesity, stress and coronary heart disease: is interleukin-6 the link? *Atherosclerosis,* Vol.148, No.2, (Februery 2000), pp. 209-214, ISSN 0021-9150.

Zakrzewska, K.E.; Cusin, I.; Sainsbury, A.; Rohner-Jeanrenaud, F. & Jeanrenaud, B. (1997). Glucocorticoids as counterregulatory hormones of leptin: toward an understanding of leptin resistance. *Diabetes,* Vol.46, No.4, (April 1997), pp. 717-719, ISSN 0012-1797.

Zukowska, Z. (2005). Atherosclerosis and angiogenesis: what do nerves have to do with it? *Pharmacological reports: PR.* Vol.57, Supplement, (June 2005), pp. 229-234, ISSN 1734-1140.

5

Dyslipidemia and Mental Illness

D. Saravane

Head of Department Medicine and Specialists
Ville-Evrard Hospital Neuilly/Marne
France

1. Introduction

Almost most mental illness, such as schizophrenia, bipolar disorder, and depression are associated with undue medical morbidity and mortality. It represents a major health problem, with 20 to 30 years shorter lifetime mortality are primarily due to premature cardiovascular disease (myocardial infarction, stroke…). The cardiovascular events are strongly linked to non modifiable risk factors such as age, gender, personal and/or family history, but also to crucial modifiable risk factors, such as overweight and obesity, dyslipidemia, diabetes, hypertension and smoking.

Although these classical risk factors exist in the general population epidemiological studies suggest that patients with severe mental illness have an increased prevalence of these risk factors.

Another point is the causes of increased metabolic and cardiovascular risk in this population are related to poverty, poor diet, sedentary and compared to the general population. The increased morbidity and mortality limited behaviour access to medical care, but also to the use of psychotropic medication. Over recent years it has become apparent that antipsychotic drugs can have a negative impact on some of the modifiable risk factors.

2. Epidemiological studies

Results of most research on the physical health of people with mental health illness suggest the morbidity and the mortality from certain physical disease is high in these populations. Patients with schizophrenia are a medically vulnerable population due to underdiagnosed medical problems, and minimal or not utilization of primary care services. Not only there is increased medical morbidity among these patients, there is also increased mortality.

Medical comorbidity in patients with bipolar disorder, is associated with an intensification of bipolar depressive symptoms and other indices of bipolar severity, as well as premature mortality. Somatic health issues remain underrecognized and suboptimally treated.

2.1 Mortality

An increasing number of studies have found higher rates of mortality in schizophrenia patients due to natural causes (Mortensen & Juel, 1993; Ruschena et al, 1998). Such increased rates of mortality due to natural causes highlight the failure to detect and manage physical health conditions in this group. In meta-analysis deaths due to natural causes accounted for

59% of the excess mortality in schizophrenia (Brown, 1997). Respiratory and cardiovascular diseases are the most common causes of natural death. The standard mortality ratio (SMR) for respiratory disease was 226 (95%CI, 209-244) and for cardiovascular disease 110 (95%CI, 105-115) (Brown, 1997). However, another study found an SMR of 1.78 for men and 0.86 for women with schizophrenia for ischemic heart disease (Lawrence et al, 2003). Analysis of standardized mortality ratios for deaths from natural causes showed an increased risk of death in patients with a wide range of psychiatric conditions, including substance misuse, schizophrenia, bipolar disorder and unipolar depression. The Standardized mortality ratios (SMR) showed that in schizophrenia it is 1.57 for all cause mortality, and cardiovascular and cancer deaths accounted for the largest number of deaths with SMRs of 1.04 and 1.00 respectively (Harris & Barraclough, 1998). Depression confers a 24% increased risk of dying within the next 6 years (Wulsin, 2000). A study published through the Centers for Disease Control and Prevention (CDC) compared the mortality of public mental health patients in 8 states with the mortality of the states' general population, for 1997 through 2000. In all the study states, mental health had a higher risk of death than the general population and died at much younger ages compared with their cohorts. In all states studied, cardiac disease was found to be the leading cause of death in mentally ill patients. And this population had lost decades of potential years of life, with average exceeding 25 years (Colton & Manderscheid, 2006).

Another indicator of the medical care is avoidable mortality. These indicators are calculated by selecting the number of avoidable causes of death considered amenable to health care (Rustein et al, 1976). A follow-up study of 30045 psychiatric in-patients born between 1912-1970 was conducted to specifically address avoidable mortality. The standardized rate ratios (SRR) for male patients with schizophrenia are 3.74 (95%CI, 2.38-5.89) and 3.99 (95%CI, 2.47-6.44) for females (Ringback Weitoft et al, 1998).

2.2 Morbidity

A study list some of the common physical conditions found in people with psychosis. These include diabetes, hyperlipidemia, cardiovascular disease, obesity, malignant neoplasms, HIV/AIDS, hepatitis, osteoporosis, hyperprolactinemia, irritable bowel syndrome and helicobacter pylori infection (Lambert et al, 2003). The prevalence of physical illness in medically screened chronic psychiatric samples has been variously reported to be 12-53% (Lyketsos et al, 2002). Another study estimate that 35% of psychiatric patients have undiagnosed physical disorder (Felker et al, 1996).Some studies have attempted to establish whether medical comorbidity exacerbates patient' psychiatric condition (Bartsch et al, 1998).

Not only do patients with mental illness die of natural causes at high rate, when medical conditions occur, these patients are much more likely to underdiagnosed and undertreated. Several studies have shown that the detection rate of physical illness among patient with mental illness is very poor. A study estimated that 45% of patients in California's public mental-health system had physical disease and, of these, 47% were undetected by the treating physician (Koran, 1989). Another study of psychiatric clinic patients revealed remarkably similar findings: 43% of patients had physical illnesses and, of these, 48% had not been diagnosed by the referring doctor, non-psychiatrist physicians had missed 33% and psychiatrists had missed 50% (Koranyi, 1979). Hall et al found that 46% of patients admitted to a research ward had an unrecognized physical illness that either caused or exacerbated their psychiatric illness; 80% had physical illnesses requiring treatment, and 4% had precancerous conditions or illnesses (Hall et al, 1981).

Research indicates that 25% to 80% of patients with schizophrenia and other mental illness have a serious medical comorbidity, yet less than half of these medical conditions are diagnosed (Cradock-O'Leary et al, 2002).

3. Causes of poor physical health in mental illness

A number of reasons exist to explain the poor detection of physical health problems in patient with mental illness. Some patients are unaware of any physical health problems, usually a consequence of cognitive deficits associated with their mental illness (Goldman, 1999). Often there is a reluctance to seek medical help and when it sought patient with mental health find it difficult to describe their problems to a medical practitioner, or present with atypical medical symptoms. Patient with schizophrenia have been shown to have a high tolerance for pain and subsequently are less likely to report this symptom (Dworkin, 1994). Another complexity concerns the effects of psychiatric illness on perceived physical health. For example, depression can lead to an increase in perceived physical symptoms and worsening of subjective health outcomes.

The management of medical conditions is a complex and problematic issue, arising largely because of the separation of medical and psychiatric health care services. The stigma of mental illness is one obvious barrier preventing psychiatric patients from receiving adequate physical health care, as some physicians may be uncomfortable in working with this patient. Another concern is managing physical conditions where patients that have an increased prevalence with psychiatric illness and where there is a general lack of treatment compliance. The challenging task of managing physical illness with this patient requires skill, patience and experience as patients often present late with complications. (Table 1)

System-Related Barriers
Lack of insurance coverage
Lack of access to health care
Stigmatization by health care providers
Lack of understanding of benefits of preventive services by health care workers
Lack of integration of medical and mental health systems
Patients–Barriers
Poverty
Non compliance
Pour communication skills
Denials of illness Related

Table 1. Barriers to health care for patients with mental illness. Adapted from Goldman.

3.1 Lifestyle risk factors

In recent years, there is a growing concern about physical illness in patients with mental illnesses, specifically the risk of cardiovascular disease. Those patients are more likely to be overweight, to smoke, to have hypertension, hyperglycemia or diabetes, and dyslipidemia (Table 2).

Estimated prevalence, % (RR)		
Modifiable risk factors	Schizophrenia	Bipolar disorder
Overweight	45–55% (1,5–2)	21–49% (1-2)
Smoking	50–80% (2-3)	54-68% (2-3)
Diabetes	10-15% (2)	8-17% (1,5-2)
Hypertension	19-58% (2-3)	35-61% (2-3)
Dyslipidemia	25-69% (≤5)	25-38% (≤3)
Metabolic syndrome	37-63% (2-3)	30-49% (1,5-2)

Table 2. Estimation prevalence and relative risk 5 (RR) of modifiable cardiovascular disease risk factors in schizophrenia and bipolar disorder compared to the general population. Adapted from Correll, 2007

3.1.1 Obesity

Excessive body weight increases the risk of morbidity from number conditions, including hypertension, dyslipidemia, type II diabetes, coronary heart disease. Excess abdominal fat is associated with dyslipidemia, hypertension and glucose intolerance. Risk of comorbid diseases has been shown to rise as BMI increases above 25 kg/m2. In psychiatric practice, weight gain is a long recognized and commonly encountered problem. A study of patients with schizophrenia reported 51% of males and 59% of females to be clinically obese, compared with 33% of people with other psychiatric disorders. This study provided an estimate of mean weight gain in patients who received standard doses of antipsychotics over 10-week period. The mean increases were 4.45 kg with clozapine, 4.15 with olanzapine, 2.92 kg with sertindole, 2.10 kg with risperidone, and 0.04 kg with ziprasidone (Allison & Casey, 2001). It is important to note that substantial weight gain is associated with both atypical (eg, clozapine, olanzapine) and conventional (eg, thioridazine, chlorpromazine) antipsychotics.

3.1.2 Smoking

The prevalence of smoking greatly exceeds that in the general population (Table 1) Heavy cigarette smoking is intimately associated with schizophrenia and it may have implications for the underlying neurobiology of the disease. Smoking is a good example of how behavior and treatment interact to increase morbidity at a number of levels. It is a risk factor for respiratory and ischemic heart disease and stroke. Cigarette smoking induces hepatic microsomal enzymes, which increase the metabolism of psychotropic medication, reducing plasma levels of antipsychotics notably olanzapine and clozapine. It may influence the patient's behavior and the treatment outcome. Therefore smokers usually require greater levels of antipsychotic medication than non-smokers to achieve similar blood levels.

3.1.3 Diabetes

It is another risk factor for coronary atherosclerosis that is associated with metabolic abnormalities that result in changes in the transport, composition and metabolism of lipoproteins.

3.1.4 Hypertension

Is a cardiovascular risk factor as it produces structural changes within the arteries. The seq uel of hypertension are greatly affected by comorbidities such as dyslipidemia, smoking, diabetes, lack of physical activity, sodium intake, and stress.

Other risk factors are attributable to unhealthy lifestyle, including social scale such as unemployment, poorer financial standing, poor diet and sedentary behaviour.

Concerning diet, a study (Mc Creadle, 2003) examined in detail the dietary intake of 102 people with schizophrenia in Scotland. Their fruit and vegetable consumption averaged 16 portions per week, less than half the recommended intake.

Brown et al, 1999 and Mc Creadle, 2003 found that patients with schizophrenia tended to take only small amounts of exercice. Factors such as features of the illness, sedative medication and lack of opportunity and general motivation may be relevant.

3.2 Medication

Psychotropic medication is associated with a host of physical complications and side effects. Old antipsychotic medication was associated with neurologic side effects, including involuntary movement disorders, such as akathisia, parkinsonism, tardive dyskinisia. New antipsychotics are more commonly use. Despite the low propensity of new antipsychotics towards extra pyramidal side effects other adverse effects associated with them include excessive weight gain, metabolic disturbances. Medical conditions attributed to the use of typical and atypical antipsychotic medication include diabetes, hyperlipidemia, and cardiovascular disease: specifically hypertension and cardiac arrhythmias, obesity (Meyer, 2002; Davidson, 2002).

4. The metabolic syndrome

Much attention has been focused on the metabolic syndrome which brings together a series of abnormal clinical and metabolic findings which are predictive of cardiovascular risk. The most commonly used definition for the metabolic syndrome are the Adult Treatment Panel III (ATP III) of the National Cholesterol Education Program (NCEP), (Jama, 2001) and the adapted ATP-III-A proposed by the American to Heart Association following the American Diabetes Association lowering of the threshold for impaired fasting glucose 100mg/dl. (Quindy et al, 2005 ; Alberti et al, 2006).

Another recent definition, by the International Diabetes Federation (Alberti et al, 2006; Sarafidis &, Nilsson, 2006) stressed the importance of waist circumference, using ethnic/race specific criteria (Table 3).

	ATP III 3 out of 5 criteria required	ATP III A 3 out of 5 criteria required	IDF waist + 2 criteria required
Waist (cm)	M>102, F>88	M>102, F>88	M≥94,F≥80
Blood pressure	≥130/85*	≥130/85*	≥130/85*
HDL cholesterol (mg/dl)	M<40, F<50	M<40,F<50	M<40,F<50
Triglycerides (mg/dl)	≥150	≥150	≥150
Fasting glucose (mg/dl)	≥110**	≥100**	≥100**

*or treated with antihypertensive medication
**or treated with insulin or hypoglycemic medication

Table 3. Definitions of metabolic syndrome: The metabolic syndrome has been shown to be an important risk factor for the development of both type 2 diabetes and cardiovascular disease.

In the study, the clinical Antipsychotic Trials of Intervention Effectiveness (CATIE), one third of patients met the NCEP criteria for metabolic syndrome at baseline (Mc Eoy et al, 2005 ; Meyer et al, 2005).

And from this study, 88% of patients with dyslipidemia were not receiving treatment, as were 62% of the hypertensive patients and 38% those with diabetes (Nasrallah et al, 2006). The presence of the metabolic syndrome increases the risk for the distribution of fat within the body is a key factor. Abdominal fat distribution, particularly visceral adiposity, increases the risk of dyslipidemia, glucose intolerance, and cardiovascular disease. Multiple organ systems are affected, including adipose, muscle, hepatic, nervous, and adrenal tissues, and the most important site of impact is the vasculature. The concept of insulin resistance is central to the metabolic syndrome. Insulin resistance is a major contributor to glucose intolerance, and the lipoprotein abnormalities seen in the metabolic syndrome are also predictable, at least in part, from the known effects of insulin to inhibit lipolysis in adipocytes. With resistance to insulin, unchecked lipolysis leads to increased delivery of free fatty acids to the liver for triglyceride synthesis and packaging into very low-density lipoprotein (VLDL) particles. Higher VLDL levels contribute to lower HDL levels because of the reciprocal exchanges between these lipoproteins mediated by cholesterol ester transfer protein. Is has been shown that blood pressure is related to insulin resistance independent of differences in age, gender, and degree of obesity(Zavaroni et al,1992). Visceral obesity is the primary determinant of insulin resistance and, as such, represents the fundamental pathophysiologic change leading to the metabolic syndrome. The risk of insulin resistance increases with adiposity, particularly the amount of visceral adiposity. Insulin resistance is associated with impaired glucose control, increase plasma triglycerides, reduced high-density lipoprotein (HDL) cholesterol, increased blood pressure, increased risk of blood clotting, and increases in markers of inflammation, all which are associated with an increase risk for cardiovascular disease. Thus, markers of insulin resistance, such as elevated fasting plasma Triglycerides, can be a key point for monitoring and evaluating a patient's risk.

5. Effects of antipsychotics treatment

Antipsychotic treatment is associated with metabolic side effects that include various degrees of weight gain, dyslipidemia and susceptibility to type 2 diabetes (Newcomer, 2005).

Elevated blood lipids, particularly triglycerides, are associated with some typical antipsychotic agents. Shortly after their introduction, phenothiazines were found to elevate serum triglyceride and total cholesterol levels. Then much was written on the effects of specific atypical drugs on lipid profiles. Both clozapine and olanzapine have been shown to cause significant hypertriglyceridemia compared with typicals. Studies have also reported a significant association between weight gain and triglyceride change for patients under atypical antipsychotic therapy (Meyer, 2001).

The atypical antipsychotics vary in their propensity to induce weight gain (Table 4): clozapine and olanzapine produce the most weight gain, quetiapine and risperidone produce intermediate weight gain, and ziprasidone and aripiprazole produce the least weight gain (Allison et al, 1999; American Diabetes Association [ADA], 2004). The differences in weight gain associated with these agents reflect their order of risk for insulin resistance, glucoregulatory dysfunction, and dyslipidemia (Haupt & Newcomer 2002; ADA, 2004).

Antipsychotic	Weight	Risk for diabetes	Worsening lipid proli B
Clozapine	+++	+	+
Olanzapine	+++	+	+
Risperidone	++	D	D
Quetiapine	++	D	D
Ziprasidone	+/-	-	-
Aripiprazole	+/-	-	-

[a]Adapted with the permission from the American Diabetes Association Abbreviation:
D = discrepant results
Symbols: + = increased effect, - = no effect

Table 4. Atypical antipsychotic drugs and metabolic disturbances[a]

Metabolic disturbances related to atypical antipsychotics may result from a direct alteration of insulin sensitivity and/or insulin secretion. Antipsychotic affinity at both histamine and muscarinie acetylcholine receptors correlates with weight gain and metabolic liability (Matsui-Sakata, 2005) and impaired parasympathic regulation of β all activity may contribute to metabolic risk (Silvestre &-Prous, 2005). Certain antipsychotic agents may directly impair glucose transporter function. Direct attenuation of glucose transporter function by antipsychotic agents would result in elevations in circulating glucose and a compensatory hypersecretion of insulin, which overtime may further reduce insulin sensitivity, triggering the cascade of events leading to metabolic syndrome and type 2 diabetes (Dwyer & Donohoe, 2003).

Some antipsychotic drugs increase appetite and this leads to adiposity. Affinity of the antipsychotic drugs for histamine-1 (H1) receptors closely correlates with weight-gaining potential and appears to involve H1 receptor-linked activation of hypothalamic AMP-kinase. Also, 5-HT2C receptor antagonism may contribute to weight gain. The H1 and 5HT2C blocking effects of antipsychotic medications may interfere with leptin-mediated appetite suppression (Reynolds,2006; Matsui-Sakata et al,2005).

Adiposity alone does not explain the potential side effects of atypical antipsychotic medications. Animal and human studies describe the adverse effect of clozapine and olanzapine on insulin and glucose metabolism (Hasnain & Vieweg, 2008). Significant insulin resistance has also been documented in non-obese patients receiving clozapine or olanzapine versus those receiving risperidone (Henderson et al, 2006). Diminished or inefficient insulin release from pancreatic beta cells as well peripheral insulin resistance may underlie the diabetogenic effect of some antipsychotic medications. Blocking muscarinic type 3 and 5-HT1A receptors may be a factor to diminished pancreatic beta-cells responsiveness and blocking 5HT2A receptor may suppress glucose uptake in muscle (Nasrallah, 2008). Some antipsychotic medications may impair and/or alter the action of insulin on adipocytes leading to progressive lipid accumulation (Vestri et al, 2007). The impaired effect of insulin on adipocytes may explain weight gain independent dyslipidemia (De leon et al, 2007, Birkenaes et al, 2008).

Another study examine whether patients taking selective serotonin reuptake inhibitors (SSRIs) are more likely to have elements of the metabolic syndrome compared with those taking no psychotropic drugs. Patients taking SSRIs had a significantly increased prevalence of obesity, abdominal fat, and hypercholesterolemia. The associations with this factors were significant after adjustment for age, gender , and several covariates. The individuals SSRIs might display differences in their side effect profile, the study performed analysis of the various SSRIs. Paroxetine was strongly associated with general and abdominal obesity but not with hypercholesterolemia, whereas citalopram was associated with neither obesity nor dyslipidemia. Patients taking sertraline, fluoxetine, or fluvoxamine, SSRIs treatment was significantly associated with abdominal obesity and with hypercholesterolemia. SSRIs induce transcriptional activation of cholesterol and fatty acid biosynthesis. The lipogenic effect could represent a common mechanism for explaining in part the lipid disturbances (Reader et al, 2006).

Weight gain is a major side effect of the main mood stabilizers. Chronic treatment with lithium is associated with increased weight, reaching more than 10kg in 20% of patients (Garland et al, 1998).Valproic acid leads to unequivocal weight gain. Lamotrigene, another anticonvulsant that acts as a mood stabilizer, is not associated with significant weight gain (Zimmermann et al, 2003).

With regard to mood stabilizers, additional factors could be involved. An insulin-like action cause by lithium at the treatment stage could increase fat deposition. In addition, edema secondary to sodium retention and subclinical hypothyroidism also contribute to weight gain (Garland et al, 1998). The mechanism by which the valproic acid causes weight gain is still little explored; an action in the sense of inhibiting oxidation of fatty acids might be involved (Isojärvi et al, 1998).

Studies are not in accordance. A controlled study, with children undergoing anticonvulsant treatment, did not find significant changes in HDL and triglycerides levels associated with use of carbamazepine or valproic acid. But, in the group taking carbamazepine, there were was significant increase in total cholesterol levels (Fanzoni et al, 1992).

Another study assessed 101 patients undergoing anticonvulsant therapy for at least 3 months. Compared with controls paired for gender and age, patients taking valproic acid presented significantly lower total cholesterol and LDL levels; patients taking carbamazepine presented significantly increased HDL and apolipoprotein A levels (Calandre et al, 1991).

6. Screening and monitoring

Identification of treatable pathology in a high-risk population, that is, screening for diabetes, dyslipidemia, hypertension is important and facilitates preventive strategies and early diagnosis. Another goal is to track metabolic disturbance in relation to antipsychotic treatment. Dyslipidemia is a general term that defines an increase in the serum concentration of various lipoproteins. Lipoproteins are usually classified into three major categories:

- Low-density lipoproteins (LDLs) are cholesterol-rich particles whose concentration is directly correlated with the risk of myocardial infarction and death.
- Very-low-density lipoproteins (VLDLs) are triglyceride-rich particles whose concentration is strongly correlated with the level of insulin resistance and inversely proportional to the serum concentration of high-density lipoproteins (HDLs).
- HDL particles are antiatherogenic lipid particles, and high serum levels of HDL are protective against coronary artery disease.

6.1 Screening

In the general population, lipid screening with a fasting lipid profile (total chol, LDL, HDL and triglyceride) is recommended for all adults aged 20 years and older, repeteated every 5 years in asymptomatic individuals (Expert Panel on Detection, Evaluation and Treatment, of High Blood Cholesterol in Adults, 2001). Adequate fasting, about 10 to 12 hours is necessary to obtain valid LDL and triglyceride levels-Target LDL levels are determined by a Framingham assessment based on age, sex, chol, HDL, systolic blood pressure, and smoking status (Wilson et al, 1998). Patients on antipsychotic treatment frequently have a metabolic dyslipidemia with elevations of triglyceride and reduced HDL (Cohn et al, 2004), along with associated features of the metabolic syndrome. Some SSRIs induced metabolic disturbance particularly hypercholesterolemia.

Treatment of metabolic dyslipidemia is a secondary goal for intervention following achievement of LDL targets. Clinical trials show that LDL-lowering therapy reduces risk for coronary heart disease (CHD). For these reasons, ATP III continues to identify elevated LDL cholesterol as the primary goal of cholesterol-lowering therapy. Those with diabetes or established cardiovascular disease are considered high risk and are treated to the most stringent LDL targets. Risk determinants in addition to LDL cholesterol include the presence or absence of CHD, other clinical forms of atherosclerotic disease , and the major risk factors other than LDL. Other major risk factors are cigarette smoking, hypertension, low HDL cholesterol, family history of premature CHD, diabetes and age. These major risks are commonly observed in patients with mental illness.

A variety of medical conditions and drugs can exacerbate hyperlipidemias. Elevations of the serum LDL cholesterol level can occur in response to hypothyroidism and nephrotic syndrome. Hypertriglyceridemia and decreased HDL levels are commonly seen with insulin resistance, diabetes, and the metabolic syndrome. This fact is usually seen in patients with mental illness. Individuals are characterized by their coronary risk profile according to the National Cholesterol Education Program Adult Treatment Panel III guidelines, as shown in Table 5.

Lipoprotein and serum concentration	Status
Low-density lipoprotein (LDL) cholesterol) (primary target of therapy) <100 mg/dl 100-129mg/dl 130-159 mg/dl ≥160 mg/dl	 Optimal Near optimal Borderline high High
Total cholesterol <200 mg/dl 200-239 mg/dl ≥ 240 mg/dl	 Desired Borderline high High
HDL cholesterol <40 ≥60	 Low High

Table 5. ATP III Classification of LDL, Total, and HDL Cholesterol (mg/dL)

6.2 Monitoring

To monitor for antipsychotic – associated metabolic disturbances, patients should be assessed before antipsychotic treatment is initiated. The results of such an assessment can also influence antipsychotic choice, particularly when patients have existing metabolic pathology or elevated risk factors. The frequency of subsequent assessments is different as it is reflected in the various antipsychotic monitoring guidelines: Mount Sinai (Chobarian et al, 2003), Australia (Lambert et al, 2004) ADA-APA(ADA,2004) Belgium (De Nayer, 2005), United Kingdom (Expert Consensus Meeting, 2004), Canada (Canadian Diabetes Association, 2005), France (Saravane et al, 2009) (Table 6).To summarize these recommendations, there are many aeras of general agreement about the importance of baseline monitoring before starting treatment and that patients should be followed more closely for the first 3 to 4 months of treatment, with subsequent ongoing reevaluation. The utility of the following tests and measures was emphasized: fasting plasma glucose, fasting lipid profile, weight and height, waist circumference, and blood pressure.

A recent study characterizes associations between the combined warnings and recommendations and baseline metabolic testing and Second-Generation Antipsychotic Drugs (SGA). A total of 109451 patients receiving Medicaid who began taking SGA was compared to a control cohort of 203527 patients who began taking albuterol but did nor receive antipsychotic medication. The main outcome measures was the monthly rates of baseline serum glucose and lipid testing for SGA-treated and propensity-matched albuterol-treated patients and monthly share of new prescriptions for each SGA drug. In a Medicaid-receiving patients, baseline glucose and lipid testing for SGA was infrequent and showed little change following the monitoring recommendations. Initial testing rates for SGA-treated patients were low: glucose, 27%; lipids, 10%. The warning was not associated with an increase in glucose testing among SGA-treated patients and was associated with only a marginal increase in lipid testing rates: 1.7%; P=. 02.(Morrato, 2010).

The important question is given the risks in patients with mental illness, how should they be monitored and how should they be treated?

Current studies indicate that patients with mental illness do not receive adequate evaluation and effective treatment of their cardio-metabolic problems. Effective communication between the primary care physician and the psychiatrist is very important for the mentally ill because of their impaired capacity to care for themselves. Such communication will improve monitoring, help early detection of metabolic disorders, and limit duplication of clinical or laboratory workup. Monitoring for metabolic side effects is primarily the responsibility of the physician prescribing antipsychotic medication and in most cases that would be a psychiatrist.

If the primary care physician observes that the patient is being prescribed such drugs without being monitored effectively, he/she should discuss this with the psychiatrist. The psychiatrist may not have the expertise to manage any abnormalities that are detected and in such situations the primary care physician will most likely take over both monitoring and management. Liaison should extend to any healthcare professionals involved in the care of patients with mental illness.

Given the serious health risks, patients taking antipsychotic drugs should receive appropriate baseline screening and ongoing monitoring.

	Mount Sinaï	Australia	ADA-APA	Belgium	UK	Canada	France
	Schizophrenia any antipsychotic	All patients any antipsychotic	All patients SGA	Schizophrenia SGA	Schizophrenia any antipsychotic	Schizophrenia	All patients any antipsychotic
Patients to monitor							
Fasting Plasma Glucose (FPG)	x	x	x	x	x	x	x
Random glucose		x			x		
Hba1c	If FPG not feasible				x		
OGTT						Follow up	
Lipids	x	x	x	x		x	x
Weight	x	x	x	x		x	x
Height	x	x	x	x		x	x
Waist circumference	x	x	x	x		x	x
Hip		x					x
Family and medical history	x	x	x	x		x	x
Ethnicity	x	x		x			
Tobacco				x			
Diet activity		x		x		x	
Signs and symptoms of diabetes	x		x	x	x	x	x
ECG							x
Blood pressure		x	x	x		x	x

Table 6. Recommended guidelines to monitor and initial workup.

6.2.1 Baseline monitoring

The recommendations are that baseline screening measures be obtained before or as soon as clinically feasible after, the initiation of any antipsychotic medication. We have to consider ethnicity, dietary habits, physical activity, support system, smoking, and alcohol and drug abuse. Keep in mind that psychotropic medications other than antipsychotic drugs such as some antidepressants and mood stabilizers may link to weight gain. The baseline assessments include:

- Personal and family history of obesity, diabetes, dyslipidemia, hypertension or cardiovascular disease
- Weight and height, so that BMI can be calculated
- Waist circumference at the level of the umbilicus
- Blood pressure
- Fasting plasma glucose
- Fasting lipid profile

If any abnormalities are identified, first, patients should be informed of their condition and supported in making lifestyle changes to adopt a healthier diet and increase physical activity. Psychiatrists should not hesitate to refer the patient to the appropriate health care professional or specialist knowledgeable about these disorders.

Even for patients free of metabolic disorders, monitor potential risk factors. Weight gain may not be dose-dependent and patients with low body mass index at baseline may be particularly vulnerable to weight gain. Glucose and lipid metabolism abnormalities may occur without weight gain.

6.2.2 Follow-up monitoring

The patient's weight should be reassessed at 4, 8, and 12 weeks after initiating or changing SGA therapy and quarterly thereafter at the time of routine visits. If a patient gains > 5% of his or her initial weight at any time during therapy, one should consider switching the medication. When switching, consideration should be given to all aspects of the individual's condition, the comparative risks and benefits of changing medications, and the individual's response to medication in managing the primary symptoms of the mental illness. In some cases, cost and availability may also be a consideration.

Fasting plasma glucose, lipid profile, and blood pressure should also be assessed 3 months after initiation of medication. Thereafter, blood pressure, plasma glucose values, lipid profile should be obtained annually or more frequently in those who have a higher baseline risk for the development of diabetes, dyslipidemia or hypertension.

7. Treatment

With all the risk factors and in the case of dyslipidemia and to reduce the global mortality of patients with mental illness we should consider lipid goal of therapy for these patients. The benefits and risks of different therapeutic agents used in the treatment of dyslipidemia and its comorbidities should be considered in the context of the patient's psychiatric condition and treatment.

7.1 Drugs

ATP III recommends a multifaceted lifestyle approach to reduce risk for coronary heart disease (CHD). This approach is designated therapeutic lifestyle changes (TLC). Some patients whose short-term or long-term risk for CHD is high will require LDL-lowering drugs in addition to TLC. When drugs are prescribed, attention to TLC should always be maintained and reinforced. Available drugs are:

- HMG-CoA reductase inhibitors: statins, their side effects are myopathy and increased liver enzymes
- Bile acid sequestrants , their side effects including gastrointestinal distress, constipation and decreased absorption of some drugs
- Nicotinic acid side effects are essentially flushing, hyperglycemia, hyperuricemia (gout), upper gastrointestinal distress and hepatotoxicity
- Fibric acids, with their side effects including dyspepsia, gallstones, myopathy, unexplained non-CHD deaths in WHO study

All these drugs reduced major coronary events, CHD deaths but we have to be carefull with their side effects and contraindications when prescribing these drugs.

Beyond the underlying risk factor, therapies directed against the lipid and nonlipid risk factors of the metabolic syndrome will reduce CHD risk.

The management of dyslipidemia in mental health is defined, as recommended by the Consensus Development Conference on Antipsychotic Drugs and Obesity and Diabetes by:

The lifestyle interventions with diet, increased physical activity and smoking cessation. They are the firs-line treatments to decrease the risk for cardiovascular disease in patient with metabolic syndrome.

7.2 Diet

Interventions that address nutrition and weight management should become a routine part of psychiatric care. Patients with mental illness did not know the components of a healthy diet. The healthy eating behavior includes:

- Cutting down fast food
- Increased healthy food items like fruits, vegetables, fish and decreased high glycemic index food items and monounsaturated fats
- Decreased processed fat free food
- Consume 4-6, but small meals
- Minimizing intake of soft drinks with sugar and with artificial sweetener

The lifestyle changes should be gradual and adapted individually for each patient. There are various educational and psychosocial programs that address the issues of health and wellness exist, like ' The Healthy Living' program (Vreeland, 2007; Hoffmann et al, 2006).

7.3 Physical activity

Patients who developed psychosis are more likely to be physically inactive (OR=3.3,95% CI 1.4-7.9) and to have poor cardio respiratory fitness (OR=2.2, 95% CI 0.6-7.8) compared with those who did not develop psychosis (Koivukangas et al, 2010). Modern guidelines on managing the physical health risks associated with schizophrenia include a recommendation about the importance of physical activity levels and fitness. This recommendation includes:

- To advise patients to engage at least 30 minutes of moderately vigorous activity on most days of the week
- Reduce sedentary behaviors such as TV watching, video/computer games
- Treating/reducing sedation and extra pyramidal effects of medications

Some studies showed that physical activity, with and without diet, resulted in modest weight loss, reduction of blood pressure and decreases in fasting plasma concentrations of glucose and insulin (Vancampfort et al, 2009).

7.4 Medication

In the general population there are many studies evaluating the impact of lipid lowering in primary and secondary prevention of coronary heart disease and stroke, but there are some concerns about its value in primary prevention, especially in vulnerable population (Vrecer et al, 2003).

Whether a low or lowered serum cholesterol level is associated with harm has been the subject of debate for a long time; ever since the unexpected finding of an increased risk of noncardiovascular mortality in early trials of lipid-lowering therapy. Subsequent research has generated conflicting evidence regarding the relation between cholesterol and violent behavior, mental illness , with positive studies imputing alterations in central serotoninergic activity as a potential underlying mechanism. A case-control study studied a cohort of 94441 individuals, 458 had newly diagnosed depression and 105 had a recorded diagnosis of suicide risk. Compared with matched control subjects, and even after adjustment for potential confounders, neither dyslipidemia nor its treatment was associated with an increase risk of depression. Similarly, no association was found between treatment and suicide risk. (Yang, 2003).

A 3-month study demonstrated that statins prescribed to patients with schizophrenia and severe dyslipidemia whilst taking antipsychotic medication led to a significant improvement in lipid profiles (Hanssens et, 2007). An earlier study with rosuvastatin proved effective in managing dyslipidemia in schizophrenic patients on antipsychotics. This study showed improvement in lipid profiles but not benefits in terms of high-density lipoprotein, waist measurement, BMI or glucose homeostasis (De Hert et al, 2006).

This last study supports the view that statins can be safely used in the short term to control abnormal lipids levels. However, there are no long-term data on its impact on either relapse or all-cause mortality, and again this is a priority for research.

The presence of metabolic syndrome is an indication for more aggressive lipid-lowering measures. Medications that raise HDL, nicotinic acid or fibrates, may be particularly beneficial in patients with metabolic syndrome, but they have not been as widely studied as medications that lower LDL-cholesterol in patients with mental illness.

The preferred initial management is still very much a lifestyle modification approach including exercise and diet.

8. Conclusion

Despite the availability of published clinical guidelines, patients with mental illness receiving medications remain vulnerable to the cardio-metabolic complications of these drugs. Implementation of a coordinated metabolic monitoring and management program for patient with mental illness will require a review of current practice and the introduction of new procedures, both of which will require time and effort on the part of the health care community.

Involvement of patient with mental illness in their treatment program will require the provision of information about their condition and medication and the development of approaches that empower, encourage, and support patients in their decisions on treatment and well-being.

The evaluation of new therapies should include detailed assessments of physical health and future risk estimates in addition to standard psychiatric outcomes. Psychiatrists have to arrange the appropriate examination and investigation of patients at risk of developing significant physical morbidity, working very closely with general practitioners and with other specialists when appropriate. We have to weight up the risk of metabolic disturbance and its potential impact on future cardiovascular risk when selecting an antipsychotic drug. We have to take a careful medical history and be prepared to monitor weight and other metabolic risk, such as glucose and lipid profile. The lipid area is significantly understudied in patients taking antipsychotic medications. Lipids may be more important than diabetes because dyslipidemia appears to occur at a higher prevalence in this patient population. Lipid levels are a significant problem because physicians are seeing hypertriglyceridemia. Knowing what we know about what causes and contributes to cardiovascular disease, we are obliged to play detective and figure out why psychiatric patients are dying sooner and more often of cardiovascular disease than the general population.

The big challenge for all is to ensure that the physical health of patients with mental illness is given the priority it deserves, helping them to face their future with the lowest possible morbidity and mortality odds stacked against them.

9. References

Alberti KGMM, Zimmet P, Shaw J. (2006). Metabolic syndrome – a new world – wide definition. A consensus statement from the International Diabetes Federation. Diabetic 25: 469–80

Allison DB, Metore JL, HEO M et al. (1999). Antipsychotic-induced weight gain: a comprehensive research synthesis. Am J Psychiatry, 156: 1686-1696

Allison DB, Casey De (2001); Antipsychotic–induced weight gain: a review of the literature. J Clin Psychiatry 6é (Suppl 7): 22-31

American Diabetes Association; American Psychiatric Association; American Association of Clinical Endocrinologists; North American Association for the Study of Obesity. Consensus development conference on antipsychotic drugs and obesity and diabetes care (2004); 27: 596-601. Available at:

http//care. Diabetejournals.org/cgi/reprint/27/2/596

American Diabetes Association, American Psychiatric Association, American Association of Clinical Endocrinologists; North American Association for the Study of Obesity. Consensus development conference on antipsychotic drugs and obesity and diabetes care. Diabetes Care (2004); 27: 596-601

Bartsch DA, Shen DL, Feinberg LE et al (1990). Screening CMHC out patients for physical illness. Hospital and Community Psychiatry 41: 786-790

Birkenaes AB, Birkeland Ja, Engh JA et al (2008). Dyslipidemia independent of body mass in antipsychotic-treated patients under real-life conditions; J Clin Psychopharmacol 28: 132-137

Brown S. (1997). Excess mortality of schizophrenia A meta – analysis. Br J. Psychiatry; 171: 502–8

Calandre EP, Rodriguez-Lopez C, Blasquez A et al, (1991). Serum lipids, lipoproteins and apolipoprotein A and B in epileptic patients treated with valproic acid and carbamazepine or Phenobarbital. Acta Neurol Scand, 83(4): 250-253

Cohn T, Prud'homme D, Streiner D et al. (2004)Characterizing coronary heart disease risk in chronic schizophrenia: high prevalence of the metabolic syndrome. Can J Psychiary, 49: 753-60

Colton CW, Manderscheid RW (2006). Congruencies in increased mortality rates, year of potential life lost, and causes of death among public mental health clients in eight states. Prev Chronic Dis, 3: A42

Consensus development conference on antipsychotic drugs and obesity and diabetes (2004) J Clin Psychiatry 65(2): 267-272

Correl CV. (2007) Balancing efficacy and safety in treatment with antipsychotics. CNS Spectr; 12 (suppl, 17) : 12–20

Canadian Diabetes Association. (2005) Positision paper: antipsychotic medications and associated risk of weight gain and diabetes. Canadian Journal of Diabetes 29:111-2

Chobanian AV, Bakris GL, Black HR, Cushman WC, Green LA, Izzo JL Jr, and others. (2003) Seventh report of the Joint National Committee on Prevenion, Detection, Evaluation, and Treatment of High Blood Pressure. Hypertension 42: 1206-52.

Cradock-O'Leary J, Young AS, Yano EM, et al (2002). Use of general medical services by VA patients psychiatric disorders. Psychiatr Serv 53: 874-878

Davidson M (2002). Risk of cardiovascular disease and sudden death in schizophrenia. J Clin Psychiatry 63 (Suppl 9): 5-11

De Hert M,Kalnicka D, van Winkel R et al. (2006). Treatment with rosuvastatin for severe dyslipidemia in patients with schizophrenia and schizoaffective disorder. J Clin Psychiatry 67/1889-96.

De Leon J, Susce MT, Johnson M et al (2007). A clinical study of the association of antipsychotics with hyperlipidemia Schizophr Res 92 : 95-102

De Nayer A, De Hert M, Scheem A, Van Gaal L, Peuskens J. (2005) Belgian consensus on metabolic problems associated with atypical antipsychotics. International Journal of Psychiatry in Clinical Pratice 9:130-7

Dworkin R (1994). Pain insensitivity in schizophrenia: A neglected phenomenon and some implications. Schizophrenia Bulletin 20: 235-248

Dwyer DS, Donohoe D: (2003) Induction of hyperglycemia in mice with atypical antipsychotic drugs that inhibit glucose uptake. 75:255-260

Expert Panel on Detection and Evaluation of Treatment of High Blood Cholesterol in Adults. Executive summary of the third report of the National Cholesterol Education Program (NCEP) expert panel on detection, evaluation and treatment of high blood cholesterol in adults (Adult Treatment Panel III)(2001). JAMA, 285: 2486-97

Expert Group. "Schizophrenia and Diabetes 2003" Expert Consensus Meeting. (2004) Dublin, 3-4 October 2003: consensus summary. Br J Psychiatry Suppl 47:S112-4

Fanzoni E, Govoni M, D'Addato S et al (1991). Total cholesterol, high-density lipoprotein cholesterol, and triglycerides in children receiving antiepileptic drugs. Epilepsia, 33(5): 932-935

Felker B, Yazel JJ, Short D (1996). Mortality and medical comorbidity among psychiatric patients. A review. Psychiatric Services 47: 1356-1363

Garland EJ, Remick RA, Zis AP: (1998) Weight gain with antidepressants and lithium. J Clin Psychopharmocol, 8(5): 323-330

Goldman L (1999). Medical illness in patients with schizophrenia Journal of Clinical Psychiatry, Suppl 21, vol 60 pp 10-15

Grundy SM, Cleeman JL, Daniels SR et al (2005). Diagnosis and management of the metabolic syndrome: an American Heart Association/National Heart, Lung and Blood Institute Scientific Statement. Circulation, 112: 2735-52

Hall RC, Gardner ER, Popkin MK et al; (1981) Unrecognized physical illness prompting psychiatric admission: a prospective study. Am J Psychiatry 138: 629-635

Hanssens L, De Hert M, van Winkel R et al. (2007) Pharmacological treatment of severe dyslipidaemia in patients with schizophrenia. Int J Clin Psychopharnacol; 22:43-9

Harris EC, Barraclough B (1998). Excess mortality of mental disorder . British Journal of Psychiatry 173: 11-53

Henderson DC, Copeland PM, Borba CP et al (2006). Glucose metabolism in patients with schizophrenia treated with olanzapine or quetiapine: a frequently sampled intravenous glucose tolerance test and minimal model analysis. J Clin Psychiatry 67: 789-797.

Hoffmann VP, Bushe C, Meyers AL et al (2008). A wellness intervention program for patients with mental illness:self-reported outcomes. J Clin Psychiatry 10(4): 329-331

Isojärvi JL, Rättyä J, Myllylä VV et al (1998). Valproate, lamitrogene, and insulin-mediated risks in women with epilepsy. Ann Neurol, 43(4): 446-451

Koran LM, Sox HC Jr, Marton KI et al (1989). Medical evaluation of psychiatric patients. Results in a state mental health system. Arch Gen Psychiatry 46: 733-740

Koranyi EK (1979). Morbidity and rate of undiagnosed physical illnesses in a psychiatric clinic population. Arch Gen Psychiatry 36: 414-419

Koivukangas J, Tammelin T, Kaakinen M et al (2010). Physical activity and fitness in adolescents at risk for psychosis within the Northern Finland 1986 Birth Cohort. Schizophr Res 116: 152-158

Lambert TJR, Velakoulis D, Pantelis C (2003).Medical comorbidity in schizophrenia. Medical Journal of Australia 178, Suppl 5: 567-570

Lambert TJ, Chapman LH. (Aust 2004) Diabetes, psychotic disorders and antipsychotic therapy: a consensus statement Med J 181:544-8

Lawrence D, Holman C, Jablensky A et al (2003). Death rate from ischemic heart disease in Western Australian psychiatric patients 1980-1998; British Journal of Psychiatry 182: 31-36

Lyketsos C, Dunn G, Kaminsky M et al (2002). Medical comorbidity in psychiatric inpatients. Relation to clinical outcomes and hospital length of stay Psychosomatics 43: 24-30

Matsui-Sakata A, Ohtani H, Sawada Y/ (2005) Receptor occupancy-based analysis of the contribution of various receptors to antipsychotic-induced weight gain and diabetes mellitus. Drug Metab Pharmacokinet 27:398-378

Mc Creadle RG (2003). Diet, smoking and cardiovascular risk in people with schizophrenia. Descriptive study. British Journal of Psychiatry, 183, 534-539

Mc Evoy JP, Meyer JM, Goff et al (2005). Prevalence of the metabolic syndrome in patients with schizophrenia: baseline results from the Clinical Antipsychotic Trials of Intervention Effectiveness (CATIE) schizophrenia trial and comparison with national estimates from NHANES III, schizophr Res, 80: 19–32

Meyer JM, Nasrallah HA, Mc Evoy JP et al (2005). The clinical Antipsychotic Trials of Intervention Effectiveness (CATIE) Schizophrenia Trial: clinical comparison of subgroups with and without the metabolic syndrome Shizophr Res, 80: 9–18

Meyer JM (2001). Effects of typical Antipsychotics on weight and serum lipid levels. J. Clin Psychiatry, 62 (suppl 27), 27–34

Morrato EH, Druss B, Hartung DM et al (2010). Metabolic testing in 3 states Medicaid programs after FDA warnings and ADA/APA recommendations for second-generation antipsychotic drugs Arch Gen Psychiatry, vol 67(1): 17-25

Mortensen P , Juel K (1993). Mortality and causes of death in first admitted schizophrenic patients. British Journal of Psychiatry 163: 183-189

Newcomer J. (2005) Second-generation (atypical) antipsychotics and metabolic effects : a comprehensive literature review? CNS Drugs, 19

Nasrallah HA (2008). Atypical antipsychotic-induced metabolic side effects: insights from receptor-binding profiles. Mol Psychiatry 13: 27-35

Nasralah HA, Meyer JM, Goff DC et al. (2006). Low rates of treatment for hypertention, dyslipidemia and diabetes in schizophrenia: data from the CATIE schizophrenia trial sample at baseline. Schizophr RES 86: 15-22

Reynolds GP, Hill MJ, Kirk SI (2006). The 5-HT2C receptor and antipsychotic induced weight gain-mechanisms and genetics, J. Psychopharmacol, 20: 15-18

Ringback Weitoft G, Gullberg A, Rosen M (1998). Avoidable mortality among psychiatric patients. Social Psychiatry and Psychiatric Epidemiology 33: 430-437

Rushena D, Mullen P, Burgess P, et al (1998). Sudden death in psychiatric patients. British Journal of Psychiatry 173: 331-336

Rutstein D, Berenberg W, Chalmers T et al (1976). Measuring the quality of medical care. A clinical method. New England Journal of Medecine 294: 582-588

Saravane D, B. Feve, Frances Y et al (2009). Drawing up guidelines for the attendance of physical health of patients with severe mental illness. L'Encéphale, 35: 330–339

Sarafidis PA, Nilsson PM (2006). The metabolic syndrome: a glance at its history. J Hypertension, 24: 621 – 626

Silvestre JS, Prous J: (2005) Research on adverse drug events, I: muscarinic M3 receptor binding affinity could predict the risk antipsychotics to induce type 2 diabetes. Methods Find Exp Clin Pharmacol 27:289-304

Vancampfort D, Knapen J, De Hert M et al (2009). Cardiometabolic effects of physical activity interventions for people with schizophrenia. Phys Ther Rev 14: 388-398

Vestri HS, Maianu L, Moellering DR et al (2007). Atypical antipsychotic drugs directly impair insulin action in adipocytes: effects on glucose transport, lipogenesis, and antilipolysis, Neuropsychopharmacology 32: 765-772

Vrecer M, Turk S, Drinovec J et al (2003). Use of statin in primary and secondary prevention of coronary heart disease and ischemic stroke. Meta-analysis of randomized trials. Int J Clin Pharmacol Ther 41: 567-577

Vreeland B (2007). Behavioral changes in patients with mental illness. J Clin Psychiatry 68 (Suppl 4): 8-13

Wilson PW, D'Agostini RB, Levy D et al (1998). Prediction of coronary heart disease using risk factor categories. Circulation 97: 1837-1847

Wulsin LR (2000). Does depression kills? Arch Intern Med 160: 1731-1732

Yang CC, Jick SS, Jick H (2003). Lipid-lowering drugs and the risk of depression and suicidal behavior. Arch Intern Med 163: 1926-1932

Zimmermann U, Kraus T, Himmerisch H et al (2003). Epidemiology, implications and mechanisms underlying drug-induced weight gain in psychiatric patients. J Psychiatr Res, 37(3): 193-220

6

Cardiovascular Risk in Tunisian Patients with Bipolar I Disorder

Asma Ezzaher[1,2], Dhouha Haj Mouhamed[1,2], Anwar Mechri[2],
Fadoua Neffati[1], Wahiba Douki[1,2], Lotfi Gaha[2]
and Mohamed Fadhel Najjar[1]
[1]Laboratory of Biochemistry-Toxicology,
[2]Research Laboratory "Vulnerability to Psychotic Disorders LR 05 ES 10",
Department of Psychiatry/Monastir University Hospital,
Tunisia

1. Introduction

Bipolar disorder (previously also labeled manic-depressive illness) is typically referred to as an episodic, yet lifelong and clinically severe affective (or mood) disorder, affecting approximately 3.5% of the population (Marmol, 2008; Simon, 2003; Wittchen et al., 2003; Woods, 2000). The term bipolar disorder, however, encompasses several phenotypes of mood disorders, i.e. mania, hypomania or cyclothymia that may present with a puzzling variety of other symptoms and disorders. According to the Fourth Edition of the Diagnostic and Statistical Manual of Mental Disorders (DSM-IV) (American Psychiatric Association, 2004), the diagnostic classificatory system used in most epidemiological studies, bipolar disorder is defined by a set of specific symptom criteria. Bipolar type I requires the presence or the history of at least one manic or mixed episode. Although, typically, patients with a manic episode also experience major depressive episodes, bipolar disorder can be diagnosed even if only one manic episode and no past major depressive episodes are present. Bipolar disorder type II differs from type I only by presence of hypomanic but no manic episodes. Hypomanic episodes differ from mania by a shorter duration (at least 4 days instead of 1 week), and less severe impairment (not severe enough to cause marked impairment in social or occupational functioning, psychiatric hospitalization, or psychotic features). The DSM-IV also includes "cyclothymia" as a bipolar spectrum disorder with hypomanic as well as depressive episodes that do not meet criteria for major depression (American Psychiatric Association, 2004).

Bipolar disorder is a chronic disease that is associated with a potentially devastating impact on patients' wellbeing and social, occupational, and general functioning (Revicki et al., 2005). The disorder ranks as the sixth leading cause of disability in the world, with an economic burden that in the US alone that was estimated more than a decade ago at $7 billion in direct medical costs and $38 billion (1991 values) in indirect costs (Wyatt et al., 1991).

A number of reviews and studies have shown that people with severe mental illness, including bipolar disorder, have an excess mortality, being two or three times as high as that in the general population. This mortality gap, which translates to a 13-30 year shortened life expectancy in severe mental illness patients, has widened in recent decades, even in countries where the quality of the health care system is generally acknowledged to be good. About 60% of this excess mortality is due to physical illness especially cardiovascular disease. Additionally, several studies have found that after suicide and accidents, cardiovascular and all vascular diseases are the main leading causes of death in these patients (De Hert et al., 2011; Garcia-Portilla et al., 2009).

Patients with bipolar disorder, especially type I, are known to suffer a considerable number of associated pathologies that may manifest at earlier ages and with higher frequency than in the general population. The most recent studies have explored cardiovascular risk and the association with metabolic and endocrine disorders fundamentally, obesity and metabolic syndrome which are clearly associated with the development of cardiovascular disease (Angst et al., 2002; Sicras et al., 2008).

Cardiovascular disease, i.e. coronary heart disease, stroke, and peripheral vascular disease, are potentially preventable diseases. Thanks to epidemiological, experimental and clinical studies, the primary determinants of cardiovascular disease have been identified, as well as the efficacy of specific interventions. The prevalence of cardiovascular disease is increasing in less urbanized, developed populations across the world, as their lifestyles change to a so called "western style", with increasing consumption of dietary saturated fat, cholesterol and salt, cigarette smoking, decreased physical activity and the rise in cardiovascular risk factors including obesity and diabetes. Other known factors that contribute to cardiovascular disease risk are stress and high alcohol intake. Among all these factors, hypercholesterolemia is the leading cause of death from cardiovascular disease. As a result, public health agencies have attempted to reduce the prevalence of hypercholesterolemia through screening and by increasing public awareness and strategies for reducing it (Muntoni et al., 2009).

The exact mechanisms increasing the incidence of cardiovascular risk in bipolar patients remain to be clarified, but they possibly include industrialisation, stress, lack of exercise, dietary lipids (that is, omega-3 fatty acid deficiency) and increasing incidence of smoking and alcohol consumption and other factors (Ezzaher et al., 2010).

This study aims to investigate the principal factors predisposing to the cardiovascular risk in Tunisian bipolar I patients (cigarette smoking, hypertension, diabetes, obesity, lipid profile, hyperhomocysteinemia and metabolic syndrome) and to determine the association between these factors and the clinical and therapeutic characteristics of bipolar I disorder.

2. Patients and methods

2.1 Subjects

This study was approved by the local ethical committee and all subjects were of Tunisian origin. Our samples included 130 patients with bipolar I disorder (37.9 ± 12.1 years) from the psychiatry department of the University Hospital of Monastir, Tunisia, 45 women (37.5 ± 13.4 years) and 85 men (38.1 ± 11.4 years). Consensus on the diagnosis, according to the Diagnostic and Statistical Manual of Mental Disorders, fourth edition (DSM-IV) criteria (American Psychiatric Association, 2004), was made by psychiatrists. The exclusion criteria were age < 18 years, other psychiatric illnesses, epilepsy or mental retardation. The control group consisted of 175 volunteer subjects without psychiatric pathology. The mean age was 40.1 ± 14.0 years, and there were 73 women (42.0 ± 14.4 years) and 102 men (38.8 ± 13.6

years). All subjects were questioned about their age, gender, previous treatments and cigarette and alcohol consumption habits.

The clinical and socio-demographic characteristics are shown in table 1. Differences between patients and controls for body mass index (BMI) (p < 0.001) and smoking status (p =0.025) were noted. Therefore, these variables were considered as potential confounder factors for this analysis.

	Patients (n = 130)		Controls (n = 175)		p
Gender: Men/Women (ratio)	85/45 (1.89)		102/73 (1.39)		0.143
Age (years) (mean ± SD)	37.9 ± 12.1		40.1 ± 14.0		0.840
BMI (kg/m²) (M ± ET)	27.1 ± 4.6		25.3 ± 4.1		< 0.001
	Nombre	%	Nombre	%	p
BMI (kg/m²)					
< 25	47	36.2	89	50.9	
[25-30[	40	30.7	72	41.1	< 0.001
≥ 30	43	33.1	14	8	
Cigarette smoking					
Yes	68	52.3	69	39.4	
No	62	47.7	106	60.6	0.025
Alcoholic beverages					
Yes	17	13.1	12	6.9	
No	113	86,9	163	93.1	0.067
Illness episode					
Depressive	21	16.2	-	-	-
Euthymic	73	56.1	-	-	-
Manic	36	27.7	-	-	-
Treatment					
Valproic acid	64	49.3	-	-	-
Lithium	12	9.2	-	-	-
Carbamazepine	10	7.7	-	-	-
Valproic acid and lithium	6	4.6	-	-	-
Antipsychotics	38	29.2	-	-	-

Antipsychotics: Haloperidol, Risperidone, Chlorpromazine, Olanzapine; BMI: body mass index

Table 1. Sociodemographic and therapeutic characteristics of studied population.

2.2 Samples
After a 12 h overnight fasting, venous blood for each patient was drawn in tubes containing lithium heparinate and immediately centrifuged. The plasma samples were stored at -20°C until the biochemical analysis.

2.3 Biochemical analysis
The methods of dosage and the normal values of the different biological parameters are shown in table 2.

Parameters	Assay	Automates	Normal values
Cholesterol	Enzymatic	Konelab 30 equipment (Thermo Electron Corporation, Ruukintie, Finland)	< 5.17 mmol/L
Triglycerides			< 1.7 mmol/L
c-HDL			Men: ≥ 1.1 mmol/L Women: ≥ 0.9 mmol/L
c-LDL			< 3.4 mmol/L
ApoA1	Immunoturbidimetry		1.2- 1.6 g/L
ApoB			0.7-1.3 g/L
Lp(a)			< 200 mg/L
Uric acid	Enzymatic		Men: 210-420 µmol/L Women: 150-360 µmol/L
Homocysteine	Fluorescence polarization (FPIA)	AxSYM® (Abbott Laboratories, Abbott Park, IL 60064, Barcelaneta, Puerto Rico)	< 15 µmol/L
Vitamin B12	Electrochemiluminescence	Elecsys 2010™ (Roche Diagnostics, Indianapolis, IN, USA)	≥ 187ng/L
Folate			≥ 3.7 µg/L
Insulin			< 17µU/mL

Table 2. Methods of dosage of the studied parameters.

2.4 Clinical evaluation
Body mass index (BMI) was calculated as weight (kg) divided by height (m²). Obesity was defined when BMI ≥ 30 kg/m² and overweight when BMI ≥ 25 kg/m² (World Health Organization, 1997).

2.5 Criteria for metabolic syndrome
Metabolic syndrome (MS) was defined according to the National Cholesterol Education Program (NCEP) Adult Treatment Panel (ATP) III modified criteria and required fulfillment of at least three of the following five components: body mass index (BMI) ≥ 28.5 kg/m², triglycerides ≥ 1.7 mmol/L, high-density lipoprotein cholesterol (c-HDL) < 1.1 mmol/L (in men) and < 0.9 mmol/L (in women), blood pressure ≥ 130 /85 mmHg and fasting glucose (≥ 6.1 mmol/L) (National Cholesterol Education Program, 2002).

2.6 HOMA-IR determination
Insulin resistance (IR) was estimated using the Homeostasis Model of Assessment equation: HOMA-IR = [fasting insulin (mU/L) × fasting glucose (mmol/L)]/22.5. IR was defined as the upper quartile of HOMA-IR. Values above 2.5 were taken as abnormal and reflect insulin resistance (Ozdemir et al., 2007). Bipolar patients with diabetes (n = 21) were excluded in the HOMA-IR analysis.

2.7 Statistical analysis

Statistical analyses were performed using SPSS 17.0 (SPSS, Chicago, IL, USA). Quantitative variables were presented as mean ± SD and comparisons were performed using the Student's t test. Qualitative variable comparisons were performed using the Chi-squared test (x^2) and Fisher's exact test (when n < 5). Comparisons between patients and controls in biological parameters were performed using analysis of variance (ANOVA) after adjustment for potential confounder factors. Odd ratios (ORs) and their 95% confidence interval (CI) were calculated and adjusted for potential confounder factors by binary logistic regression. The statistical significance level was set at $p < 0.05$. All variables with a p value < 0.25 between the two studied groups (patients and controls) were considered as potential confounder factors for this analysis.

3. Results

Table 3 shows the comparisons of biological variables between bipolar I patients and controls.

Biological variables	Patients (n = 130)	Controls (n = 175)	p	p*
Triglycerides (mmol/L)	1.95 ± 1.55	1.23 ± 0.81	< 0.001	< 0.001
Cholesterol (mmol/L)	4.42 ± 0.99	4.37 ± 1.26	0.707	0.856
c-LDL (mmol/L)	2.14 ± 1.10	2.37 ± 1.38	0.118	0.047
c-HDL (mmol/L)				
Men (85/102)	1.04 ± 0.37	0.98 ± 0.29	0.192	0.017
Women (45/73)	1.17 ± 0.36	1.21 ± 0.48	0.542	0.702
ApoA1 (g/L)	1.20 ± 0.23	1.40 + 0.67	< 0.001	0.028
ApoB (g/L)	0.82 ± 0.28	0.83 ± 0.24	0.784	0.777
ApoB/Apo A1	0.71 ± 0.26	0.65 ± 0.25	0.086	0.314
Lp(a) (mg/L)	243 ± 223	87 ± 129	< 0.001	< 0.001
Homocysteine (µmol/L)	15.8 ± 8.9	11.5 ± 5.0	< 0.001	< 0.001
Vitamin B12 (ng/L)	356 ± 198	360 ± 190	0.837	0.819
Folate (µg/L)	3.3 ± 0.9	5.1 ± 2.8	< 0.001	<0.001
Uric acid (µmol/L)				
Men (85/102)	311 ± 99	250 ± 107	0.001	0.005
Women (45/73)	246 ± 97	197 ± 73	0.012	0.408

* Lipid profile parameters, folatemia, vitamin B12 and uric acid were adjusted for gender, BMI, cigarette smoking, alcoholic beverages, diabetes and hypertension
*Hcys was adjusted for gender, BMI, cigarette smoking, alcoholic beverages, diabetes, hypertension, folatemia and vitamin B12

Table 3. Comparisons of biological variables between bipolar I patients and controls.

Compared with controls, patients had significantly higher triglycerides (1.95 ± 1.55 Vs 1.23 ± 0.81 mmol/L; p < 0.001), Lp(a) (243 ± 223 Vs 87 ± 129 mg/L; p < 0.001), homocysteine levels (15.8 ± 8.9 Vs 11.5 ± 5.0 µmol/L; p < 0.001) and uric acid (311 ± 99 Vs 250 ± 107 µmol/L; p = 0.001 in men; 246 ± 97 Vs 197 ± 73 µmol/L; p = 0.012 in women), and significantly lower ApoA1 (1.20 ± 0.23 Vs 1.40 ± 0.67 g/L; p < 0.001) and folate (3.3 ± 0.9 Vs 5.1 ± 2.8 µg/L; p < 0.001) levels. After adjustment for potential confounder factors, these differences remained significant for all of these parameters except for uric acid which is remained significantly higher only for men (table 3).

Table 4 reports the association between bipolar I disorder and cigarette smoking, alcoholic beverages, obesity, diabetes, hypertension, lipid profile parameters, hyperhomocysteinemia, hypofolatemia, hypovitamin B12 and, hyperuricemia.

Parameters	Patients (n = 130)	Controls (n = 175)	OR	IC 95%	p	OR*	p*
Cigarette smoking	52.3%	39.4%	1.68	1.06-2.66	**0.025**	-	-
Alcoholic beverages	13.1%	6.9%	2.04	0.94-4.44	0.067	-	-
Obesity (BMI ≥ 30 kg/m²)	33.1%	8%	5.68	2.94-10.96	**< 0.001**	8.69	**< 0.001**
Diabetes ≥ 6.1 mmol/L	16.1%	9.7%	1.79	0.90-3.55	0.092	1.60	0.325
Hypertension (≥ 130/85 mm Hg)	5.4%	16%	0.34	0.15-0.78	0.008	0.43	0.136
Hypercholesterolemia (≥ 5.17 mmol/L)	26.2%	26.9%	0.96	0.57-1.61	0.891	0.99	0.987
Hypertriglyceridemia (≥ 1.7 mmol/L)	53.1%	17.7%	4.10	2.44-6.90	**< 0.001**	3.71	**< 0.001**
HyperLDL (≥ 3.4 mmol/L)	13.1%	26.9%	0.39	0.22-0.73	0.002	0.48	< 0.001
¥HypoHDL	59.2%	58.3%	1.00	0.63-1.59	0.975	0.78	0.359
HyperLp(a) (≥ 200 mg/L)	47.7%	14.8%	5.25	3.04-9.07	**< 0.001**	4.48	**< 0.001**
Hyperhomocysteinemia (≥15 µmol/L)	39.2%	18%	2.80	1.66-4.72	**< 0.001**	1.95	**0.038**
Hypovitamin B12 (< 187 ng/L)	21.2%	14.9%	0.69	0.34-1.38	0.296	0.62	0.215
Hypofolatemia (< 3.7 µg/L)	66.2%	36.2%	3.44	2.13-5.54	**< 0.001**	3.69	**< 0.001**
£Hyperuricemia	10.8%	4.4%	2.05	0.71-5.91	0.176	1.58	0.439

* Lipid profile parameters, folatemia, vitamin B12 and uric acid were adjusted for gender, BMI, cigarette cigarette smoking, alcoholic beverages, diabetes and hypertension; * Hcys was adjusted for gender, BMI, cigarette smoking, alcoholic beverages, diabetes, hypertension, folatemia and vitamin B12; *Diabetes was adjusted for gender, BMI, cigarette smoking, alcoholic beverages, hypertension and dyslipidemia; *Obesity was adjusted for gender, cigarette smoking, alcoholic beverages, hypertension, diabetes and dyslipidemia; *Hypertension was adjusted for gender, cigarette smoking, alcoholic beverages, diabetes and dyslipidemia; \ c-HDL <1.1 mmol/L (in men) and < 0 .9 (in women); £ uric acid: 210-420 µmol/L (in men) and 150-360 µmol/L (in women)

Table 4. Association between bipolar I disorder and cigarette smoking, alcoholic beverages, obesity, diabetes, hypertension, lipid profile parameters, hyperhomocysteinemia, hypofolatemia, hypovitamin B12, and hyperuricemia.

We showed significant association between bipolar I disorder and some cardiovascular risk factors: obesity (33.1% Vs 8%, OR = 5.68, IC 95% = 2.94-10.96; p < 0.001), hyperLp(a) (47.7% Vs 14.8%, OR = 5.25, IC 95% = 3.04-9.07; p < 0.001), hypertriglyceridemia (53.1% Vs 17.7%, OR = 4.10, IC 95% = 2.44-6.90; p < 0.001), hypofolatemia (66.2% Vs 36.2%, OR = 3.44, IC 95% = 2.13-5.54; p < 0.001), hyperhomocysteinemia (39.2% Vs 18%, OR = 2.80, IC 95% = 1.66-4.72; p < 0.001) and cigarette smoking (52.3% Vs 39.4%, OR = 1.68, IC 95% = 1.06-2.66; p = 0,025). After adjustment for potential confounder factors, these associations remained significant (table 4).

Alcoholic beverage, diabetes and hyperuricemia were not significantly associated with this illness but we showed that they were more frequents in patients than controls (13.1% Vs 6.9%, p = 0.067; 16.1% Vs 9.7%, p = 0.325; 10.8% Vs 4.4%, p = 0.439; respectively). Additionally, the risk of diabetes and hyperuricemia were respectively multiplied by 1.5 in patients (16.1% Vs 9.7%, OR = 1.60, IC 95% = 0.62-4.12; p = 0.325; 10.8% Vs 4.4%, OR = 1.58, IC 95% = 0.49-5.08; p = 0.439) and the risk of alcoholic beverage by two (13.1% Vs 6.9%, OR = 2.04, IC 95% = 0.94-4.44; p = 0.067) (table 4).

On the contrary, this disease was not associated with hypertension (5.4% Vs 16%, OR = 0.43, IC 95% = 0.14-1.29; p = 0.136) nor with hyperLDL (13.1% Vs 26.9%, OR = 0.48, IC 95% = 2.53-7.95; p < 0.001) (table 4).

Fig.1. illustrates the receiver Operating Characteristic (ROC) of three index of atherogenicity as predictive factors of cardiovascular risk.

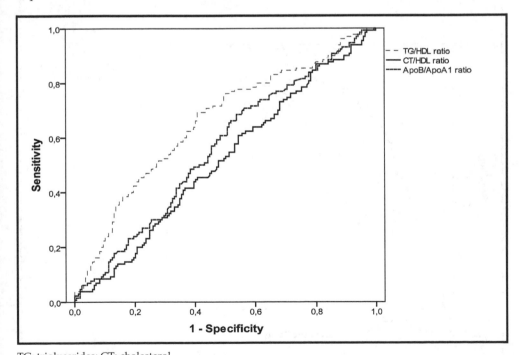

TG: triglycerides; CT: cholesterol

Fig. 1. Receiver Operating Characteristic (ROC) of three index of atherogenicity as predictive factors of cardiovascular risk.

The specificity and sensibility of three index of atherogenicity as predictive factors of cardiovascular risk are shown in table 5.

Parameters	AUC (95% CI)	Cut off	Specificity	Sensibility	p
TG/HDL	0.65 [0.59-0.71]	1.12	0.63	0.62	< 10⁻³
CT/HDL	0.52 [0.44-0.57]	3.93	0.53	0.57	0.661
ApoB/ApoA1	0.56 [0.49-0.62]	0.66	0.54	0.55	0.070

TG: triglycerides; CT: cholesterol; AUC; Area under the curve

Table 5. Specificity and sensibility of three index of atherogenicity as predictive factors of cardiovascular risk

Fig. 2. Illustrates the Receiver Operating Characteristic (ROC) of Lp(a) and homocysteine as predictive factors of cardiovascular risk.

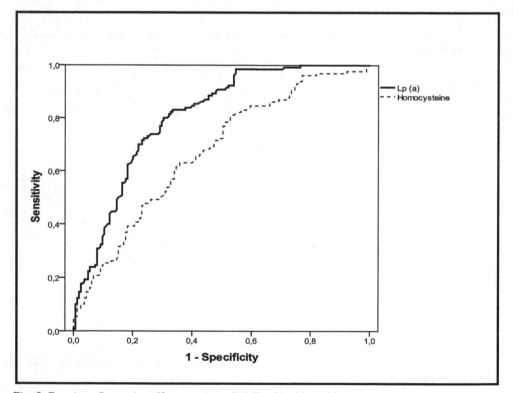

Fig. 2. Receiver Operating Characteristic (ROC) of Lp(a) and homocysteine as predictive factors of cardiovascular risk.

Table 6 reports the specificity and sensibility of Lp(a) and homocysteine as predictive factors of cardiovascular risk.

Parameters	AUC (95% CI)	Cut off	Specificity	Sensibility	p
Lp(a) (mg/L)	0.80 [0.75-0.85]	168	0.75	0.74	< 10^{-3}
Homocysteine (µmol/L)	0.52 [0.44-0.57]	13.4	0.60	0.62	< 10^{-3}

AUC; Area under the curve

Table 6. Specificity and sensibility of Lp(a) and homocysteine as predictive factors of cardiovascular risk.

TG/HDL ratio and Lp(a) were found as the best predictive factors of cardiovascular risk in terms of sensibility (0.62, 0.74; respectively) and specificity (0.63, 0.75; respectively) at threshold of 1.12 and 168 mg/L, respectively (tables 5, 6; fig 1, 2).

The prevalence of metabolic syndrome (modified NCEP-ATP III) and its profile in bipolar I patients are shown in table 7.

	N	%
Total of the association of 5 criteria	**2**	**5.9**
Diabetes, Obesity, Hypertriglyceridemia, Low c-HDL	1	
Diabetes, Obesity, Low c-HDL, High blood pressure	1	
Diabetes, Hypertriglyceridemia, Low c-HDL, High blood pressure	1	
Total of the association of 4 criteria	**3**	**8.8**
Obesity, Hypertriglyceridemia, Low c-HDL	15	
Diabetes, Low c-HDL, Hypertriglyceridemia	6	
Obesity, Hypertriglyceridemia, Diabetes	4	
Obesity, Hypertriglyceridemia, High blood pressure	2	
Diabetes , High blood pressure, Obesity	1	
Hypertriglyceridemia, Low c-HDL, High blood pressure	1	
Total of the association of 3 criteria	**29**	**85.3**
At least three or more criteria	**34**	**100**

Table 7. Prevalence of metabolic syndrome (modified NCEP-ATP III) and its profile in bipolar I patients.

The prevalence of metabolic syndrome in bipolar I patients was 26.1% (N = 34). The highest prevalence of this syndrome was obtained by the association between obesity, low c-HDL and hypertrilyceridemia (44.1 %) (Table 7).

Table 8 reports the Prevalence of the components of metabolic syndrome in the total sample of bipolar I patients.

Criteria	N (%)
c-HDL < 1.1 mmol/L (men) and < 0 .9 (women)	77(59.2)
TG ≥ 1.7 mmol/L	69(53.1)
BMI ≥ 28.5 kg/m²	44 (33.8)
Fasting blood glucose ≥ 6.1 mmol/L	21 (16.1)
Blood pressure ≥ 130/85 mm Hg	7(5.4)

Table 8. Prevalence of the components of metabolic syndrome in the total sample (N=130).

The prevalence of individual diagnostic components, in the total sample, was as follows: 59.2% for low c-HDL, 53.1% for hypertriglyceridemia, 33.8% for obesity (BMI $\geq$ 28.5 kg/m²), 16.1% for high fasting glucose and 5.4% for hypertension (Table 8).

Table 9 reports the characteristics of patients with or without metabolic syndrome.

Variables	With MS [N= 34 (26.1%)] N (%)	Without MS [N= 96 (73.9%)] N (%)	p values
Gender			
Men	21 (24.7)	64 (75.3)	0.60
Women	13 (28.9)	32 (71.1)	
Illness episode			
Depressive	4 (19)	17 (81)	0.651[a]
Euthymic	19 (26)	54 (74)	
Manic	11 (30.5)	25 (69.5)	
Treatment			
Antipsychotics	10 (26.3)	28 (73.7)	
Mood stabilizers	24 (26.1)	68 (74.9)	
Lithium	4 (33.3)	8 (66.7)	0.9574[a]
Valproic acid	17 (26.6)	47 (73.4)	
Carbamazepine	2 (20)	8 (80)	
Lithium and valproic acid	1 (16.7)	5 (83.3)	
	Mean ± SD	Mean ± SD	p
Age (years)	40.4 ± 8.8	37.0 ± 12.7	0.11
HOMA-IR	6.0 ± 4.3*	2.4 ± 1.7**	< 0.001
Uric acid (μmol/L)	335 ±117	272 ± 92	< 0.001

* n = 23 (11 diabetic patients were excluded);
** n = 86 (10 diabetic patients were excluded
[a]Statistical analysis was detected using Fisher's exact test

Table 9. Characteristics of patients with or without metabolic syndrome.

We found that gender was not associated with metabolic syndrome, 24.7% in men and 28.9% in women. As to age, we found that patients with metabolic syndrome were older than metabolic syndrome free patients (40.4 ± 8.8 years Vs 37.0 ± 12.7 years), but this difference was not significant (table 9).

Our present data showed that there is no difference in metabolic syndrome prevalence between patients receiving antipsychotic and mood stabilizers treatment. However, we noted that patients treated with lithium had the highest prevalence of metabolic syndrome (table 9).

Our study failed to show any significant association between metabolic syndrome and illness episode, whereas, manic patients had the highest prevalence of this disorder (30.5%) (table 9).

Patients with metabolic syndrome had significantly higher levels of uric acid (p < 0.001) than metabolic syndrome free patients (table 9).

Concerning HOMA-IR analysis, after diabetic patients exclusion (n = 21), we noted that patients with metabolic syndrome had significantly higher levels of HOMA-IR (p < 0.001) than metabolic syndrome free patients (table 9).

The variations of lipid profile parameters according to the illness episode and therapeutic characteristics of bipolar I patients are shown in table 10.

	Triglycerides (mmol/L)	Cholesterol (mmol/L)	c-HDL (mmol/L) Men	Women	c-LDL (mmol/L)	Lp (a) (mg/L)	ApoB/Apo A1
Patients (n = 130)	1.95 ± 1.55	4.42 ± 0.99	1.04 ± 0.37	1.17 ± 0.36	2.14 ± 1.10	243 ± 223	0.71 ± 0.23
Illness episode							
Depressive (n = 21)	1.95 ± 1.32	4.49 ± 0.96	1.12 ± 0.28	0.99 ± 0.36	2.14 ± 1.09	158 ± 91	0.82 ± 0.41
Euthymic (n = 73)	1.94 ± 1,80	4.53± 0.96	1.05 ± 0.41	1.26 ± 0.33	2.18 ± 1.04	268 ± 242	0.68 ± 0.19
Manic (n = 36)	1.97 ± 1.25	4.14 ± 1.0	0.98 ± 0.32	1.10 ± 0.11	2.08 ± 1.25	240 ± 228	0.70 ± 0.26
Treatment							
Valproic acid (n = 64)	1.78 ± 1.20	4.25 ±1.00	1.05 ± 0.40	1.13 ± 0.24	2.11 ± 1.12	240 ± 232	0.70 ± 0.24
Lithium (n = 12)	1.43 ± 0.95	4.40 ± 0.85	1.10 ± 0.36	0.86 ± 0.49	2.17 ± 0.82	170 ± 93	0.78 ± 0.29
Carbamaze pine (n = 10)	2.24 ± 3.25	4.60 ± 1.10	0.97 ± 0.33	1.44 ± 0.40	1.75 ± 0.74	293 ± 221	0.66 ± 0.22
AVP and Li (n =6)	2.33 ± 1.07	3.93 ± 0.40	1.10 ± 0.28	0.79	2.10 ± 1.22	153 ± 69	0.76 ± 0.23
Anti-psychotics (n = 38)	2.26 ± 1.64	4.74 ± 1.00	1.03 ± 0.36	1.26 ± 0.40	2.30 ± 1.23	271 ± 248	0.71 ± 0.30

AVP: valproic acid; Li: lithium

Table 10. Variations of lipid profile parameters according to the illness episode and therapeutic characteristics of bipolar I patients.

Our study failed to show any significant association between lipid profile parameters, illness episode and treatment, while euthymic patients were found to have the highest levels of Lp(a) and depressive patients had the highest levels of ApoB/ApoA1 ratio (table 10). Additionally, we showed that women taking lithium had the lowest c-HDL values and patients taking carbamazepine had the highest values of Lp(a) (table 10).

Table 11 reports the variations of uric acid, homocysteine, folate and vitamin B12 concentrations according to the illness episode and therapeutic characteristics of bipolar I patients.

	Uric acid (µmol/L)		Homocysteine (µmol/L)	Folate (µg/L)	Vitamin B12 (ng/L)
	Men (n = 85)	Women (n = 45)			
Patients (n = 130)	311 ± 99	246 ± 97	15.8 ± 8.9	3.3 ± 0.9	356 ± 198
Illness episode					
Depressive (n = 21)	228 ± 79	205 ± 128	15.2 ± 6.7	3.4 ± 1.3	481 ± 299[a]
Euthymic (n = 73)	309 ± 110	271 ± 95	16.1 ± 10.1	3.4 ± 0.7	322 ± 165
Manic (n = 36)	327 ± 87	217 ± 57	15.5 ± 7.7	3.3 ± 1.2	352 ± 158
Treatment					
Valproic acid (n = 64)	328 ± 91	279 ± 109	16.3 ± 10.0	3.5 ± 0.9	361 ± 91
Lithium (n = 12)	331 ± 79	219 ± 88	17.1 ± 12.7	2.8 ± 0.6	399 ± 79
Carbamazepine (n = 10)	278 ± 160	207± 61	16.9 ± 9.4	3.2 ± 0.8	240 ± 160*
AVP and Li (n = 6)	343 ± 76	288	15.5 ± 2.9	3.0 ± 0.8	518 ± 236*
Antipsychotics (n = 38)	269 ± 96	218 ± 83	14.2 ± 5.9	3.4 ± 1.5	338 ± 233

AVP: valproic acid; Li: lithium; *Carb Vs AVP/Li, p = 0.04; [a]F_{2-130} = 5.688, p = 0.004

Table 11. Variations of uric acid, homocysteine, folate and vitamin B12 concentrations according to the illness episode and therapeutic characteristics of bipolar I patients.

We found a significant association between vitamin B12 values and illness episode (F_{2-130} = 5.688, p = 0.004). Manic patients had lower values of this parameter than depressive patients. Moreover, we showed that vitamin B12 was significantly associated with the therapeutic characteristics. Indeed, patients taking carbamazepine had significantly lower values of this parameter than those taking valproic acid and lithium (p = 0.04) (table 11).

In patients, there was no significant change in homocysteine, folate and uric acid values in relation to illness episodes and the treatment, whereas the lowest values of uric acid were seen in depressive patients (both in men and women) compared to manic patients and in men taking antipsychotics and women taking carbamazepine compared to the other groups (table 11).

The distribution of BMI according to the illness episode and therapeutic characteristics is shown in table 12.

Our study failed to show any significant association between the BMI and to the illness episode and, therapeutic characteristics. However, we found that obesity was more frequent in depressive patients than in those with manic episode (38.1% Vs 27.8%). In addition, obesity and overweight were more frequent (72% and 52%; respectively) in patients taking valproic acid or lithium (table 12).

BMI (kg/m²) Characteristics	BMI ≥ 30 n = 43 (%)	25 ≤ BMI < 30 n = 40 (%)	BMI < 25 n = 47 (%)
Illness episode			
Depressive (n = 21)	8 (38.1)	4 (19.1)	9 (42.8)
Euthymic (n = 73)	25 (34.2)	23 (31.5)	25 (34.3)
Manic (n = 36)	10 (27.8)	13 (36.1)	13 (36.1)
Treatment			
Valproic acid (n = 64)	25 (39.1)	17 (26.6)	22 (34.3)
Lithium (n = 12)	6 (50)	4 (33.3)	2 (16.7)
Carbamazepine (n = 10)	2 (20)	5 (50)	3 (30)
AVP and Li (n = 6)	2 (33.3)	3 (50)	1 (16.7)
Antipsychotics (n = 38)	8 (21.1)	11 (28.9)	19 (50)

AVP: valproic acid; Li: lithium

Table 12. Distribution of BMI according to the illness episode and therapeutic characteristics.

4. Discussion

Our study showed that patients had significantly higher levels of triglycerides and Lp(a), and significantly lower levels of ApoA1 than control subjects. Furthermore, bipolar I disorder was showed to have significant association with hyperLp(a) (47.7% Vs 14.8%, OR = 4.48, IC 95% = 2.53-7.95; $p < 0.001$) and hypertriglyceridemia (53.1% Vs 17.7%, OR = 3.71, IC 95% = 2.13-6.46; $p < 0.001$).

In patients, the TG/HDL ratio and Lp(a) were found as the best predictive factors of cardiovascular risk in terms of sensibility (0.62, 0.74; respectively) and specificity (0.63, 0.74; respectively) at threshold of 1.12 and 168 mg/L, respectively. These results reflect a high risk of cardiovascular disease and may explain the high rates of morbidity and mortality in this population. Several studies have found mortality rates between 1.5 and 2.5 times higher in bipolar patients than the general population. After suicide and accidents, cardiovascular and all vascular diseases are the leading causes of death in these patients, with standardized mortality ratios ranging from 1.47 to 2.6. (Garcia-Portilla et al., 2009; Sicras et al., 2008).

The exact mechanisms increasing the incidence of cardiovascular risk in bipolar patients remain to be clarified, but they possibly include industrialisation, stress, lack of exercise, dietary lipids (that is, omega-3 fatty acid deficiency), increasing incidence of smoking and alcohol consumption and other factors (Ezzaher et al., 2010). These hypotheses will be, in part, justified later in this study.

Several investigators have been hypothesized that abnormalities in fatty acid composition may play a role in psychiatric disorders (Horrobin & Bennett, 1999). Maes et al. (1996, 1999) reported that patients with major depression had a significantly elevated ratio of ecosapentaenoic acid (EPA; 20: 5n-3)/docosahexaenoic acid (DHA; 22: 6n-3), lower level of EPA and total n-3 Omega-3 polyunsaturated fatty acids, in both serum cholesteryl esters and phospholipids when compared to patients with minor depression and normal controls. Similar findings were revealed in terms of fatty acid compositions of the erythrocyte membrane (Adams et al., 1996; Edwards et al., 1998; Peet et al., 1998; Chiu et al., 2003).

Moreover, many prospective and case-control studies have shown a positive association between serum triglycerides and coronary artery disease risk and demonstrated the importance of fasting triglycerides level as an independent risk factor. A number of clinical trials including the Framingham Heart Study have concluded that a low HDL cholesterol level predicts the risk for coronary artery disease independently of other risk factors. Each 1 mg/dL decrease in HDL cholesterol has been shown to increase risk for coronary artery disease by 2% in men and 3% in women. The Veterans Affairs High-Density Lipoprotein Cholesterol Interventional Trial, investigating the impact of fibrate therapy on cardiovascular risk, demonstrated that 6% increase in HDL cholesterol was associated with a 22% decrease in coronary events (Kabakci et al., 2008). In addition, Lp(a) has been shown to be an independent risk factor for atherosclerosis (Hakim et al., 2008) and has been found to exert a broad variety of pro-atherogenic and pro-thrombotic properties (von Eckardstein et al., 2001). Elevated plasma Lp(a) has been shown also to be associated with premature cardiovascular disease, premature cerebrovascular disease and premature peripheral vascular disease (Valentine et al., 1996).

The underlying mechanism for the altered lipid status in bipolar patients is unclear. A possible explanation might be found in the patient's nutritional status, the decrease in physical activity and the medications used (Ezzaher et al., 2010). Additionally, Chung et al. (2007) reported that bipolar disorder is associated with perturbations in lipid profile which play an important role in the pathophysiology of mood disorders, particularly in bipolar disorders. Indeed, cholesterol is one component of circulating lipoprotein particles that, besides handling cholesterol, carries micronutrients such as vitamins A and E as well as triglycerides and phospholipids. The latter compounds give rise to substrates such as fatty acids and choline, which are used in both the structural lipids of neuronal membranes and intercellular communication. Therefore, higher levels of one or more compounds of lipoprotein particles circulating in the bloodstream may produce subtle but measurable enhancements of mental processes by influencing the supply of fat-soluble micronutrients, specific fatty acids, or structural lipids (Ezzaher et al., 2010).

Our study failed to found any significant association between lipid profile parameters and illness episode, while euthymic patients were found to have the highest levels of Lp(a). Additionally, depressive patients had the highest levels of ApoB/Apo A1 ratio. However, some authors (Sagud et al., 2009) showed that serum cholesterol and LDL values were significantly lower in manic patients and others (Chung et al., 2007) showed that there was no difference in mean serum level of cholesterol or triglycerides among patients with manic, mixed, or depressive episode. These differences could be due to ethnicity and eating habits.

About therapeutic characteristics, any significant association was shown between lipid profile parameters and treatment, while, women taking lithium had the lowest c-HDL values and patients taking carbamazepine had the highest values of Lp(a). The mechanism(s) by which these drugs exert weight gain are not well known, but are presumed to involve increased energy intake (e.g., overeating), decreased energy expenditure (e.g., reduced resting metabolic rate, reduced physical activity, or reduced diet-induced thermogenesis), or a combination of the two (Malhotra & McElroy, 2002).

Additionally, we found that the prevalence of metabolic syndrome was 26.1% among patients, 24.7% in men and 28.8% in women. These prevalences were definitely higher than those reported in the Tunisian general population (13% in men and 18% in women) using a previous criteria (Bouguerra et al., 2006).

Compared with other studies, the prevalence of metabolic syndrome in our patients is included between those in Spanish patients (22.4%), Italian patients (25.3%) and US patients (30%) (Garcia-Portilla et al., 2008; Salvi et al., 2008; Fagiolini et al., 2005). The increasing prevalence of metabolic syndrome is important because it confers greater cardiovascular morbidity and mortality. Prospective observational studies have demonstrated an association between metabolic syndrome and development of type II diabetes (Hanson et al., 2002; Resnick et al., 2003; Klein et al., 2002; Sattar et al., 2003), cardiovascular disease (Lakka et al., 2002; Kip et al., 2004), and stroke (Kurl et al.,2006).

Our study showed that the highest prevalence of metabolic syndrome was obtained by the association between obesity, low c-HDL and hypertriglyceridemia. Moreover, the most individual components of this syndrome, in the total sample of patients, was low c-HDL (59.2%), hypertriglyceridemia (53.1%) and obesity (BMI $\geq$ 28.5 kg/m²) (33.8%), confirming in part the higher risk of dyslipidemia and obesity in bipolar I patients and in other hand the higher risk of cardiovascular disease in this population.

We found no significant difference in the prevalence of metabolic syndrome among gender and age. This is in line with results reported by Yumru et al., (2007).

We noted that there was no significant change in the prevalence of metabolic syndrome in relation to illness episode; however, manic patients had the highest prevalence. This may explain the high risk of cardiovascular disease in manic patients compared with depressive one (Murray et al., 2009). Additionally, Angst et al. (2002) showed that individuals with bipolar I disorder are at greater risk for cardiovascular mortality than individuals with bipolar II disorder. However, the difference in cardiovascular mortality between the two bipolar subtypes reflects the manic symptom burden, which predicts cardiovascular mortality independently of diagnosis and cardiovascular risk factors at intake. The results suggest that mania, either directly (through factors intrinsic to illness) or indirectly (through other mediators or associated variables), may itself influence cardiovascular disease.

Our study failed to show any significant association between metabolic syndrome and treatment. However, we noted that patients treated with lithium had the highest prevalence of metabolic syndrome. The increased risk to develop metabolic syndrome during treatment with lithium is in part related to its propensity to induce weight gain. According to Casey, lithium has been shown to stimulate appetite and increase calorie intake through different mechanisms.

HOMA-IR is significantly higher in patients with metabolic syndrome than others. This increase in HOMA-IR values reflects an insulin resistance and is associated with two to three fold increases in cardiovascular disease independent of classical risk factors (Toalson et al., 2004). In addition, uric acid levels were significantly higher in patients with metabolic syndrome. According to Vuorinen-Markkola et al. (1994), hyperuricemia forms another consistent feature of the metabolic syndrome what led to the suggestion of uric acid being a new component of the syndrome.

In addition, Chien et al., (2008) reported that metabolic syndrome induces high oxidative stress and the accompanying hyperuricemia worsens this stress. Furthermore, uric acid stimulates vascular smooth muscle proliferation, induces endothelial dysfunction, decreases endothelial nitric oxid production, and consequently, makes peripheral tissue resistant to insulin effects and results in endothelial dysfunction (Chien et al., 2008). High levels of uric acid are associated with increased renal glomerular pressure and sodium reabsorption, enhanced by high insulin concentrations (Alkerwi et al., 2009). In addition, hyperuricemia was associated with insulin resistance markers, including triglycerides, microalbuminuria and impaired glucose tolerance. These disturbances contribute to increase cardiovascular risk (Chien et al., 2008). This insulin- resistance causes steatosis, which is associated with hyper secretion of hepatic enzymes (Fromenty et al., 2004).

In men, uric acid was significantly higher in patients than controls. Additionally, the risk of hyperuricemia in bipolar I patients was approximately multiplied by 1.5 (10.8% Vs 4.4%, OR = 1.58, IC 95% = 0.49-5.08; p = 0.439). Many, but not all, epidemiological studies have suggested that high plasma uric acid is a risk factor for cardiovascular diseases. This raised level of plasma uric acid, parallel to an increased risk of cardiovascular diseases, could be either primary or secondary to the underlying causes of the cardiovascular diseases. However, the specific role of plasma uric acid in this constellation remains uncertain, although it may be involved in the platelet adhesiveness, aggregation, or inflammation and it may be implicated in the genesis of hypertension. In contrast, there is some evidence that the increase of plasma uric acid is protective against the cardiovascular diseases, since uric acid acts as an endogenous antioxidant, and the higher plasma uric acid levels found in cardiovascular diseases patients suggest that any protective antioxidant effect of uric acid is hidden by other negative effects in these pathogeneses (Haj mouhamed et al., 2010).

Additionally, Torres et al. (2007), reported that hyperuricemia which implicated in the oxidative stress plays an important role in the pathophysiology of bipolar disorders. The idea that the purinergic system might be involved in bipolar disorder dates back to Kraepelin, who was the first to describe an association between manic symptoms, uric acid excretion, hyperuricemia, and gout. In fact, the purinergic system modulates sleep, motor activity, cognition, attention, behavior, and mood. Even in the absence of a psychiatric diagnosis, individuals with higher uric acid levels are more likely to show higher drive, disinhibition, hyperthymia, or irritable temperament (Lorenzi et al., 2010). Similarly, diseases characterized by purinergic turnover dysfunction and uric acid overproduction (e.g., Lesch–Nyhan syndrome) are associated with impulsive/aggressive behavior, disinhibition, and increased sexual drive (Salvadore et al., 2010).

Among clinical and therapeutic characteristics, we found that there was no significant change in uric acid values in relation to illness episodes and the treatment. This finding is not in agreement with the previous studies that reported that plasma uric acid levels were higher only during the manic phase of bipolar disorder but not during the depressive or euthymic phases (De Berardis et al., 2008). Additionally, lithium was found to low uric acid plasma levels and to have uricosuric effects in mania. Carbamazepine and phenytoin similarly decreased uric acid levels; in contrast, valproate appeared to have the opposite effect. However, it is important to note that the effect of these drugs on uric acid levels in relationship to clinical improvement in patients with bipolar disorder has not been systematically evaluated (Salvadore et al., 2010).

Compared with controls, patients had significantly higher levels of homocysteine and significantly lower levels of folatemia. Additionally, significant associations were showed between bipolar I disorder and hyperhomocysteinemia (39.2% Vs 18%, OR = 1.95, IC 95% = 1.04-3.69; p = 0.038) and hypofolatemia (66.2% Vs 36.2%, OR = 3.69, IC 95% = 2.20-6.19; p < 0.001). Homocysteine is an intermediary metabolite of the essential amino acid methionine. Folate and vitamin B12 are required for remethylation of homocysteine to methionine (Hankey & Eikelboom, 1999).

According to Reynolds (2006), hyperhomocysteinaemia has long been identified as a risk factor for vascular disease and the lowering of homocysteine concentrations by the treatment with folic acid, or possibly vitamin B12 and vitamin B6 which might reduce the risk of both cardiovascular and cerebrovascular diseases. Moreover, the association between increased circulating homocysteine concentrations and premature vascular thrombotic events in individuals with hereditary homocystinuria is well established. This process may include platelet activation, smooth muscle cell proliferation, and enhanced leukocyte binding to the endothelium. In recent years, a relationship between milder degrees of hyperhomocysteinaemia and vascular disease has emerged, and this has been the subject of intense research. Hyperhomocysteinemia can be caused by a wide range of disorders, the most important of which are genetic defects of the enzymes involved in homocysteine metabolism and/or deficiencies of their co-factors: folate (former vitamin B9), vitamin B12 and vitamin B6 (Haj mouhamed et al., 2011).

Our study showed a significant association between bipolar I disorder and hyperhomocysteinemia. The exact mechanisms underlying the hyperhomocysteinemia in this disease are not completely understood and controversed among studies. Several hypotheses have been postulated including nutritional folate and vitamin B deficiency, and/or reduced glomerular filtration rate in bipolar patients (Vuksan-Ćusa et al., 2011). En effect, we found a significant association between this disease and hypofolatemia. Furthermore, some authors (Atmaca et al., 2005) showed that at a high concentration, homocysteine is considered to be a neurotoxic substance, causing activation of NMDA (N-methyl D-aspartate) receptors and leading to excitotoxicity. By impairing the neural plasticity and promoting neuronal degeneration, homocysteine could contribute to the pathogenesis of neurodegenerative and psychiatric disorders (Ipcioglu et al., 2008). Additionally, homocysteine is a methyl donor when activated to S-adenosylmethionine. So aberrant DNA methylation due to hyperhomocysteinemia also may be involved in the pathogenesis of bipolar disorder as well as schizophrenia (Mill et al., 2008).

In the other hand, folate appears to influence the synthesis rate of tetrahydrobiopterin, a cofactor in the hydroxylation of phenylalanine and tryptophan, rate-limiting steps in the biosynthesis of dopamine, norepinephrine, and serotonin, neurotransmitters postulated to play a role in the monoamine hypothesis of affective disorders. In addition, methyl tetrahydrofolate has been shown to bind to presynaptic glutamate receptors, where it may potentially modulate the release of other neurotransmitters, including the monoamines (Atmaca et al., 2005).

Moreover, some studies showed that lower folatemia in patients with psychiatric disorders can be due to their nutritional status (Reif et al., 2005). Indeed, poor appetite as a symptom of bipolar disorder could lead to decreased intake of B vitamins which could then lead to elevated homocysteine concentrations (Tolmunen et al., 2004).

We found a significant association between vitamin B12 values and illness episode. Manic patients had lower values of this parameter than depressive patients. This can be explained by the eating habits of bipolar patients. Indeed, Parikh et al. (2000) found that manic episode is often associated with weight loss.

About therapeutic characteristics, we showed that only vitamin B12 was significantly associated with the medication use. Indeed, patients taking carbamazepine had significantly lower values of this parameter than those taking valproic acid and lithium. These findings are not in agreement with others studies. In fact, Derkes and Westphal (2005) showed that carbamazepine can cause elevated homocysteine concentrations. Although, according to Ozbek et al (2008), homocysteine, folate and vitamin B12 were not related to drug usage. Additionally, Osher et al (2008) reported that there were no significant differences in homocysteine levels between patients receiving versus not receiving lithium, neuroleptic or valproate. However, Sener et al. (2006) suggested that carbamazepine, as enzyme inducer, can directly modulate the activity of different liver enzymes. Liver enzyme induction may cause depletion of the cofactor involved, folic acid, pyridoxal 5′-phosphate and vitamin B12, leading to the alterations in homocysteine status.

Our study showed that bipolar I patients are so much more likely to be smokers than controls (52.3% Vs 39.4%, OR = 1.68, IC 95% = 1.06-2.66; p = 0.025). An association between smoking and bipolar I disorder has been established and prevalence rates for lifetime and current smoking have been shown to be as high as 82.5% and 68.8% respectively (Lasser et al., 2000). The possible explanations for the high rates of smoking include an increased genetic vulnerability, a greater susceptibility to addiction because of a greater subjective experience of reward or pleasure, or that tobacco helps relieve some of the symptoms related to a behavioural disorder. For example, cigarette smoking may be an attempt to self-medicate symptoms of depression, anxiety, boredom or loneliness. Other possible explanations for continuing to smoke include increased withdrawal symptoms and reduced side effects from psychiatric medication (Williams & Ziedonis, 2004). Additionally, it has been reported that nicotine stimulates the brain to release dopamine, which is associated with pleasurable feelings, and smokers quickly develop regular smoking patterns. Eventually, smokers need increasing levels of nicotine to feel 'normal'. In the other hand, cigarette smoking is known to contribute to many diseases, including cancer, chronic obstructive pulmonary disease, stroke, cardiovascular diseases, and peptic ulcers. Investigators have attempted to elucidate the mechanisms of the pathogenesis associated with cigarette smoking, but the conclusions were not consistent. A basic hypothesis is that free radicals cause oxidative damage to macromolecules such as lipids, proteins, and DNA. Therefore, these radicals play an important role in the pathogenesis of these diseases (Haj mouhamed et al., 2010).

In this study, the prevalence of obesity is higher in patients with bipolar I disorder than in controls. Moreover, the risk of obesity in these patients is approximately multiplied by nine (33.1% Vs 8%, OR = 8.69, IC 95% = 3.61-20.87; p < 0.001).

In bipolar I patients, the prevalences of obesity and overweight were respectively 33.1 % and 30.7 %. These findings were similar to those reported by Elmslie et al (2000) and Fagiolini et al (2002) (36 % and 32 %). However, higher values were reported by McElroy et al (2004) (44 % and 20 %).

For this population, we found that the prevalence of obesity greatly exceeded that found in controls (12.3%) and in the general population (20%) (Haddad et al., 2006). Obesity in patients with bipolar I disorder thus constitutes a major public health problem and suggests that the development and testing of specific interventions that target the obesity epidemic in this particular population are urgently needed. Bipolar disorder and obesity both have tremendous impact on the physical and mental well-being of affected individuals. Therefore, both illnesses should be treated with a coordinated intensive and multifaceted treatment (Fagiolini et al., 2003).

Moreover, the risk of obesity in these patients is approximately multiplied by nine (33.1% Vs 8%, OR = 8.69, IC 95% = 3.61-20.87; p < 0.001). This could be one of the missing factors in understanding the relationship between psychiatric disorders and increased cardiovascular risk. In fact, some studies have reported that psychiatric disorders, particularly bipolar disorder, are significantly associated with adverse cardiovascular events and coronary heart disease (Garcia-Portilla et al., 2009). The mechanisms through which obesity leads to coronary heart disease remain hotly debated, but the accumulation, particularly, of visceral fat is widely favoured as the primary mechanism, leading, through the release of fatty acids and other mediators, to insulin resistance, dyslipidaemia, and a pro-inflammatory state. However, obesity in general, and central obesity in particular (ie. excessive visceral intra-abdominal fat) have been under-recognised as risk factors for coronary heart disease in the population, where most attention has been placed on smoking and cholesterol (Pinkney, 2001).

According to Raji et al (2009), the cardiovascular afflictions including obesity, diabetes, hypertension and stroke increase the risk for cognitive decline and dementia, but it is unknown whether these factors, specifically obesity and type 2 diabetes mellitus, are associated with specific patterns of brain atrophy. Obesity and type 2 diabetes mellitus may amplify the risk for dementia by worsening cerebral atrophy even in cognitively intact individuals, raising their vulnerability to future Alzheimer's disease neuropathology.

The same authors, mostly in subjects younger than 65 years, suggest also that increased body tissue fat content (adiposity) is correlated with atrophy in the temporal cortex, frontal lobes, putamen, caudate, precuneus, thalamus, and white matter. It is unknown, but of great interest, whether high tissue fat content, as measured by BMI, is associated with differences in brain structure in cognitively normal elderly (Raji et al., 2009).

Additionally, some studies showed that obesity has psychosocial consequences, including discrimination and stigmatization, which may contribute to the severity of bipolar disorder by negatively impacting patients' general physical health and functioning, quality of life, self-esteem, and psychological well-being. Obese patients have an increased risk of sleep apnea, which causes sleep disruptions and may lead to mood destabilization in patients with bipolar disorder. Obesity may also impact effectiveness of pharmacotherapies by altering the distribution and elimination of medications. Truncal obesity, which is most common, increases the risk of type 2 diabetes mellitus, dyslipidemia, hypertension, stroke, ischemic heart disease, and early death (Cheymol, 2000; Fagiolini et al., 2003; Plante & Winkelman, 2008).

In addition, obesity was more frequent in depressive patients than in those with manic episode (38.1% Vs 27.8%). Previous studies reported that patients who had depressive symptomatology were more likely to have excessive caloric and cholesterol intake, to smoke and to be inactive than non-depressed subjects. Another explanation might involve biological mechanisms: it is ascertained that hypothalamic–pituitary- adrenal (HPA) axis dysregulation and high cortisol blood levels lead to increased visceral fat. HPA axis dysregulation has been a common finding in both unipolar and bipolar disorders; recently, some studies reported that increased cortisol blood levels correlated to the amount of intra-abdominal fat in major depression (Maina et al., 2008).

About therapeutic characteristics, we found that obesity and overweight were more frequent (72% and 52%; respectively) in patients taking valproic acid or lithium. These findings are in line with those reported by De Hert et al. (2011). Moreover, Casey et al. (2005) reported that lithium have been shown to stimulate appetite through different mechanisms. The "carbohydrate craving" that is thought to be one of the mechanisms of increased calorie intake in people taking lithium is well known. In addition, it is believed that valproate also stimulates weight gain through a variety of mechanisms, especially the development of insulin resistance and diabetes mellitus type 2. In this line, our study found that this type of diabetes is frequent in patients (16.2%). Additionally, the risk of diabetes is multiplied by 1.5 in patients (16.2% Vs 9.7%, OR = 1.60, IC 95% = 0.62-4.12; p = 0.325).

Previous studies suggested that patients with both bipolar disorder and comorbid diabetes have more lifetime psychiatric hospitalizations than patients with bipolar patients without diabetes. The association between these two disorders underscores the importance of screening for diabetes in patients with bipolar illness, particularly because early detection and initiation of treatment to control glycemia may prevent diabetes-related complications. Moreover, other studies have demonstrated cerebrovascular lesions involving small intraparenchymal cerebral vessels and focal infarctions in patients with diabetes. These lesions predominantly occur in areas providing blood supply to the base of the pons, thalamus, and basal ganglia. Diabetes has been implicated as a risk factor for subcortical white-matter lesions observed on magnetic resonance imaging (MRI) scans; similar MRI findings have been noted in patients with bipolar disorder. Cerebral microvascular disease may lead to greater frequency of manic episodes, another reason to minimize diabetes-related complications in patients with comorbid bipolar disorder (Cassidy et al., 1999; Holman et al., 2008).

Alcoholic beverage was not significantly associated with this illness but we showed that it was more frequent in patients than controls (13.1% Vs 6.9%, OR = 2.04, IC 95% = 0.94-4.44; p = 0.067). It has been well documented that bipolar disorder and alcoholism commonly co-occur. In fact, the lifetime prevalence of alcohol abuse and drug abuse in people with bipolar disorder are known to be three to nine times more frequent that of the general population (Merikangas et al., 2007; Regier et al., 1990; ten Have et al., 2002).

Additionally, some studies showed that the feelings of depression and anxiety associated with bipolar can be a factor that leads to alcoholism. People with bipolar disorder may use alcohol or other drugs to self medicate these feelings, especially in instances where the person has not been diagnosed. However, alcohol makes the symptoms of bipolar disorder worse. Anyone who shows symptoms of bipolar disorder should seek the advice of medical professionals (Le Strat, 2010).

Some studies have shown that alcohol directly contributes to heart disease and stroke. Heavy drinking raises levels of triglycerides circulating in the bloodstream leading to diabetes and blocked or narrowed arteries that carry blood to the heart. If coronary arteries are clogged with fats, blood cannot flow freely, resulting in heart disease or stroke. Additionally, alcohol directly contributes to heart failure by damaging the heart muscle and arteries. Cardiomyopathy, or an enlargement of the heart muscle, results from long-term alcohol use. An enlarged heart no longer works efficiently and fails to provide enough oxygenated blood to other organs of the body. Furthermore, alcohol is associated with cardiac arrhythmia (irregular heartbeat), sudden cardiac death, stroke and atrial fibrillation (Pearson, 1996).

In our patients, hypertension was not associated with bipolar disorder (5.4% Vs 16%, OR = 0.43, IC 95% = 0.14-1.29; p = 0.136). De Heart et al. (2010) explained the decrease of hypertension frequency in individuals with a mental illness by changes in lifestyle of patients such as reducing salt intake.

Several methodological limitations should be considered when interpreting these findings. First, larger sample sizes of groups would be beneficial. Second, our work is a cross-sectional study that does not permit to follow up biological parameters. Third the sample of bipolar patients may not be representative of more heterogeneous populations. Finally, the diagnosis of controls was made by psychiatrists but without formal use of structured instruments to exclude psychiatric disorders in controls.

5. Conclusion

Our results demonstrate that Tunisian bipolar I patients are exposed to higher cardiovascular risk. In fact, they had perturbations in lipid profile: significantly higher values of triglycerides and Lp(a), and significantly lower values of ApoA1, significantly hyperhomocysteinemia and hyperuricemia (in men), significantly hypofolatemia and high prevalence of metabolic syndrome. Obesity, hyperLp(a), hypertriglyceridemia, hypofolatemia, hyperhomocysteinemia and cigarette smoking were the main cardiovascular risk factors associated with bipolar I disorder. Indeed, the risk of obesity was increased approximately for nine once, hyperLp(a), hypertriglyceridemia and hypofolatemia approximately for four once and the other factors approximately for tow once. The TG/HDL ratio and Lp(a) were found as the best predictive factors of cardiovascular risk in terms of sensibility and specificity at threshold of 1.12 and 168 mg/L, respectively.

Our findings noted a significant association between vitamin B12 values and illness episode. Manic patients had lower values of this parameter than depressive patients. Moreover, we showed that vitamin B12 was significantly associated with the therapeutic characteristics. Indeed, patients taking carbamazepine had significantly lower values of this parameter than those taking valproic acid and lithium. Additionally, there was no significant change in homocysteine, folate, uric acid values and metabolic syndrome in relation to illness episode and the treatment, whereas the patients with metabolic syndrome had significant higher levels of HOMA-IR and uric acid than metabolic syndrome free.

Therefore, bipolar I patients require specific care, particularly for lipid profile, vitamin status and weight; the effectiveness of this care will be evaluated during follow-up period Clinicians should track the effects of treatment on physical and the biological parameters, and should facilitate access to appropriate medical care.

6. Acknowledgement

The authors thank the patients and control subjects for their assistance in this study.

7. References

Alkerwi, A.; Boutsen, M.; Vaillant, M.; Barre, J.; Lair, ML.; Albert, A.; Guillaume, M. & Dramaix, M. (2009). Alcohol consumption and the prevalence of metabolic syndrome: A meta-analysis of observational studies. *Atherosclerosis*, 204, 624-635.

American Psychiatric Association. (2004). *Diagnostic and Statistical Manual of Mental Disorders*, 4th edition. American Psychiatric Association,Washington DC.

Angst, F.; Stassen, HH.; Clayton, PJ. & Angst, J. (2002). Mortality of patients with mood disorders: follow-up over 34-38 years. *Journal of Affective Disorders*, 68, 167-181.

Atmaca, M.; Tezcan, E.; Kululu, M.; Kirtas, O. & Ustunda, B. (2005). Serum folate and homocysteine levels in patients with obsessive-compulsive disorder. *Psychiatry and Clinical Neurosciences*, 59, 616-620.

Bouguerra, R.; Ben Salem, L.; Alberti, H.; Ben Rayana, C.; El Atti, J.; Blouza, S. Gaigi, S.; Achour, A.; Ben Slama, C. & Zouari, B. (2006). Prevalence of metabolic abnormalities in the Tunisian adults: a population based study. *Diabetes & Metabolism*, 32, 215-221.

Casey, DE. (2005). Metabolic issues and cardiovascular disease in patients with psychiatric disorders. *The American Journal of Medicine*, 118, 15-22.

Cassidy, F.; Ahearn, E. & Carroll, BJ. (1999). Elevated frequency of diabetes mellitus in hospitalized manic-depressive patients. *The American Journal of Psychiatry*, 156, 9, 1417-1420.

Cheymol, G. (2000). Effects of obesity on pharmacokinetics implications for drug therapy. *Clinical Pharmacokinetics*, 39,3, 215-231.

Chien, KL.; Hsub, HC.; Lee, YT. & Chen, MF. (2008). Renal function and metabolic syndrme components on cardiovascular and all-cause mortality. *Atherosclerosis*, 197, 860-867.

Chung, KH.; Tsai, SY. & Lee, HC. (2007). Mood symptoms and serum lipids in acute phase of bipolar disorder in Taiwan. *Psychiatry and Clinical Neurosciences*, 61, 428-433.

De Brardis, D.; Conti, CM.; Campanella, D.; Carano, A.; Di Giuseppe, B.; Valchera, A.; Tancredi, L.; Serroni, N.; Pizzorno, AM.; Fulcheri, M.; Gambi, F.; Sepede, G.; Moschetta, FS.; Salerno, RM. & Ferro, FM. (2008). Evaluation of plasma antioxidant levels during different phases of illness in adult patients with bipolar disorder. *Journal of Biological Regulators & Homeostatic Agents*, 22, 195-200.

De Hert, M.; Correll, CU.; Bobes, J.; Cetkovich-Bakmas, M.; Cohen, D.; Asai I.; Detraux J.; Gautam S.; Möller HJ.; Ndetei, DM.; Newcomer, JW.; Uwakwe R. & Leucht S. (2011). Physical illness in patients with severe mental disorders. I. Prevalence, impact of medications and disparities in health care. *World Psychiatry*, 10, 52-77.

De Hert, M.; Dekker, JM.; Wood, D.; Kahl, KG.; Holt, RIG. & Möller, HJ. (2010). Maladie cardiovasculaire et diabète chez les sujets souffrant d'une maladie mentale sévère. Déclaration de position de l'European Psychiatric Association (EPA), soutenue par l'European Association for the study of Diabetes (EASD) et l'European Society of Cardiology (ESC). *European Psychiatry*, in press.

Dierkes, J. & Westphal S. (2005). Effect of drugs on homocysteine concentrations. *Seminars in Vascular Medicine*, 5(2), 124-139.

Elmslie, JL.; Silverstone, JT.; Mann, JL.; Williams, SM. & Romans, SE. (2000). Prevalence of overweight and obesity in bipolar patients. *The Journal of Clinical Psychiatry*, 61, 179-184.

Ezzaher, A.; Haj Mouhamed, D.; Mechri, A.; Neffati, F.; Douki, W.; Gaha, L. & Najjar, MF. (2010). Lower paraoxonase 1 activity in Tunisian bipolar I patients. *Annals of General Psychiatry*, 9, 36.

Fagiolini, A.; Frank, E.; Houck, PR.; Mallinger, AG.; Swartz, HA.; Buysse, DJ.; Ombao H. & Kupfer, DJ. (2002). Prevalence of obesity and weight change during treatment in patients with bipolar I disorder. *The Journal of Clinical Psychiatry*, 63, 528-533.

Fagiolini, A.; Kupfer, DJ.; Houck, PR.; Novick, DM. & Frank, E. (2003). Obesity as a correlate of outcome in patients with bipolar I disorder. *The American Journal of Psychiatry*, 160, 1, 112-117.

Fagiolini, A.; Frank, E.; Scott, JA.; Turkin, S. & Kupfer, DJ. (2005). Metabolic syndrome in bipolar disorder: findings from the bipolar disorder center for Pennsylvanians. *Bipolar Disorders*, 7, 424-430.

Fromenty, B.; Robin, MA.; Igoudjil, A.; Mansouri, A. & Pessayre, D. (2004). The ins and outs of mitochondrial dysfunction in NASH. *Diabetes & Metabolism*, 30, 121-138.

Garcia-Portilla, MP.; Saiz, PA.; Benabarre, A.; Sierra, P.; Perez, J.; Rodriguez, A.; Livianos, L.; Torres, P. & Bobes, J. (2008). The prevalence of metabolic syndrome in patients with bipolar disorder. *Journal of Affective Disorders*, 106, 197-201.

Garcia-Portilla, MP.; Saiz, PA.; Bascaran, MT.; Martinez, S.; Benabarre, A.; Sierra, P.; Torres, P.; Montes, JM.; Bousoño, M. & Bobes, J. (2009). Cardiovascular risk in patients with bipolar disorder. *Journal of Affective Disorders*, 115, 1-7.

Haddad, FG.; Brax, H.; Zein, E. & Abou el Hessen, T. (2006). L'obésité et les pathologies associées dans un centre de soins au Liban. *Journal Médical Libanais*, 54, 152-155.

Haj Mouhamed, D.; Ezzaher, A.; Neffati, F.; Douki, W.; Gaha, L. & Najjar, MF. (2010). Effect of cigarette smoking on plasma uric acid concentrations. *Environmental Health and Preventive Medicine*, 1-6.

Haj Mouhamed, D.; Ezzaher, A.; Neffati, F.; Douki, W. & Najjar, MF. (2011). Effect of cigarette smoking on plasma homocysteine concentrations. *Clinical Chemistry and Laboratory Medicine*, 49, 3, 479-483.

Hakim, NA.; Hafizan, MT.; Baizurah, MH. & Zainal, AA. (2008). Serum lipoprotein(a) levels in patients with atherosclerotic peripheral vascular disease in Hospital Kuala Lumpur. *Asian Journal of Surgery*, 31, 1, 11-15.

Hankey, GJ. & Eikelboom, JW. Homocysteine and vascular disease. (1999). *Lancet*, 354, 407-413.

Hanson, RL.; Imperatore, G.; Bennet, PH. & Knowler, WC. (2002). Components of the "metabolic syndrome" and incidence of type 2 diabetes. *Diabetes*, 51, 3120.

Holman, RR.; Paul, SK.; Bethel, MA.; Matthews, DR. & Neil, HA. (2008). 10-year follow-up of intensive glucose control in type 2 diabetes. *The New England Journal of Medicine*, 359, 15, 1577-1589.

Ipcioglu, OM.; Ozcan, O.; Gultepe, M.; Ates, A.; Basoglu, C. & Cakir, E. (2008). Reduced urinary excretion of homocysteine could be the reason of elevated plasma homocysteine in patients with psychiatric illnesses. *Clinical Biochemistry*, 41, 831-835.

Kabakci, G.; Koylan, N.; Ilerigelen, B.; Kozan, O. & Buyukozturk, K. (2008). Impact of dyslipidemia on cardiovascular risk stratification of hypertensive patients and association of lipid profi le with other cardiovascular risk factors: results from the ICEBERG study. *Journal of Integrated Blood Pressure Control*, 1, 5-13.

Kessler, RC.; Berglund, P.; Demler, O.; Jin, R.; Merikangas, KR. & Walters, EE. (2005). Lifetime prevalence and age-of-onset distributions of DSM-IV disorders in the National Comorbidity Survey Replication. *Archives of General Psychiatry*, 62, 593-602.

Kip, KE.; Marroquin, OC.; Kelley, DE.; Johnson, BD.; Kelsey, SF.; Shaw, LJ.; Rogers, WJ. & Reis, SE. (2004). Clinical importance of obesity versus the metabolic syndrome in cardiovascular risk in women: a report from the Women's Ischemia Syndrome Evaluation (WISE) study. *Circulation*, 109, 706.

Klein, BE.; Klein, R. & Lee, KE. (2002). Components of the metabolic syndrome and risk of cardiovascular disease and diabetes in Beaver Dam. *Diabetes Care*, 25, 1790.

Kurl, S.; Laukkanen, JA.; Niskanen, L.; Laaksonen, D.; Sivenius, J.; Nyyssönen, K. & Salonen, JT. (2006). Metabolic syndrome and the risk of stroke in middle-aged men. *Stroke*, 37, 806-811.

Lakka, HM.; Laaksonen, DE.; Lakka, TA. Niskanen, LK.; Kumpusalo, E.; Tuomilehto, J. & Salonen, JT. (2002). The metabolic syndrome and total cardiovascular disease mortality in middle-aged men. *The Journal of the American Medical Association*, 288, 2709.

Lasser, K.; Boyd, JW.; Woolhandler, S.; Himmelstein, DU.; McCormick, D. & Bor, DH. (2000). Smoking and mental illness: A population-based prevalence study. *The Journal of the American Medical Association*, 284, 2606-2610.

Le Strat, Y. Trouble bipolaire et comorbidités addictives. (2010). *Annales medico-psychologiques*, 168, 584-587.

Lorenzi, TM.; Borba, DL.; Dutra, G. & Lara, DR. (2010). Association of serum uric acid levels with emotional and affective temperaments. *Journal of Affective Disorders*, 121, 161-164.

Maina, G.; Salvi, V.; Vitalucci, A.; D' Ambrosio, V. & Bogetto, F. (2008). Prevalence and correlates of overweight in drug-naïve patients with bipolar disorder. *Journal of Affective Disorders*, 110, 149-155.

Malhotra, S. & McElroy, S. (2002). Medical management of obesity associated with mental disorders. *The Journal of Clinical Psychiatry*, 63, 24-32.

Marmol, F. (2008). Lithium: bipolar disorder and neurodegenerative diseases possible cellular mechanisms of the therapeutic effects of lithium. *Progress in Neuro-Psychopharmacology & Biological Psychiatry*, 32, 1761-1771.

McElroy, SL.; Kotwal, R.; Malhotra, S.; Nelson, EB.; Keck, PE. & Nemeroff, CB. (2004). Are mood disorders and obesity related a review for the mental health professional. *The Journal of Clinical Psychiatry*, 65, 634-651.

Merikangas, KR.; Akiskal, HS.; Angst, J.; Greenberg, PE.; Hirschfeld, RM.; Petukhova, M. & Kessler, RC. (2007). Lifetime and 12-month prevalence of bipolar spectrum disorder in the national comorbidity survey replication. *Archives of General Psychiatry*, 64, 543-552.

Mill J, Tang T, Kaminsky Z.; KhareT.; Yazdanpanah, S.; Bouchard, L.; Jia, P.; Assadzadeh, A.; Flanagan, J.; Schumacher, A.; Wang SC. & Petronis, A. (2008). Epigenomic profiling reveals DNA-methylation changes associated with major psychosis. *The American Journal of Human Genetics*, 82, 696-711.

Muntoni, S.; Atzori, L.; Mereu, R.; Manca, A.; Satta, G.; Gentilini, A.; Bianco, P.; Baule, A.; Baule, GM. & Muntoni, S. (2009). Risk factors for cardiovascular disease in Sardinia from 1978 to 2001: A comparative study with Italian mainland. *The European Journal of Internal Medicine*, 20, 373-377.

Murray, DP.; Weiner, M.; Prabhakar, M. & Fiedorowicz, JG. (2009). Mania and mortality: why the excess cardiovascular risk in bipolar disorder?. *Current Psychiatry Reports*, 11, 475- 480.

National Cholesterol Education Program (NCEP). (2002). Expert panel on detection, evaluation, and treatment of high blood cholesterol in adults (Adult Treatment Panel III). Third Report of the National Cholesterol Education Program (NCEP). Expert panel on detection, evaluation, and treatment of high blood cholesterol in adults (Adult Treatment Panel III) final report. *Circulation*, 106, 3143-3421.

Osher, Y.; Bersudsky Y.; Silver H.; Sela, BA. & Belmaker, RH. (2008). Neuropsychological correlates of homocysteine levels in euthymic bipolar patients. *Journal of Affective Disorders*, 105, 229-233.

Ozbek, Z.; Kucukali, CI.; Ozkok, E.; Orhan, N.; Aydin, M.; Kilic, G.; Sazci, A. & Kara, I. (2008). Effect of the methylenetetrahydrofolate reductase gene polymorphisms on homocysteine, folate and vitamin B12 in patients with bipolar disorder and relatives. *Progress in Neuro-Psychopharmacology & Biological Psychiatry*, 32: 1331-1337.

Ozdemir, A.; Yalinbas, B.; Selamet, U.; Eres, M.; Turkmen, F.; Kumbasar, F.; Murat, B.; Keskin, AT. & Barut, Y. (2007). The effect of hepatitis C virus infection on insulin resistance in chronic haemodialysis patients. *Yonsei Medical Journal*, 48, 274-280.

Parikh, S.; Parker, C.; Cooke, R.; Krüger, S.; McIntyre, R.; Kusznir, A.; Bartha, C.; Ashton, L.; Damianakis, M.; Mancini, D. & Zetes-Zanatta, L. (2000). *Le trouble bipolaire. Guide d'information*, Camh, Ontario, Canada.

Pearson, TA. (1996). Alcohol and heart disease. *Circulation*, 94, 3023-3025.

Pinkney, J. (2001). Implications of obesity for diabetes and coronary heart disease in clinical practice. *British Journal of Diabetes & Vascular Disease*, 1, 103-106.

Plante, DT. & Winkelman, JW. (2008). Sleep disturbance in bipolar disorder: therapeutic implications. *The American Journal of Psychiatry*, 165, 7, 830-843.

Regier, DA.; Farmer, ME.; Rae, DS.; Keith, SJ.; Judd, LL. & Goodwin, FK. (1990). Comorbidity of mental disorders with alcohol and other drug abuse. Results from the Epidemiologic Catchment Area (ECA) study. *The Journal of the American Medical Association*, 264, 2511-2518.

Reif, A.; Pfuhlmann, B. & Lesch, KP. (2005). Homocysteinemia as well as methylenetetrahydrofolate reductase polymorphism are associated with affective psychoses. *Progress in Neuro-Psychopharmacology & Biological Psychiatry*, 29: 1162-1168.

Resnick, HE.; Jones, K.; Ruotolo, G.; Jain, AK.; Henderson, J.; Lu, W. & Howard, BV. (2003). Insulin resistance, the metabolic syndrome, and risk of incident cardiovascular disease in nondiabetic American Indians: the Strong Heart study. *Diabetes Care*, 26, 861.

Revicki, DA.; Matza, LS.; Flood, E. & Lloyd, A. (2005). Bipolar disorder and health-related quality of life: review of burden of disease and clinical trials. *Pharmacoeconomics*, 23, 6, 583-594.

Reynolds, E. (2006). Vitamin B12, folic acid and the nervous system. *Lancet Neurology*, 5, 949-960.

Sagud, M.; Mihaljevic-Peles, A.; Pivac, N.; Jakovljevic, M. & Muck-Seler, D. (2007). Platelet serotonin and serum lipids in psychotic mania. *Journal of Affective Disorders*, 61, 428-433.

Salvadore, G.; Viale, CI.; Luckenbaugh, DA.; Zanatto, V.; Portela, LV.; Souza, DO.; Zarate, CA. & Machado-Vieira, R. (2010). Increased uric acid levels in drug-naïve subjects with bipolar disorder during a first manic episode. *Progress in Neuro-Psychopharmacology & Biological Psychiatry*, 34, 819-821.

Salvi, V.; Albert, U.; Chiarle, A.; Soreca, I.; Bogetto, F. & Maina, G. (2008). Metabolic syndrome in Italian patients with bipolar disorder. *General Hospital Psychiatry*, 30, 318-323.

Sattar, N.; Gaw, A.; Scherbakova, O.; Ford, I.; O'Reilly, DSJ.; Haffner, SM.; Isles, C.; Macfarlane, PW.; Packard, CJ.; Cobbe, SM. & Shepherd, J. (2003). Metabolic syndrome with and without C-reactive protein as a predictor of coronary heart disease and diabetes in the West of Scotland Coronary Prevention Study. *Circulation*, 108, 414.

Sener, U.; Zorlu, Y.; Karaguzel, O.; Ozdamar, O.; Coker, I. & Topbas, M. (2006). Effects of common anti-epileptic drug monotherapy on serum levels of homocysteine, Vitamin B12, folic acid and Vitamin B6. *Seizure*, 15, 79-85.

Sicras, A.; Rejas, J.; Navarro, R.; Serrat, J. & Blanca, M. (2008). Metabolic syndrome in bipolar disorder: a cross-sectional assessment of a Health Management Organization database. *Bipolar Disorders*, 10, 1-10.

Simon, GE. (2003). Social and economic burden of mood disorders. *Biological Psychiatry*, 54, 208-215.

Ten Have, M.; Vollebergh, W.; Bijl, R. & Nolen, WA. (2002). Bipolar disorder in the general population in the Netherlands (prevalence, consequences and care utilisation): data from the Netherlands Mental Health Survey and Incidence Study (NEMESIS). *Journal of Affective Disorders*, 68, 203-213.

Toalson, P., Ahmed, S., Hardy, T. & Kabinoff, G. (2004). The metabolic syndrome in patients with severe mental illnesses. *Primary care companion to the Journal of clinical psychiatry*, 6, 152-158.

Tolmunen, T.; Hintikka, J.; Voutilainen, S.; Ruusunen, A.; Alfthan, G.; Nyyssönen, K.; Viinama·ki, H.; Kaplan, GA. & Salonen, JT. (2004). Association between depressive symptoms and serum concentrations of homocysteine in men: a population study[1-3]. *The American Journal of Clinical Nutrition*, 80, 1574-1578.

Torres, IJ.; Boudreau, VG. & Yatham, LN. (2007). Neuropsychological functioning in euthymic bipolar disorder: a meta-analysis. *Acta psychiatrica Scandinavica. Supplementum*, 434, 17-26.

Valentine, RJ.; Kaplan, HS.; Green, R.; Jacobsen, DW.; Myers, SI. & Clagett, GP. (1996). Lipoprotein (a), homocysteine, and hypercoagulable states in young men with premature peripheral on arthrosclerosis: A prospective controlled analysis. *Journal of Vascular Surgery*, 23, 53-63.

von Eckardstein, A.; Schulte, H.; Cullen, P. & Assmann, G. (2001). Lipoprotein(a) further increases the risk of coronary events in men with high global cardiovascular risk. *Journal of the American College of Cardiology*, 37, 2, 434-439.

Vuksan-Ćusa, B.; Jakovljević, M.; Sagud, M.; Mihaljević Peleš, A.; Marčinko, D.; Topić, R.; Mihaljević, S. & Sertić, J. (2011). Metabolic syndrome and serum homocysteine in patients with bipolar disorder and schizophrenia treated with second generation antipsychotics. *Psychiatry Research*, 189(1), 21-25.

Vuorinen-Markkola, H. & Yki-Jarvinen, H. (1994). Hyperuricemia and insulin resistance. *The Journal of Clinical Endocrinology & Metabolism*, 78, 25-29.

Williams, JM. & Ziedonis, D. (2004). Addressing tobacco among individuals with a mental illness or an addiction. *Addictive Behaviors*, 29, 1067-1083.

Wittchen, HU.; Mühlig, S. & Pezawas, L. (2003). Natural course and burden of bipolar disorders. *International Journal of Neuropsychopharmacology*, 6, 145-154.

Woods, SW. (2000). The economic burden of bipolar disease. *Journal of Clinical Psychiatry*, 61, 38- 41.

World Health Organisation. (1997). *Obesity: Preventing and Managing the Global Epidemic (publication WHO/NÛT/NCD/98.1)*, Geneva, Switzerland.

Yumru, M.; Savas, HA.; Kurt, E.; Kaya, MC.; Salek, S.; Savas, E. Oral, ET. & Atagun, I. (2007). Atypical antipsychotics related metabolic syndrome in bipolar patients. *Journal of Affective Disorders*, 98, 247-252.

Wyatt, RJ. & Henter, I. (1995). An economic evaluation of manic-depressive illness-1991. *Social Psychiatry and Psychiatric Epidemiology*, 30, 213-219.

Edwards, R.; Peet, M.; Shay, J. & Horrobin, D. (1998). Omega-3 polyunsatu- rated fatty acid levels in the diet and in red blood cell membranes of depressed patients. *Journal of Affective Disorders*, 48, 149-155.

Peet, M.; Murphy, B.; Shay, J. & Horrobin, DF. (1998). Depletion of omega-3 fatty acid levels in red blood cell membranes of depressive patients. *Biological Psychiatry*, 43, 315-319.

Maes, M.; Smith, R.; Christophe, A.; Cosyns, P.; Desnyder, R. & Meltzer, HJ. (1996). Fatty acid composition in major depression: decreased omega 3 fractions in cholesteryl esters and increased C20:4 omega 6/C20:5 omega 3 ratio in cholesteryl esters and phospholipids. *Journal of Affective Disorders*, 38, 35-46.

Maes, M.; Christophe, A.; Delanghe, J.; Altamura, C.; Neels, H. & Meltzer, HT. (1999). Lowered omega-3 polyunsaturated fatty acids in serum phospholipids and cholesteryl esters of depressed patients. *Psychiatry Research*, 85, 275-291.

Chiu, CC.; Huang, SY.; Suc, KP.; Luc, ML.; Huanga, MC.; Chen, CC. & Shen, WW. (2003). Polyunsaturated fatty acid deficit in patients with bipolar mania. *European Neuropsychopharmacology*, 13, 99-103.

7

Cholesterol and Triglycerides Metabolism Disorder in Malignant Hemopathies

Romeo-Gabriel Mihăilă
"Lucian Blaga" University of Sibiu
Romania

1. Introduction

The aim of this chapter is to achieve a synthesis of the major studies existing in the literature on correlations between lipid metabolism and malignant hemopathies. We will expose the fundamental research data and their impact on clinical treatment. The purpose of this review is to help the clinicians to understand better the pathological disorders of the lipid metabolism and use the existing therapeutic arsenal to improve the treatment outcomes. The research and the recognition of the presence of dyslipidemia is useful, as well as monitoring them during oncological therapy. The treatment of dyslipidemia may not be only an option when a patient with malignant hemopathy has acquired multidrug resistance. It can contribute to reversing this resistance, but it can also have adverse effects that must be recognized, followed and treated.

There are numerous studies in literature, but the connection between blood levels of various lipid fractions and hematologic malignancies is still unknown (Cvetkovic et al., 2009). Various epidemiological studies have found that between blood lipids and various neoplastic diseases there are correlations, thus the question is whether in the pathogenesis of cancer are not involved various lipid disorders (Moschovi M et al., 2004). At the same time it is believed that in patients with metabolic syndrome (MS), blood lipid levels may have correlations with the risk of cancer (Ulmer H et al., 2009).

2. The lipid profile evolution under cancer treatment

Cvetkovic & al. studied 47 patients with malignant non-Hodgkin's lymphoma (NHL) and found that before the treatment, compared with patients in the control group, blood levels of phospholipids, cholesterol (CH) and high density lipoprotein-cholesterol (HDL-cholesterol) had significantly lower values. After chemotherapy (3 or 6 cycles) the blood lipid levels reached even lower values in patients where the disease progressed, as opposed to those who achieved complete remission or whose disease was stationary, cases in which lipids increased progressively. (Cvetkovic et al., 2009).

In an other study conducted in Poland on the lipid levels of 238 patients with different hematological malignant diseases Kuliszkiewicz-Janus M et al. found that HDL-cholesterol values were significantly different from those of patients in the control group when the disease was in active phase, but in the remission phase the difference was statistically significant only in patients with NHL and acute leukemia (Kuliszkiewicz-Janus et al., 2008).

In a health investigation conducted on 156,153 subjects, with 5079 incident cancers in men and 4738 cancers in women, and a mean of 10.6 years of survey, there was an inverse association between serum triglyceride (TG) levels and NHL (2). But in the study conducted by Kuliszkiewicz-Janus M et al., the TG value increased in the active disease period in all the hematological malignancies besides NHL (Kuliszkiewicz-Janus et al., 2008).

Mihăilă R and al. made a cross-sectional research on all the patients with chronic lymphocytic leukemia (CLL) existing in a county department of hematology and a group of volunteer subjects from the medical staff with no malignant pathology. They found an augmentation of TG values in the patients with CLL (p <0.00001), an argument for a possible link between the MS and chronic lymphoproliferations. Hypercholesterolemia present in the patients with CLL from the above study may have consequences regarding the multiple drug resistance, subject to further future study. (Mihăilă et al., 2010)

Nearly all the children with ALL when diagnosed and during chemotherapy revealed a predictable model of serum dyslipidemia that consisted of very low levels of HDL-cholesterol, and elevated TG, and low-density lipoprotein cholesterol (LDL-cholesterol), that regained normal values during the remission period (Moschovi et al., 2004).

In patients with secondary hemophagocytic syndrome an augmentation of TG was observed when diagnosed or during the disease period and TG values decreased when the disease improved under treatment (Okamoto et al., 2009). In patients with aggressive T cell lymphoma, fasting TG level was higher in those with hemophagocytic syndrome group than in the patients who had no hemophagocytic syndrome (Tong et al., 2008).

3. The consequences of treatments with antineoplastic drugs

In children with acute lymphoblastic leukemia (ALL), treated with asparaginase dyslipidemia was frequently observed (Cohen et al., 2010).

A child heterozygote for apolipoprotein E 3/4 and with ALL who received pegasparaginase, presented an important aumentation of serum TG value, which normalized after continuous insulin infusion (Lawson et al., 2011). Another patient with a heterozygote type of familial lipoprotein lipase defect syndrome developed an important increase of serum TG value that was treated by three plasma exchanges with frozen plasma (Nakagawa et al., 2008).

An adult patient with ALL also had an acute pancreatitis because of an important hypertriglyceridemia that appeared after asparaginase administration (Kfoury-Baz et al., 2008), as well as a 10 years old boy who had been previously treated with asparaginase and corticosteroids (Ridola et al., 2008), both successfully treated by plasmapheresis sessions (Kfoury-Baz et al., 2008; Ridola et al., 2008).

In a group of children and adolescent patients recently diagnosed with ALL during treatment a progresive increase of serum CH values to 274+/-124 mg/dl was observed. In this group of patients the average value of TG during tratment was 459+/-526 mg/dl. Two patients had hypertriglyceridemia-related complications: a thrombosis of saggital sinus and an infarct of the left frontal lobe. The observed dyslipidemia disappeared in all children after the asparaginase administration (Cohen et al., 2010).

A prospective study assessed the lipid levels in children with ALL. At diagnosis, there was a significantly low level of total CH and HDL-cholesterol and at the same time a high level of TG. The patients were treated with the ALLIC 2002 protocol (including L-asparaginase), during which the values of total CH and HDL-cholesterol augmented, but they still remained lower than for the control group. The main serum TG level was significantly higher as compared to that of witnesses (Zalewska-Szewczyk et al., 2008).

A retrospective analysis showed that imatinib mesylate, used for the treatment of patients with chronic myeloid leukemia, led to a diminishing of serum CH and TG values (Franceschino et al., 2008). In a Romanian patient with chronic myeloid leukemia who received usual-dose of imatinib mesylate, a rapid and sustained normalization of serum CH, TG, low- and high-density lipoproteins and glucose values was found (Gologan et al., 2009). In some types of leukemia it was found that Kit receptor tyrosine kinase is overexpressed in a pathological manner, also that CH depletion was able to prevent Kit-mediated activation of the phosphatidylinositol 3-kinase downstream target Akt, which inhibits cell proliferation (Jahn et al., 2007).

The treatment of cutaneous lymphomas with T cells using bexarotene can produce a serum TG augmentation, as in the three cases reported. The treatment with fenofibrate is recommended, but if adverse effects occure or a statin is needed to reduce hypertriglyceridemia, omega-3 fatty acids may be a therapeutic solution during the bexarotene administration. (Musolino et al., 2009)

4. Is the metabolic syndrome a risk factor for some malignant hemopathies?

The main risk factors for excess weight and obesity are high caloric diet and sedentary lifestyle. A study conducted in a county hospital in Transylvania examined the presence of MS in all 56 patients with NHL existing in its records and a control group of 64 consecutive patients with non-cancerous diseases in the same hospital (control group). Patients with NHL had significantly more frequently arterial hypertension, significantly higher body mass index values, and a significantly higher number of components of the MS as compared to those of the control group. This observation advocates the idea that excess weight may be a risk factor for this type of neoplasia. (Mihăilă et al., 2009)

In a group of 170 non-Hispanic white pediatric cancer survivors, among males, body adiposity was more important in survivors than in witnesses, as was trunk fat. The survivors had higher values of CH, TG, LDL-cholesterol than the witnesses, and the first watched TV more hours than controls (Miller TL et al., 2010). It was observed that the young survivors of ALL, disease which they had in their childhood, especially those who received cranial radiotherapy, are likely to develop hyperlipidemia, insulin resistance, obesity, arterial hypertension and even MS soon after the treatment (Trimis et al., 2007).

After an average period of 37 months after the end of type ALL-BFM 90 chemotherapy protocol, out of 52 patients almost half were overweight, nearly 6% - obese, more than half had at least one risk factor for MS, and about 6% had MS (Kourti et al., 2005).

It was found that the consequences of treatment performed for ALL during childhood may become manifest when subjects reach adulthood. Cranial irradiation favors more the appearance of MS: 60% of those who had been so treated had at least two of the five components of MS when they become adults, and only 20% of those who had not been irradiated. The pathogenetic mechanism that explains the metabolic effects of cranial irradiation implies growth hormone (GH) deficiency, lower level of insulin-like growth factor 1, fasting hyperinsulinemia, abdominal obesity and hyperlipidemia, especially in women (Gurney et al., 2006). In another study, ALL survivors who received cranial irradiation developed more frequently MS than those nonirradiated (23% towards 7%), probably because of higher prevalence of excess weight and arterial hypertension (van Waas et al., 2010).

In a study conducted on a group of 184 adults who had ALL in their childhood, the overall prevalence of MS has been even higher - 9.2%. Peripheral stem cell allografts after total body irradiation favored the occurrence of hypertriglyceridemia, low HDL-cholesterol and increased fasting glucose level (Oudin et al., 2011).

In Sweden a group of adults was analysed; they survived after ALL during childhood and were submitted to radio-and chemotherapy. Those who received treatment for 5 years with GH compared with those not treated so for 8 years, showed significant changes in HDL-cholesterol, glucose and apolipoprotein B / apolipoprotein A1 ratio, and MS was significantly less frequent. (Follin et al., 2010)

Another study conducted in Sweden on adults who had childhood leukemia, found an augmentation of total body fat, especially of trunk adiposity and an evolution towards an unfavorable lipid spectrum. These observations were correlated with low levels of endocrine secretion of GH, a consequence of previous cranial irradiation. (Jarfelt et al., 2005)

An interesting combination of diseases was described in a 54 years old woman: after being diagnosed with chronic neutrophilic leukemia a liver biopsy was made. The histopathological diagnosis was of nonalcoholic steatohepatitis (NASH) with neutrophilic infiltrate. The authors consider that the leukemia cells that infiltrated the liver contributed to the emergence of NASH. The administration of cytosine arabinoside contributed to a significant decrease in fat degeneration. (Yoshida et al., 2004)

There are few studies on the metabolism of chylomicrons in patients with cancer. The study of a group of patients with Hodgkin and nonHodgkin lymphoma, as compared to a healthy control group, led to the observation that after an intravenous administration of a chylomicron-like emulsion, the levels of CH, TG and VLDL were significantly higher in patients with lymphoma because of the profound disturbance of the chylomicrons lipolysis and their removal deficit. (Gonçalves et al., 2003)

A very interesting observation was achieved in a line of promyelocytic leukemia NB4 cells: the administration of peroxisome proliferator-activated receptor gamma ligands was able not only to induce differentiation but also to favor lipogenesis in NB4 cells. This fact suggests a close link between differentiation and lipogenesis process in human myeloid cells thus stimulated. (Yasugi et al., 2006).

5. Cholesterol metabolism disorder

It is known that cell membranes contain lipid rafts, belonging to CH-rich microdomains. These components of the cell membrane are involved in intracellular signal transduction processes mediated by the receptor and in the self-renewal of ES cells. (Lee et al., 2010) The administration of methyl-beta-cyclodextrin, that is a CH-sequestering agent useful for the lipid raft destruction, is able to restore the activity of large conductance background K(+) channels. This favors the activation by stretch. (Nam et al., 2007) The depletion of CH from the cell membranes leads to lipid rafts destruction, that are responsible for bloking the translocation of leukemia inhibitory factor receptor and gp 130 (Port et al., 2007).

A group of Russian researchers studied the role of membrane CH in a line of human leukaemia K562 cells regarding the regulation of mechanosensitive cation channels activated by stretch. They consider that the above-mentioned suppression of this channel activation in leukemia cell line by methyl-beta-cyclodextrin is produced by F-actin rearrangement due to lipid raft destruction. (Morachevskaya et al., 2007)

In the regulation of lipid and CH metabolism liver X receptors are also involved, they are nuclear receptors. They can modulate the proliferation and survival of both normal and malignant B and T lymphocytes. (Geyeregger et al., 2009)

The correlation between increasing CH in lipid domains and the possible cancerosus cell transformation is very interesting (Ajith et al., 2008). It is believed that CH is important for cell proliferation, because low serum CH values may be the result of high cellular CH need of cancerous cells. Low serum CH values correlate with elevated levels of CH in lymphocytes. Evidence of low levels of CH in the culture medium is due to the development of lymphoma cells, which would consume more CH for their own proliferation. The experimental administration of mevastatin in vitro, which inhibits CH synthesis, did not determine a significant variation of the concentration of CH in the culture medium, while cell growth diminished. (Pugliese et al., 2010)

Low serum CH levels are also frequently found in acute leukemia patients. These patients have significantly lower serum values of CH, HDL-cholesterol, and LDL-cholesterol. A possible explanation for the low levels of HDL-cholesterol in the patients with acute leukemia could be an increased expression of a possible selective site for HDL-cholesteryl ester. (Gonçalves et al., 2005)

Malignant, proliferative cells have an intense metabolism of CH, while decreased intake of CH is responsible for decreasing cell proliferation. In a human line of promyelocytic HL-60 cells, an inhibition of cell cycle progression from G2 phase can be obtained by an enzymatic inhibition of CH synthesis at a stage before 7-dehydrocholesterol production. Drugs such as zaragozic acid or SKF 104976 can induce the expression of antigen 11c, a cluster of differentiation. These products have a comparable action to all-trans retinoic acid, which induces monocyte differentiation. (Sánchez-Martín et al., 2007)

Chronic lymphocytic leukemia (CLL) is a heterogenous malignant hemopathy. In these patients, in the presence of UM-IGHV, which is a negative prognostic factor, there are increased levels of CH and lactate and low levels of glycerol and 3-hydroxybutyrate. (MacIntyre et al., 2010)

CD5 antigen is responsible for CH synthesis and even for adipogenesis. It is known that malignant cells from CLL are undergoing a process of continuous stimulation due to CD5 activation and cell survival. (Gary-Gouy et al., 2007) A continuous activation of an antiapoptotic pathway explains the CLL cells survival. Apolipoprotein E4-very low density lipoproteins is responsible for the high level of apoptosis in CLL cells. Lipoprotein lipase is the enzyme that metabolizes very low density lipoproteins to low-density lipoprotein. It was observed that an increase of lipoprotein lipase mRNA levels is present in CLL patients with shorter survival. (Weinberg et al., 2008)

CH synthesis is also increased in patients with T-ALL who are glucocorticoid resistant (Beesley et al., 2009).

The growth of a promyelocytic leukemia cell line – HL-60 can be experimentally supressed by sodium cholesteryl sulfate, cholesteryl bromide, and cholesteryl-5alpha. The first two are responsible for the cell arrest in S and G2/M phases, and the last product – in the G2/M phase. (Ishimaru et al., 2008)

It was found that in xenotransplanted severely combined immunodeficient mice the most abundant bone marrow CH amounts are located in leukemia-rich sites. In vitro, in leukemic cells CH is able to stimulate FLT-1 expression and VEGF production. Human leukemic cells from patients with AML are significantly richer in CH than normal cells and this CH augmentation represents a marker of aggressive evolution. (Casalou et al., 2011)

6. Experimental and clinical observations on cholesterol metabolism disorder

ABCA1 and ApoA-I are responsible for the efflux of CH in human monocyte leukemia cell line derived foam cells. This decrease of the concentration of CH can be enhanced by administration of rosiglitazone. (Lü et al., 2010) Animals fed on alternate days have showed lower incidence of lymphomas, after tumor inoculation have had higher survival, and some types of cells have proliferated more slowly. It seems that this diet in humans would favor increased levels of HDL-cholesterol and lower those of triacylglycerol. (Varady et al., 2007)

It was found that ether phospholipid edelfosine is able to accumulate and selectively destroy mantle cell lymphoma and CLL cells, underlining the importance of the action on lipid rafts and Fas/CD95 for the therapy of these lymphoproliferations. CH depletion is involved in lipid raft disruption and in the diminishing of drug captation. (Mollinedo et al., 2010)

Some clinical observations on the presence of dyslipidemia in patients with malignant hemopathies are presented in Table 1.

Author	Disease	Dyslipidemia
Inamoto et al., 2005	ALL + cholestasis from graft versus host disease	hypercholesterolemia
Lim et al., 2007	NHL	serum HDL-cholesterol decrease
Gokhale et al., 2007	NHL	serum total CH level was significantly higher in patients who completed the treatment for NHL than in those who completed ALL therapy
Garg et al., 2011	intravascular large B cell lymphoma	low serum levels of HDL-cholesterol
Helman et al., 2011	MALT + obesity	hypercholesterolemia

MALT = mucosa-associated lymphoid tissue lymphoma

Table 1. Examples of dyslipidemia in patients with malignant hemopathies.

7. The cholesterol and the treatment with anti-CD20 monoclonal antibodies

It has been noted that the loss of CH is responsible for the decrease in the number of sites that can fix some monoclonal antibodies, including CD20. CH depletion or Shiga-like toxin binding have been causes of disruption of CD20 localization, but not of CD77 in lipid rafts. (Jarvis et al., 2007)

DXL625 is an anti-CD20 monoclonal antibody, capable of causing independently in vitro apoptosis of a lymphoma B cells line. This apoptosis is inhibited by the loss of membrane CH or of chelation of extracellular calcium, fact that underlines the role of lipid raft and calcium in this process. (Bingaman et al., 2010)

Many lymphoproliferations with B cells have indication of treatment with rituximab, an anti-CD20 antibody. The inhibitor therapeutic effect of rituximab occurs at the same time as the decrease of CH deposits from lipid rafts, with decreased B-cell receptor relocation to lipid rafts structures, and with the disruption of the expression of BCR immunoglobulin, lowering it. (Kheirallah et al., 2010)

The first monoclonal antibody that was approved for the treatment of B-cell lymphoproliferative malignancies was rituxan, a chimeric monoclonal anti-CD20 antibody. It has been observed that the monoclonal antibody attachment to CD20 produces a redistribution of these antigens to lipid rafts, which are specialized membrane microdomains. If rituxan is not used, the CD20 antigen affinity to lipid rafts is small. Intracellular calcium entry and apoptosis have been completely eliminated experimentally by extracting CH, which has led to the destruction of the integrity of lipid raft structures and to the dissociation of CD20 antigen from a fraction that is resistant to Triton X-100. From this it results that for the activation of caspase induced by CD20- lipid rafts appear to have an essential role. (Janas et al., 2005)

In multidrug resistance two populations of P-glycoprotein (P-gp) are involved. One is located in the membrane regions that are resistant to detergent; it has optimal P-gp ATPase activity; the verapamil can activate it and the orthovanadate can inhibit it almost entirely. The other population is located in another part of the membrane; it has less activity than P-gp ATPase of the first population; the verapamil can inhibit it, and its sensitivity to the orthovanadate is less. The first population of Pgp is surrounded by deposits of CH that may have the role to stimulate the P-gp ATPase activity, but the CH near the second population of Pgp does not seem to have such a role. (Barakat et al., 2005)

Rituximab induced apoptosis may be diminished by depletion of membrane deposits of CH, which does not allow the association to the detergent-insoluble lipid rafts of the antigen hypercrosslinked CD20. Under the action of rituximab, the antibody-bound CD20, found in lipid rafts in a high-affinity structure, activates src family kinases, interfering with the signal-transmission mechanism, which it inhibits. (Unruh et al., 2005)

Besides their CH-lowering effects, statins have pleiotropic effects, including the antileukemic ones observed in vitro and in vivo (Sassano et al., 2009), but they disrupt the binding (Winiarska et al., 2008) and the antitumour activity of rituximab (Ennishi et al., 2010), as a consequence of the changing of the antigen CD20 conformation (Ennishi et al., 2010; Winiarska et al., 2008). Statins interfere with the detection of CD20 as well as the antilymphomatous function of the rituximab (Winiarska et al., 2008). But in a study that analyzed the progression-free survival in 3 years and overall survival in a group of patients with diffuse large B-cell lymphoma, including some patients who were taking statins, it was found that there were no statistically significant differences, fact that advocates the idea that statins used in clinical treatment do not alter the prognosis of patients with diffuse large B-cell lymphoma under R-CHOP treatment. (Ennishi et al., 2010)

8. Statins as adjuvant treatment in malignant hemopathies

After chemotherapy, the blasts of acute myeloid leukemia (AML) respond by increasing cellular content of CH, which increases resistance to treatment. (Kornblau et al., 2007) Statins are pharmacologic inhibitors of 3-hydroxy-3-methylglutaryl-CoA reductase (HMG-CoA reductase) - the regulatory enzyme of CH synthesis (Nonaka et al., 2009; Sassano et al., 2007). In vitro, they block HMG-CoA reductase and by this they contribute to restore sensitivity to chemotherapy. (Kornblau et al., 2007) HMG-CoA regulates not only the synthesis of CH but also that of the higher isoprenoids, as geranylgeranyl pyrophosphate (Fuchs et al., 2008). By the inhibition of the prenylation processes, in vitro, statins reduce cellular proliferation and stimulate apoptosis of cancerous cells (Nonaka et al., 2009; Sassano et al., 2007). It was found that simvastatin inhibits geranylgeranylation processes of small

GTPases Rab5B and Rac1 in certain leukemic cells (for example, adult T-cell leukemia). (Nonaka et al., 2009)

The excessive proliferation inhibition induced by simvastatin results from the induction of apoptosis, cell cycle arrest in phase G2 / M, and accumulation of p21 protein. Simvastatin is able to remove resistance to apoptosis that occurs during treatment with bortezomib, by reducing geranylgeranyl pyrophosphate synthesis and cell survival mechanism dependant on this. (Fuchs et al., 2008) In IgM secreting cell lines and cells from Waldenstrom macroglobulinaemia, simvastatin showed antiproliferative and cytotoxic effects and stimulated the apoptosis. Simvastatin had a synergistic effect with bortezomib, dexamethasone and fludarabine by augmenting their cytotoxicity. (Moreau et al., 2008).

A group of 23 patients with lymphoproliferative diseases, for which statins had not been contraindicated, was treated for 3 days with simvastatin at a dose of 120 mg/day. Serum CH level and that of total lipids decreased significantly (p<0.001 and, respectively, p = 0.016). Serum ALT decreased unsignificantly, while that of AST increased, the growth was close to the statistical significance limit, but was not higher than the upper normal level. Flowcytometric dosage of annexine V showed that simvastatin induced early and late apoptosis increase (p = 0.007, respectively, p = 0.003). By its effect on apoptosis, simvastatin could be an adjuvant treatment for patients with lymphoproliferative disorders. (Mihăilă et al., 2009)

By their CH-lowering effect, statins are promising drugs for the treatment of lymphomas (63 Winiarska et al., 2008). A female patient suffering from NHL with large B-cells whose primary location was the mammary gland had hypercholesterolemia, hypertriglyceridemia and was hypertensive. During the treatment with R-CHOP and radiotherapy that followed (30 Gy), she received lovastatin (20 mg/day) and verapamil. After the first 30 days of treatment, both CH and TG were normalized, and after the whole treatment, the patient has been in complete remission that persists today. (Mihăilă et al, 2008) Lovastatin was administered to the patient not only because she was dyslipidemic, but also because the literature claims that the drug is useful in malignant lymphomas, leukemias and multiple myeloma by its pleiotropic effects. In 1998 the first article about a farnesyltransferase inhibitor (L-744, 832) was published, inhibitor that proved to be effective in mice with mammary carcinomas and lymphomas (Mangues et al., 1998). Lovastatin acts by inhibition of geranylgeranylation, followed by reduction of intracellular signaling mechanisms, which results in reduction of time and dose-dependency of the viability of lymphoma cells in vitro. This is the result of apoptosis stimulation as well as of the decrease of lymphoma cells proliferation, the latter by induction of G1 arrest in cell cycle (van de Donk et al., 2003).

In a rat lymphoma model lovastatin administration during radiotherapy led to cell cycle arrest in different phases, which justified the continuation of the treatment with this drug in the female patient during radiotherapy; the experimental model mentioned, the combination of lovastatin with radiotherapy resulted in a synergistic action (Rozados et al., 2005, as cited in Mihăilă et al., 2008). Lovastatin administration did not preclude the response to polychemoterapy that included rituximab. In fact, although it is only one case, the experimental findings do not always overlap with clinical outcomes. The authors consider that the combination of lovastatin with verapamil favored the response to anticancer treatment and prevented the possible multidrug resistance (Mihăilă et al., 2008). The combination of lovastatin + R-CHOP did not lead to adverse effects. Six years after the end of therapy, the patient is still in complete remission.

In a cell line of acute promyelocytic leukemia (NB4) atorvastatin and fluvastatin showed to be potent stimulators of cell differentiation and apoptosis (Sassano et al., 2007). When to the treatment with idarubicin and high-dose cytarabine of patients with AML pravastatin was added, CR / CRp was observed in 11 of 15 new patients, out of which 8 of 10 had unfavorable cytogenetics, and 9 of 22 patients who received rescue medication that pravastatin did not influence the length of neutropenia, of thrombocytopenia or of the toxicity of chemotherapy. (Kornblau et al., 2007)

Statins are active also in acute promyelocytic leukemia cells, where they augment the antileukemic response that depends on all-trans retinoic acid (ATRA). The c-Jun NH_2-terminal kinase pathway is required for leukemic cells differentiation induced by statins. Statins also intervene in modulating ATRA-dependent transcription. This was revealed by the selective expression of a large number of genes (400) when atorvastatin was administered together with ATRA. (Sassano et al., 2009) This drug combination could be a solution for reversing the ATRA-resistance of leukemic cells (Sassano et al., 2007).

Unlike the subgroup of normal and AML cells CD34 (-), the CD34 (+) is more sensitive to lovastatin. Both populations of cells were strongly inhibited when lovastatin was added to chemotherapy. Leukemic cell samples from different patients with AML had heterogeneous sensitivity to lovastatin. Fifty percent of the patients with unfavorable treatment response had cytogenetic examination with poor prognosis and significantly more blasts in the peripheral blood. (de Jonge-Peeters et al., 2009)

It was observed that high expression of CXCR4 correlates with a shorter survival time of patients with AML. In some models of cancer hypoxia it leads to the increase of CXCR4. On the other hand, increased $pO_{(2)}$ causes depletion of CH, which alters lipid rafts and leads to structural changes, which result in increased rejection of CXCR4 microparticles. (Fiegl et al., 2009) Atorvastatin administred in doses of 16 mg/kg body wt showed to be effective in the inhibition of ascites tumor growth and induced apoptosis of a cell line of Daltons' Lymphoma Ascites that was transplanted into mice (Ajith et al., 2008).

In vitro, simvastatin induced apoptosis of CLL cells, found in short term culture and contributed to lower BCL-2/BAX report; it was found that its effect of apoptosis induction is tumor-specific and does not affect normal lymphocytes. The association of simvastatin with fludarabine or cladribine synergistically induces DNA damages, and these lead to apoptosis. The proportion of cells found in apoptosis induced by simvastatin +/- chemotherapy was not correlated with the expression of negative prognostic markers of the disease (ZAP-70 and CD38) or its stage in the RAI classification. (Podhorecka et al., 2010)

The interaction of adhesion molecules, with fundamental role in cellular interaction processes, including those concerning EBV-transformed B cells is blocked by some statins. These drugs also inhibit intracellular activation of NF-kappaB and contribute to the emergence of transformed B-cell apoptosis. In mice with severe combined immune deficiency, simvastatin caused delayed emergence of the lymphomas induced by EBV. (Cohen et al., 2005)

Both the simvastatin and the tipifarnib have cytotoxic effect on AML cell lines and their associated administration has a synergistic effect. This combination administered to CD34(+) AML cells resulted in the increase of the inhibitory effect only on normally responsive AML cells; however, the combination administred to CD34(-) AML cells had augmented inhibitory effect in all cells. (van der Weide et al., 2009)

It was observed that statins are able to decrease the expression of BCL-2, an antiapoptotic molecule, favoring the appearance of apoptosis of CD4(+) CD28(null) T cells - a T aggressive and long-lasting lymphocyte subpopulation, which can infiltrate the atheromatous plaques, contributing to the their destabilization, which facilitates the instalation of major coronary accidents. (Link et al., 2011)

9. ABC transporters and cholesterol homeostasis

In many neoplastic diseases, increased expression of proteins on which depends the multidrug resistance correlates with the presence of refractory disease. A small proportion of AML leukemia cells is responsible for the tumor proliferation and expansion. These are leukemic stem cells, primitive cells, which are frequently in a quiescent state. When they leave the quiescent state and progress along the cell cycle, these cells are characterized by the ability of self-renewal and express some ATP-binding cassette (ABC) transporters. It was observed that when some ABC transporters have a high expression in leukemia cells, the prognosis of patients with AML is reserved as the response to treatment is inadequate. (de Jonge-Peeters et al., 2007)

The most studied transporter is the P-glycoprotein transporter (P-gp) - an ABC transporter responsible for unidirectional transmembrane translocation of the substrate (Gayet et al., 2005). P-gp is frequently involved in the emergence of multidrug resistance during chemotherapy (Shu & Liu, 2007). The multidrug resistance gene encodes this membrane transporter. Not only P-gp occurs in CH homeostasis at the cellular level, but also the synthesis of CH and CH-esters affects ATP-ase (Bucher et al., 2007) and the transmembrane transport by P-gp (Bucher et al., 2007; Shu & Liu, 2007). The lipid structure of the cell membranes also depends on the P-gp function (Dos Santos et al., 2007).

The ATP-ase activity of P-gp is controlled linearly by CH of the membrane structure. On the other hand, the decrease of membrane CH correlates with the non-linear decrease of the daunorubicin efflux induced by P-gp. An effective way to raise awareness of ALL CEM resistant to chemotherapy cells consists of partial depletion of the CH from cell membrane structure, that lowers the daunorubicin efflux by P-gp. (Gayet et al., 2005)

CH is able to increase basal activity of P-gp ATP-ase and increase P-gp sensitivity to progesterone and verapamil, modulators of this transporter. (Bucher et al., 2007) LDL-cholesterol can enlarge P-gp expression. In an experiment conducted in vitro, HMG-CoA reductase inhibitors were added to a primitive leukemia cells line (KG1a) and the observation was that lovastatin caused a decrease of 26% of P-gp expression, and pravastatin - a decrease of 16 %. (Connelly-Smith et al., 2007) But the CH derived from LDL was also able to restore sensitivity to chemotherapy of a human lymphoblastic leukemia cell line. It seems that the mechanism explaining this return is the restoration of the membrane CH and the reducing of the P-gp-associated ATPase to the same level. (Shu & Liu, 2007) The changes of the membrane CH quantity may be responsible for P-gp inhibition. It was observed that disassembly of lipid rafts can be produced both by the decrease of the CH content and by its increase. For a normal capacity of P-gp transport it is necessary to maintain accurate properties of membrane structures known as lipid raft. (Dos Santos et al., 2007)

In a clinical trial involving patients with CLL the P-gp expression of lymphocytes from peripheral blood was determined flowcytometricaly. Those patients whose lymphocytes expressed P-gp were treated for 6 days with 80 mg lovastatin daily, then a new sample of peripheral blood was examined flowcytometricaly. Lymphocytes of six of the 27 studied patients expressed P-gp; about 20% of them were positive. Following the administration of lovastatin only 7.33% of them also expressed P-gp (p = 0.016). Compared to the proportion of positive lymphocytes at baseline, the decline was of 63.35%. During the study, CH decreased statistically significantly, with 20.43%. There was no observation of the appearance of possible drug adverse effects. In conclusion, the 6 days therapy with lovastatin was able to reduce significantly the CH and the number of lymphocytes in the membranes where P-gp is expressed, so that this statin could contribute through its pleiotropic effects to reduce multidrug resistance, especially when it is followed by chemotherapy. (Mihăilă et al., 2010)

This drug efflux pump can be inhibited by verapamil, too, the research made in vitro proved that it can reduce multidrug resistance. In such a study conducted in two patients with leukemic lymphoma resistant to treatment, verapamil was able to increase the intracellular amount of doxorubicin (Tidefelt et al., 1994).

It was found that verapamil was able to overcome the P-gp - mediated resistance to doxorubicin and vincristine in a canine cell line of B cell lymphoma (GL-1) (Uozurmi et al., 2005, as cited in Mihăilă et al., 2008). These experimental findings were not confirmed by parallel administration of chemosensitizer verapamil to chemotherapy (cyclophosphamide, doxorubicin, vincristine, and dexamethasone) in patients with medium and high level NHL found in advanced stages. This drug combination did not increase the therapeutic response and did not extend the survival in these patients as compared to those treated only with the mentioned chemotherapy (without verapamil) (Gaynor et al., 2001, as cited in Mihăilă et al., 2008), but it cannot be excluded that it could be effective in some patients who develop multidrug resistance. But, in metastatic breast carcinoma that has become resistant to anthracyclines verapamil has showed that it is able to increase the survival of patients (Belpomme et al., 2000, as cited in Mihăilă et al., 2008). In the case of the patient described above with hypertension and primary mammary NHL, the evolution has been favorable under the combination of verapamil to chemo- and radiotherapy, that has resulted in a event-free survival of 6 years (up to the present day) (Mihăilă et al., 2008).

In another study, 45 patients with proliferative haematological disorders were included in one of the following two groups: A - those who had hypertension and who received verapamil + chemotherapy, and B - those with normal blood pressure, who received only chemotherapy. Group A included 7 patients with chronic lymphoproliferations and 2 with chronic myleoproliferations; under treatment, both systolic and diastolic pressure decreased significantly in all patients in the group. Initially the serum CH level was higher than in the patients in group B (p = 0.004), while other biological tests did not vary significantly between group A and B. No adverse effects were observed during the study. The fact that the initial blood CH was higher in in patients in group A suggests that malignant cells of patients in group B captured more blood CH that contributed to their proliferation. Although the average survival was not significantly different between group A and B, in group A there were more patients with stable disease (77.78% versus 44.44% - p<0.0001) while in group B more patients had progressive disease (30.56 % versus 11.11% - p<0.0001). The deaths due to progressive disease were significantly more numerous in group B. The authors consider that verapamil is useful not only because of its antihypertensive effect, but also due to its pleiotropic effects through which it could influence the evolution of neoplasia by inhibiting P-gp function and the efflux of drugs from lymphoma or leukemia cells. (Mihăilă et al., 2008)

10. Conclusions

Various epidemiological studies have found that between blood lipids and various neoplastic diseases there are some correlations.

Some authors found that in patients with newly diagnosed NHL the blood levels of CH, phospholipids and HDL-cholesterol had lower values than those of controls and the values of CH increased progressively after chemotherapy if the disease reached complete remission or was stationary, unlike those with disease progression, that their blood lipid levels were even lower.

Nearly all the children with ALL when diagnosed and during chemotherapy revealed a predictable model of serum dyslipidemia that consisted of very low levels of HDL-cholesterol, and elevated TG, and LDL-cholesterol, that regained normal values during the remission period.

In children with ALL, treated with asparaginase, hypertriglyceridemia was frequently observed and it can be cause of acute pancreatitis and thrombosis.

Imatinib mesylate, used for the treatment of patients with chronic myeloid leukemia, led to a diminishing of serum CH and TG values and CH depletion can inhibit cell proliferation.

The young survivors of ALL, disease which they had in their childhood, especially those who received cranial radiotherapy, are likely to develop hyperlipidemia, insulin resistance, obesity, arterial hypertension and even MS soon after the treatment.

Cranial irradiation favors more the appearance of MS by GH deficiency, lower level of insulin-like growth factor 1, fasting hyperinsulinemia, abdominal obesity and hyperlipidemia, especially in women.

It is believed that CH is important for cell proliferation, because low serum CH values may be the result of high cellular CH need of cancerous cells. Low serum CH values correlate with elevated levels of CH in lymphocytes. Malignant, proliferative cells have an intense metabolism of CH, while decreased intake of CH is responsible for decreasing cell proliferation.

An increase of lipoprotein lipase mRNA levels is present in CLL patients with shorter survival.

CD5 antigen is responsible for CH synthesis and even for adipogenesis. It is known that malignant cells from CLL are undergoing a process of continuous stimulation due to CD5 activation and cell survival.

The loss of CH is responsible for the decrease in the number of sites that can fix some monoclonal antibodies, including CD20. Statins interfere with the detection of CD20 antigen as well as the antilymphomatous function of the rituximab, but this effect was not showed in some clinical studies.

Statins reduce cellular proliferation and stimulate apoptosis of cancerous cells. By their pleiotropic effects, statins can be useful in the treatment of different diseases, like NHL, CLL, multiple myeloma and AML, as adjuvant therapy.

The association of simvastatin with fludarabine or cladribine synergistically induces DNA damages, and these lead to apoptosis.

Statins are active also in acute promyelocytic leukemia cells, where they augment the antileukemic response that depends on all-trans retinoic acid.

The ATP-ase activity of P-gp, frequently involved in the emergence of multidrug resistance during chemotherapy, is controlled linearly by CH of the membrane structure. The changes of the membrane CH quantity may be responsible for P-gp inhibition.

This drug efflux pump can be inhibited by statins and verapamil.
By their pleiotropic effects, statins are useful not only for dyslipidemia treatment, but also in antineoplastic therapy.

11. Acknowledgment

I am deeply grateful to my teacher - Melinda Erzse - who was kind to check the English text and make the appropriate corrections.

12. References

Ajith, T.A.; Anu, V., & Riji, T. (2008). Antitumor and apoptosis promoting properties of atorvastatin, an inhibitor of HMG-CoA reductase, against Dalton's Lymphoma Ascites tumor in mice. *J Exp Ther Oncol*. Vol.7, No.4, (October-December 2008), pp.291-298, ISSN: 1359-4117.

Barakat, S.; Gayet, L., Dayan, G., Labialle, S., Lazar, A., Oleinikov, V., Coleman, A.W., & Baggetto, L.G. (2005). Multidrug-resistant cancer cells contain two populations of P-glycoprotein with differently stimulated P-gp ATPase activities: evidence from atomic force microscopy and biochemical analysis. *Biochem J*. Vol.388, Pt.2, (June 2005), pp.563-571.

Beesley, A.H.; Firth, M.J., Ford. J., Weller, R.E., Freitas, J.R., Perera, K.U., & Kees, U.R. (2009). Glucocorticoid resistance in T-lineage acute lymphoblastic leukaemia is associated with a proliferative metabolism. *Br J Cancer*. Vol.16, No.100(12), (June 2009), pp.1926-1936.

Bingaman, M.G.; Basu, G.D., Golding, T.C., Chong, S.K., Lassen, A.J., Kindt, T.J., & Lipinski C.A. (2010). The autophilic anti-CD20 antibody DXL625 displays enhanced potency due to lipid raft-dependent induction of apoptosis. *Anticancer Drugs*. 2010 Jun; Vol.21, No.5, (June 2010), pp.532-542.

Bucher, K.; Belli, S., Wunderli-Allenspach, H., & Krämer, S.D. (2007). P- glycoprotein in proteoliposomes with low residual detergent: the effects of cholesterol. *Pharm Res*. Vol.24, No.11, (November 2007), pp.1993-2004.

Casalou, C.; Costa, A., Carvalho, T., Gomes, A.L., Zhu, Z., Wu, Y., & Dias, S. (2011). Cholesterol Regulates VEGFR-1 (FLT-1) Expression and Signaling in Acute Leukemia Cells. *Mol Cancer Res*. Vol.9, No.2, (February 2011), pp.215-224.

Cohen, H.; Bielorai, B., Harats, D., Toren, A., & Pinhas-Hamiel, O. (2010). Conservative treatment of L-asparaginase-associated lipid abnormalities in children with acute lymphoblastic leukemia. *Pediatr Blood Cancer*. Vol.54, No.5, (May 2010), pp.703-706.

Cohen, J.I. (2005). HMG CoA reductase inhibitors (statins) to treat Epstein-Barr virus- driven lymphoma. *Br J Cancer*. Vol.92, No.9, (May 2005), pp.1593-1598.

Connelly-Smith, L.; Pattinson, J., Grundy, M., Shang, S., Seedhouse, C., Russell, N., & Pallis, M. (2007). P-glycoprotein is downregulated in KG1a-primitive leukemia cells by LDL cholesterol deprivation and by HMG-CoA reductase inhibitors. *Exp Hematol*. Vol.35, No.12, (December 2007), pp.1793-1800.

Cvetkovic, Z.; Cvetkovic, B., Petrovic, M., Ranic, M., Debeljak-Martarcic, J., Vucic, V., & Glibetic, M. (2009). Lipid profile as a prognostic factor in cancer patients. *J BUON*. Vol.4, No.3, (July-September 2009), pp.501-506.

de Jonge-Peeters, S.D.; Kuipers, F., de Vries, E.G., & Vellenga, E. (2007). ABC transporter expression in hematopoietic stem cells and the role in AML drug resistance. *Crit Rev Oncol Hematol*. Vol.62, No.3, (June 2007), pp.214-226.

de Jonge-Peeters, S.D.; van der Weide, K., Kuipers, F., Sluiter, W.J., de Vries, E.G., & Vellenga, E. (2009). Variability in responsiveness to lovastatin of the primitive CD34+ AML subfraction compared to normal CD34+ cells. *Ann Hematol*. Vol.88, No.6, (June 2009), pp.573-580.

Dos Santos, S.M.; Weber, C.C., Franke, C., Müller, W.E., & Eckert, G.P. (2007). Cholesterol: Coupling between membrane microenvironment and ABC transporter activity. *Biochem Biophys Res Commun*. Vol.354, No.1, (March 2007), pp.216-221.

Ennishi, D.; Asai, H., Maeda, Y., Shinagawa, K., Ikeda, K., Yokoyama, M., Terui, Y., Takeuchi, K., Yoshino, T., Matsuo, K., Hatake, K., & Tanimoto, M. (2010). Statin-independent prognosis of patients with diffuse large B-cell lymphoma receiving rituximab plus CHOP therapy. *Ann Oncol*. Vol.21, No.6, (June 2010), pp.1217-221.

Fiegl, M.; Samudio, I., Clise-Dwyer, K., Burks, J.K., Mnjoyan, Z., & Andreeff, M. (2009). CXCR4 expression and biologic activity in acute myeloid leukemia are dependent on oxygen partial pressure. *Blood*. Vol.113, No.7, (February 2009), pp.1504- 1512.

Follin, C.; Thilén, U., Osterberg, K., Björk, J., & Erfurth, E.M. (2010). Cardiovascular risk, cardiac function, physical activity, and quality of life with and without long-term growth hormone therapy in adult survivors of childhood acute lymphoblastic leukemia. *J Clin Endocrinol Metab*. Vol.95, No.8, (August 2010), pp.3726-3735.

Franceschino, A.; Tornaghi, L., Benemacher, V., Assouline, S., & Gambacorti-Passerini, C. (2008). Alterations in creatine kinase, phosphate and lipid values in patients with chronic myeloid leukemia during treatment with imatinib. *Haematologica*. Vol.93, No.2, (February 2008), pp.317-318.

Fuchs, D.; Berges, C., Opelz, G., Daniel, V., & Naujokat, C. (2008). HMG-CoA reductase inhibitor simvastatin overcomes bortezomib-induced apoptosis resistance by disrupting a geranylgeranyl pyrophosphate-dependent survival pathway. *Biochem Biophys Res Commun*. Vol.374, No.2, (September 2008), pp.309-314.

Garg, A.; Hosfield, E.M., & Brickner, L. (2011). Disseminated intravascular large B cell lymphoma with slowly decreasing high-density lipoprotein cholesterol. *South Med J*. Vol.104, No.1, (January 2011), pp.53-56.

Gary-Gouy, H.; Sainz-Perez, A., Marteau, J.B., Marfaing-Koka, A., Delic, J., Merle-Beral, H., Galanaud, P., & Dalloul, A. (2007). Natural phosphorylation of CD5 in chronic lymphocytic leukemia B cells and analysis of CD5-regulated genes in a B cell line suggest a role for CD5 in malignant phenotype. *J Immunol*. Vol.179, No.7, (October 2007), pp.4335-4344.

Gayet, L.; Dayan, G., Barakat, S., Labialle, S., Michaud, M., Cogne, S., Mazane, A., Coleman, A.W., Rigal, D., & Baggetto, L.G. (2005). Control of P-glycoprotein activity by membrane cholesterol amounts and their relation to multidrug resistance in human CEM leukemia cells. *Biochemistry*. Vol.44, No.11, (March 2005), pp.4499- 4509.

Geyeregger, R.; Shehata, M., Zeyda, M., Kiefer, F.W., Stuhlmeier, K.M., Porpaczy, E., Zlabinger, G.J., Jäger, U., & Stulnig, T.M. (2009). Liver X receptors interfere with cytokine-induced proliferation and cell survival in normal and leukemic lymphocytes. *J Leukoc Biol*. Vol.86, No.5, (November 2009), pp.1039-1048.

Gokhale, C.D.; Udipi, S.A., Ambaye, R.Y., Pai, S.K., & Advani, S.H. (2007). Post-therapy profile of serum total cholesterol, retinol and zinc in pediatric acute lymphoblastic leukemia and non-Hodgkin's lymphoma. *J Am Coll Nutr.* Vol.26, No.1, (February 2007), pp.49-56.

Gologan, R.; Constantinescu, G., Georgescu, D., Ostroveanu, D., Vasilache, D., Dobrea, C., Iancu., D., & Popov, V. (2009). Hypolipemiant besides antileukemic effect of imatinib mesylate. *Leuk Res.* Vol.33, No.9, (September 2009), pp.1285-1287.

Gonçalves, R.P.; Hungria, V.T., Chiattone, C.S., Pozzi, D.B., & Maranhão, R.C. (2003). Metabolism of chylomicron-like emulsions in patients with Hodgkin's and with non-Hodgkin's lymphoma. *Leuk Res.* Vol.27, No.2, (February 2003), pp.147-153.

Gonçalves, R.P.; Rodrigues, D.G., & Maranhão, R.C. (2005). Uptake of high density lipoprotein (HDL) cholesteryl esters by human acute leukemia cells. *Leuk Res.* Vol.29, No.8, (August 2005), pp.955-959.

Gurney, J.G.; Ness, K.K., Sibley, S.D., O'Leary, M., Dengel, D.R., Lee, J.M., Youngren, N.M., Glasser, S.P., & Baker, K.S. (2006). Metabolic syndrome and growth hormone deficiency in adult survivors of childhood acute lymphoblastic leukemia. *Cancer.* Vol.107, No.6, (September 2006), pp.1303-1312.

Helman, R.; Teixeira, P.P., Mendes, C.J., Szegö, T., & Hamerschlak, N. (2011). Gastric MALT Lymphoma and Grade II Obesity: Gastric Bypass Surgery as a Therapeutic Option. *Obes Surg.* Vol.21, No.3, (March 2011), pp.407-409.

Inamoto, Y.; Teramoto, T., Shirai, K., Tsukamoto, H., Sanda, T., Miyamura, K., Yamamori, I., Hirabayashi, N., & Kodera, Y. (2005). Severe hypercholesterolemia associated with decreased hepatic triglyceride lipase activity and pseudohyponatremia in patients after allogeneic stem cell transplantation. Int J *Hematol.* Vol.82, No.4, (November 2005), pp.362-366.

Ishimaru, C.; Yonezawa, Y., Kuriyama, I., Nishida, M., Yoshida, H., & Mizushina, Y. (2008). Inhibitory effects of cholesterol derivatives on DNA polymerase and topoisomerase activities, and human cancer cell growth. *Lipids.* Vol.43, No.4, (April 2008), pp.373-382.

Jahn, T.; Leifheit, E., Gooch, S., Sindhu, S., & Weinberg, K. (2007). Lipid rafts are required for Kit survival and proliferation signals. *Blood.* 2007 Vol.110, No.6, (September 2007), pp.1739-1747.

Janas, E.; Priest, R., Wilde, J.I., White, J.H., & Malhotra, R. (2005). Rituxan (anti-CD20 antibody)-induced translocation of CD20 into lipid rafts is crucial for calcium influx and apoptosis. *Clin Exp Immunol.* Vol.139, No.3, (March 2005), pp.439-46.

Jarfelt, M.; Lannering, B., Bosaeus, I., Johannsson, G., & Bjarnason, R. (2005). Body composition in young adult survivors of childhood acute lymphoblastic leukaemia. *Eur J Endocrinol.* Vol.153, No.1, (July 2005), pp.81-89.

Jarvis, R.M.; Chamba, A., Holder, M.J., Challa, A., Smith, D.C., Hodgkin, M.N., Lord, J.M., & Gordon, J. (2007). Dynamic interplay between the neutral glycosphingolipid CD77/Gb3 and the therapeutic antibody target CD20 within the lipid bilayer of model B lymphoma cells. *Biochem Biophys Res Commun.* 2007 Vol.355, No.4, (April 2007), pp.944-949.

Kfoury-Baz, E.M.; Nassar, R.A., Tanios, R.F., Otrock, Z.K., Youssef, A.M., Albany, C., Bazarbachi, A., & Salem, Z.M. (2008). Plasmapheresis in asparaginase-induced hypertriglyceridemia. *Transfusion*. Vol.48, No.6, (June 2008), pp.1227-1230. Kheirallah, S.; Caron, P., Gross, E., Quillet-Mary, A., Bertrand-Michel, J., Fournié, J.J., Laurent, G., & Bezombes, C. (2010). Rituximab inhibits B-cell receptor signaling. *Blood*. Vol.115, No.5, (February 2010), pp.985-994.

Kornblau, S.M.; Banker, D.E., Stirewalt, D., Shen, D., Lemker, E., Verstovsek, S., Estrov, Z., Faderl, S., Cortes, J., Beran, M., Jackson, C.E., Chen, W., Estey, E., & Appelbaum, FR. (2007). Blockade of adaptive defensive changes in cholesterol uptake and synthesis in AML by the addition of pravastatin to idarubicin + high- dose Ara-C: a phase 1 study. *Blood*. Vol.109, No.7, (April 2007), pp.2999-3006. Kourti, M.; Tragiannidis, A., Makedou, A., Papageorgiou, T., Rousso, I., & Athanassiadou, F. (2005). Metabolic syndrome in children and adolescents with acute lymphoblastic leukemia after the completion of chemotherapy. *J Pediatr Hematol Oncol*. Vol.27, No.9, (September 2005), pp.499-501.

Kuliszkiewicz-Janus, M.; Małecki, R., & Mohamed, A.S. (2008). Lipid changes occuring in the course of hematological cancers. *Cell Mol Biol Lett*. Vol.13, No.3, (September 2008), pp.465-474, ISSN 1689-1392.

Lawson, E.B.; Gottschalk, M., & Schiff, D.E. (2011). Insulin infusion to treat severe hypertriglyceridemia associated with pegaspargase therapy: a case report. *J Pediatr Hematol Oncol*. Vol.33, No.2, (March 2011), pp.e83-86.

Lee, M.Y.; Ryu, J.M., Lee, S.H., Park, J.H., & Han, H.J. (2010). Lipid rafts play an important role for maintenance of embryonic stem cell self-renewal. *J Lipid Res*. Vol.51, No.8, (August 2010), pp.2082-2089.

Lim, U.; Gayles, T., Katki, H.A., Stolzenberg-Solomon, R., Weinstein, S.J., Pietinen, P., Taylor, P.R., Virtamo, J., & Albanes, D. (2007). Serum high-density lipoprotein cholesterol and risk of non-Hodgkin lymphoma. *Cancer Res*. Vol.67, No.11, (June 2007), pp.5569-5574.

Link, A.; Selejan, S., Hewera, L., Walter, F., Nickenig, G., & Böhm, M. (2011). Rosuvastatin induces apoptosis in CD4(+)CD28 (null) T cells in patients with acute coronary syndromes. *Clin Res Cardiol*. Vol.100, No.2, (February 2011), pp.147- 158.

Lü, Z.; Gou, L.P., Chen, L., Xie, B., & Qin, J. (2010). [Effect of lovastatin and rosiglitazone on cholesterol reverse transportation in foam cell]. *Zhonghua Nei Ke Za Zhi*. Vol.49, No.8, (August 2010), pp.696-699.

MacIntyre, D.A.; Jiménez, B., Lewintre, E.J., Martín, C.R., Schäfer, H., Ballesteros, CG., Mayans, J.R., Spraul, M., García-Conde, J., & Pineda-Lucena, A. (2010). Serum metabolome analysis by 1H-NMR reveals differences between chronic lymphocytic leukaemia molecular subgroups. *Leukemia*. Vol.24, No.4, (April 2010), pp.788-797.

Mangues, R.; Corral, T., Kohl, N.E., Symmans, W.F., Lu, S., Malumbres, M., Gibles, J.B., Oliff, A., & Pellicer, A. (1998). Antitumor effect of a farnesyl protein transferase inhibitor in mammary and lymphoid tumors overexpressing N-ras in transgenic mice. *Cancer Res*. Vol.58, (March 1998), pp.1253-1259.

Mihăilă, R.; Rezi, E.C., Cătană, A., Flucuş, O., Deac, M., & Mihăilă, R. (June 2008). Can Verapamil influence the evolution of the malignant haemopathies? The 13th Congress of the European Hematology Association, Copenhagen, Denmark, June, 12-15, 2008; In: *Haematologica – the Hematology Journal*. Abstract Book: 518, ISSN 0390-6078.

Mihăilă, R.; Rezi, E.C., & Deac, M. (2008). Primary mammary non-Hodgkin malignant lymphoma. *Archives of the Balkan Medical Union*, Vol.43, No.4, (December 2008), pp.289-292, ISSN 0041-6940.

Mihăilă, R.; Mocanu, L., Rezi, E.C., Cătană, A., Flucuș, O., Bera, L., Mihăilă, R., & Deac, M. (June 2009). The role of simvastatin in inducing apoptosis at patients with malignant haemopathies. The 14th Congress of the European Hematology Association, Berlin, June 4-7, 2009; In: *Haematologica – the Hematology Journal*. Abstract Book: 1194, ISSN 0390-6078.

Mihăilă, R.; Rezi, E.C., Isăilă, R., Boca, G., Mihăilă, R., & Deac, M. (June 2009). Is obesity a risk factor for nonHodgkin malignant lymphomas? The 14th Congress of the European Hematology Association, Berlin, June 4-7, 2009. In: *Haematologica – the Hematology Journal*, 2010, S2; Abstract Book: 1725, ISSN 0390-6078.

Mihăilă, R.; Cocișiu, G., Bera, L., Cătană, A., Flucuș, O., Rezi, E.C., Mihăilă, R., & Ciută, D. (June 2010). Study concerning the association between chronic lymphocytic leukemia and dyslipidemia. The 15th Congress of the European Hematology Association, Barcelona, Spain, June 10-13, 2010. In *Haematologica – the Hematology Journal*, 2010, S2; Abstract Book: 526-527, ISSN 0390-6078.

Mihăilă, R.; Mocanu, L., Cocișiu, G., Ciută, D., & Mihăilă, R. (2010). Effect of lovastatin on multidrug resistance to patients with chronic lymphocytic leukemia. *Archives of the Balkan Medical Union*, Vol.45, No.3, (September 2010), pp. 186-188. ISSN 0041-6940

Miller, T.L.; Lipsitz, S.R., Lopez-Mitnik, G., Hinkle, A.S., Constine, L.S., Adams, M.J., French, C., Proukou, C., Rovitelli, A., & Lipshultz, S.E. (2010). Characteristics and determinants of adiposity in pediatric cancer survivors. *Cancer Epidemiol Biomarkers Prev.* Vol.19, No.8, (August 2010), pp.2013-2022.

Mollinedo, F.; de la Iglesia-Vicente, J., Gajate, C., Estella-Hermoso de Mendoza, A., Villa-Pulgarin, J.A., de Frias, M., Roué, G., Gil, J., Colomer, D., Campanero, M.A., & Blanco- Prieto, M.J. (2010). In vitro and In vivo selective antitumor activity of Edelfosine against mantle cell lymphoma and chronic lymphocytic leukemia involving lipid rafts. *Clin Cancer Res.* Vol.16, No.7, (April 2010), pp.2046-2054, ISSN: 1557-3265.

Morachevskaya, E.; Sudarikova, A., & Negulyaev, Y. (2007). Mechanosensitive channel activity and F-actin organization in cholesterol-depleted human leukaemia cells. *Cell Biol Int.* Vol.31, No.4, (April 2007), pp.374-381.

Moreau, A.S.; Jia, X., Patterson, C.J., Roccaro, A.M., Xu, L., Sacco, A., O'Connor, K., Soumerai, J., Ngo, H.T., Hatjiharissi, E., Hunter, Z.R., Ciccarelli, B., Manning, R., Ghobrial, I.M., Leleu, X., & Treon, S.P. (2008). The HMG-CoA inhibitor, simvastatin, triggers in vitro anti-tumour effect and decreases IgM secretion in Waldenstrom macroglobulinaemia. *Br J Haematol.* Vol.142, No.5, (September 2008), pp.775-785.

Moschovi, M.; Trimis, G., Apostolakou, F, Papassotiriou, I., & Tzortzatou-Stathopoulou, F. (2004). Serum lipid alterations in acute lymphoblastic leukemia of childhood. *J Pediatr Hematol Oncol.* Vol.26, No.5, (May 2004), pp.289-293.

Musolino, A.; Panebianco, M., Zendri, E., Santini, M., Di Nuzzo, S., & Ardizzoni, A. (2009). Hypertriglyceridaemia with bexarotene in cutaneous T cell lymphoma: the role of omega-3 fatty acids. *Br J Haematol.* Vol.145, No.1, (April 2009), pp.84-86.

Nakagawa, M.; Kimura, S., Fujimoto, K., Atumi, H., Imura, J., Chikazawa, Y., Imamura, H., Okuyama, H., Yamaya, H., Fukushima, T., Nakagawa, A., Asaka, M., & Yokoyama, H. (2008). A case report of an adult with severe hyperlipidemia during acute lymphocytic leukemia induction therapy successfully treated with plasmapheresis. *Ther Apher Dial*. Vol.12, No.6, (December 2008), pp.509-513.

Nam, J.H.; Lee, H.S., Nguyen, Y.H., Kang, T.M., Lee, S.W., Kim, H.Y, Kim, S.J., Earm, Y.E., & Kim, S.J. (2007). Mechanosensitive activation of K+ channel via phospholipase C-induced depletion of phosphatidylinositol 4,5-bisphosphate in B lymphocytes. *J Physiol*. Vol.582, No.3, (August 2007), pp.977-990.

Nonaka, M.; Uota, S., Saitoh, Y., Takahashi, M., Sugimoto, H., Amet, T., Arai, A., Miura, O., Yamamoto, N., & Yamaoka, S. (2009). Role for protein geranylgeranylation in adult T-cell leukemia cell survival. *Exp Cell Res*. 2009 Jan 15; Vol.315, No.2, (January 2009), pp.141-150.

Okamoto, M.; Yamaguchi, H., Isobe, Y., Yokose, N., Mizuki, T., Tajika, K., Gomi, S., Hamaguchi, H., Inokuchi, K., Oshimi, K., & Dan, K. (2009). Analysis of triglyceride value in the diagnosis and treatment response of secondary hemophagocytic syndrome. *Intern Med*. Vol.48, No.10, (October 2009), pp.775-781, ISSN: 1349-7235

Oudin, C.; Simeoni, M.C., Sirvent, N., Contet, A., Begu-Le Corroller, A., Bordigoni, P., Curtillet C, Poirée M, Thuret I, Play B, Carazza Massot M, Chastagner P, Chambost H, Auquier, P., & Michel, G. (2011). Prevalence and risk factors of the metabolic syndrome in adult survivors of childhood leukemia. *Blood*. Vol.117, No.17, (April 2011), pp.4442-4448.

Podhorecka, M.; Halicka, D., Klimek, P., Kowal, M., Chocholska, S., & Dmoszynska, A. (2011). Simvastatin and purine analogs have a synergic effect on apoptosis of chronic lymphocytic leukemia cells. *Ann Hematol*. Vol.89, No.11, (November 2010), pp.1115-1124.

Port, M.D.; Gibson, R.M., Nathanson, N.M. (2007). Differential stimulation-induced receptor localization in lipid rafts for interleukin-6 family cytokines signaling through the gp130/leukemia inhibitory factor receptor complex. *J Neurochem*. Vol.101, No.3, (May 2007), pp.782-793.

Pugliese, L.; Bernardini, I., Pacifico, N., Peverini, M., Damaskopoulou, E., Cataldi, S., & Albi, E. (2010). Severe hypocholesterolaemia is often neglected in haematological malignancies. *Eur J Cancer*. Vol.46, No.9, (June 2010), pp.1735-1743.

Ridola, V.; Buonuomo, P.S., Maurizi, P., Putzulu, R., Annunziata, M.L, Pietrini, D., & Riccardi, R. (2008). Severe acute hypertriglyceridemia during acute lymphoblastic leukemia induction successfully treated with plasmapheresis. *Pediatr Blood Cancer*. Vol.50, No.2, (February 2008), pp.378-380.

Sánchez-Martín, C.C.; Dávalos, A., Martín-Sánchez, C., de la Peña, G., Fernández-Hernando, C., & Lasunción, M.A. (2007). Cholesterol starvation induces differentiation of human leukemia HL-60 cells. *Cancer Res*. Vol.67, No.7, (April 2007), pp.3379-3386.

Sassano, A.; Katsoulidis, E., Antico, G., Altman, J.K., Redig, A.J., Minucci, S., Tallman, M.S., & Platanias, L.C. (2007). Suppressive effects of statins on acute promyelocytic leukemia cells. *Cancer Res*. Vol.67, No.9, (May 2007), pp.4524-4532.

Sassano, A.; Lo Iacono, M., Antico, G., Jordan, A., Uddin, S., Calogero, R.A., & Platanias, L.C. (2009). Regulation of leukemic cell differentiation and retinoid-induced gene expression by statins. *Mol Cancer Ther*. Vol.8, No.3, (March 2009), pp.615-625.

Shu, Y. & Liu, H. (2007). Reversal of P-glycoprotein-mediated multidrug resistance by cholesterol derived from low density lipoprotein in a vinblastine-resistant human lymphoblastic leukemia cell line. *Biochem Cell Biol.* Vol.85, No.5, (October 2007), pp.638-646.

Tidefelt, U.; Juliusson, G., Elmhorn-Rosenborg, A., Peterson, C., & Paul, C. (1994). Increased intracellular concentrations of doxorubicin in resistant lymphoma cells in vivo by concomitant therapy with verapamil and cyclosporin A. *Eur J Haematol.* Vol.52, (May 1994), pp.276-282, ISSN 1600-0609

Tong, H.; Ren, Y., Liu, H., Xiao, F., Mai, W., Meng, H., Qian, W., Huang, J., Mao, L., Tong, Y., Wang, L., Qian, J., & Jin, J. (2008). Clinical characteristics of T-cell lymphoma associated with hemophagocytic syndrome: comparison of T-cell lymphoma with and without hemophagocytic syndrome. *Leuk Lymphoma.* Vol.49, No.1, (January 2008), pp.81-87.

Trimis, G.; Moschovi, M., Papassotiriou, I., Chrousos, G., & Tzortzatou-Stathopoulou, F. (2007). Early indicators of dysmetabolic syndrome in young survivors of acute lymphoblastic leukemia in childhood as a target for preventing disease. *J Pediatr Hematol Oncol.* Vol.29, No.5, (May 2007), pp.309-314.

Ulmer, H.; Borena, W., Rapp, K., Klenk, J., Strasak, A., Diem, G., Concin, H., & Nagel, G. (2009). Serum triglyceride concentrations and cancer risk in a large cohort study in Austria. *Br J Cancer.* Vol.101, No.7, (October 2009), pp.1202-1206.

Unruh, T.L.; Li, H., Mutch, C.M., Shariat, N., Grigoriou, L., Sanyal, R., Brown, C.B., & Deans, J.P. (2005). Cholesterol depletion inhibits src family kinase-dependent calcium mobilization and apoptosis induced by rituximab crosslinking. *Immunology.* Vol.116, No.2, (October 2005), pp.223-232.

van de Donk, N.W.; Schotte, D., Kamphuis, M.M., van Marion, A.M., van Kessel, B., Bloem, A.C., & Lokhorst, H.M. (2003). Protein geranylgeranylation is critical for the regulation of survival and proliferation of lymphoma tumor cells. *Clin Cancer Res.* Vol.9, (November 2003), pp.5735-5748, ISSN: 1557-3265

van der Weide, K.; de Jonge-Peeters, S.D., Kuipers, F., de Vries, E.G., & Vellenga, E. (2009). Combining simvastatin with the farnesyltransferase inhibitor tipifarnib results in an enhanced cytotoxic effect in a subset of primary CD34+ acute myeloid leukemia samples. *Clin Cancer Res.* Vol.15, No.9, (May 2009), pp.3076-3083.

van Waas, M.; Neggers, S.J., Pieters, R., & van den Heuvel-Eibrink, M.M. (2010). Components of the metabolic syndrome in 500 adult long-term survivors of childhood cancer. *Ann Oncol.* Vol.21, No.5, (May 2010), pp.1121-1126, ISSN 1569-8041

Varady, K.A. & Hellerstein, M.K. (2007). Alternate-day fasting and chronic disease prevention: a review of human and animal trials. *Am J Clin Nutr.* Vol.86, No.1, (July 2007), pp.7-13.

Weinberg, J.B.; Volkheimer, A.D., Mihovilovic, M., Jiang, N., Chen, Y., Bond, K., Moore, J.O., Gockerman, J.P., Diehl, L.F., de Castro, C.M., Rizzieri, D.A., Levesque, M.C., Dekroon, R., & Strittmatter, W.J. (December 2008). Apolipoprotein E genotype as a determinant of survival in chronic lymphocytic leukemia. *Leukemia.* 2008 Dec; Vol.22, No.12, (December 2008), pp.2184-2192.

Winiarska, M.; Bil, J., Wilczek, E., Wilczynski, G.M., Lekka, M., Engelberts, P.J., Mackus, W.J., Gorska, E., Bojarski, L., Stoklosa, T., Nowis, D., Kurzaj, Z., Makowski, M., Glodkowska, E., Issat, T., Mrowka, P., Lasek, W., Dabrowska-Iwanicka, A., Basak, G.W., Wasik, M., Warzocha, K., Sinski, M., Gaciong, Z., Jakobisiak, M., Parren, P.W., & Golab, J. (2008). Statins impair antitumor effects of rituximab by inducing conformational changes of CD20. *PLoS Med*. Vol.5, No.3, (March 2008). Pp.e64.

Yasugi, E.; Horiuchi, A., Uemura, I., Okuma, E., Nakatsu, M., Saeki, K., Kamisaka, Y., Kagechika, H., Yasuda, K., & Yuo, A. (2006). Peroxisome proliferator-activated receptor gamma ligands stimulate myeloid differentiation and lipogenensis in human leukemia NB4 cells. *Dev Growth Differ*. Vol.48, No.3, (April 2006), pp.177-188.

Yoshida, C.; Kojima, H., Iijima, T., Katsura, Y., Shimizu, S., Suzukawa, K., Mukai, H.Y., Hasegawa, Y., Abei, M., & Nagasawa, T. (2004). Association of non-alcoholic steatohepatitis (NASH) with chronic neutrophilic leukemia. *Eur J Haematol*. Vol.72, No.3, (March 2007), pp.225-228.

Zalewska-Szewczyk, B.; Matusiak, I., Wyka, K., Trelińska, J., Stolarska, M., & Młynarski, W. (2008). [Changes in the lipid profile in children with acute lymphoblastic leukaemia - the influence of the disease and its treatment]. *Med Wieku Rozwoj*. Vol.12, No.4, Pt.2, (October-December 2008), pp.1035-1040.

8

Dyslipidemia in Patients with Lipodystrophy in the Use of Antiretroviral Therapy

Rosana Libonati, Cláudia Dutra, Leonardo Barbosa,
Sandro Oliveira, Paulo Lisbôa and Marcus Libonati
Tropical Medicine Center, Federal University of the Pará, Pará
Brasil

1. Introduction

Dyslipidemia is a change in serum lipids levels, which is associated with increased risk of cardiovascular events when are found elevated (American Heart Association, 2002, Sposito et al., 2007). Before introduction of antiretroviral therapy (HAART), patients with acquired immunodeficiency syndrome (AIDS) developed a dyslipidemia characterized by isolated elevation of triglycerides (TG) and decrease in total cholesterol (TC) and its fractions (Gkrania-Klotsas & Klotsas, 2007; Mulligan, 2003). With the advent of HAART, especially with the use of protease inhibitors (PI), this situation changed to a lipid profile with elevated TG, TC, lipoproteins of very low and low density (VLDL-C and LDL-C) and decrease in high density lipoprotein (HDL-C), leaving these patients at risk for developing diabetes, hypertension and other complications (Chen et al., 2002; Furtado et al., 2007; Garg, 2000; Gkrania-Klotsas & Klotsas, 2007; Kotler, 2008; Mulligan, 2003; Sattler, 2008; Segarra-Newnham, 2002; Schering & Tovar, 2006; Yu et al., 2005).

Studies estimate that the prevalence of dyslipidemia in patients with HIV (Human Immunodeficiency Virus) during use of antiretroviral therapy can vary from 33% to 82% and may be influenced by several factors including study type, sample type and time of HAART (Gkrania-Klotsas & Klotsas, 2007; Schering & Tovar, 2006; Yu et al., 2005).

2. HIV lipodystrophy syndrome

According to UNAIDS and World Health Organization (WHO) (2009) there was a large increase in the prevalence of HIV carriers in the world, reaching 33.4 million in 2008, value explained by the maintenance of annual incidence and the increase of the survival (Lihn et al. 2003; Mallewa et al., 2008). However, was noted a illness pattern change of these patients which ever left to be affected by a clinical feature characteristic of opportunistic diseases to develop HIV lipodystrophy syndrome (HIVLS) (Kramer et al., 2009; Ministry of Health of Brazil, 2008; Samaras et al., 2009; Stankov & Behrens, 2010).

Body composition abnormalities have been reported in 40-50% of HIV-positive outpatients. This proportion is higher in patients receiving antiretroviral therapy. The rate of lipodystrophy can be high depending on the characteristics of the cohort (sex, age and possibly race), the type and duration of antiretroviral therapy (Grinspoon & Carr, 2005).

The HIVLS presents three distinct forms according to distribution pattern: lipoatrophy, with fat loss in limbs, face and buttocks; lipohypertrophy, with localized increase of abdominal, breast and dorsocervical subcutaneous cellular tissue, besides visceral deposit and lipoma formation; and the mixed form with signs of both syndromes earlier (Sattler, 2008; Mello et al., 2008) (Figure 1).

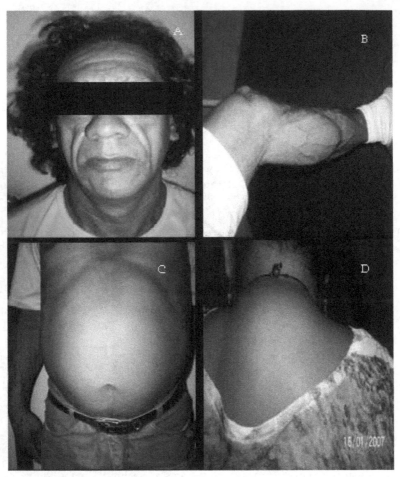

Legend: A) facial lipoatrophy with facial furrows accentuated, bony prominence, and loss of Bichat's fat (malar fat). B) Lipoatrophy of the lower limbs with prominent veins. C) Visceral lipohypertrophy, with increased waist circumference and little subcutaneous tissue. D) Dorsocervical lipohypertrophy. Photos of the collection of Dr. Rosana Libonati.

Fig. 1. Morphological changes in HIV patients with lipodystrophy syndrome, Pará, Brazil.

In addition to fat distribution alterations, metabolic changes are expressed as a mixed dyslipidemia with hypertriglyceridemia, total hypercholesterolemia, low density lipoprotein (LDL-C) elevation, reduction of high density lipoprotein (HDL-C), besides the induction of insulin resistance culminating in establishment of type II diabetes (Furtado et.,

2007; Chen et al., 2002; Garg, 2000; Sattler, 2008, Yu et al., 2005). The changes in the concentrations of plasma lipids are more observed in patients receiving protease inhibitors (PI) (Yu et al., 2005).

Prospective studies investigating body composition in patients starting HAART for the first time have showed increases in fat during the initial months of treatment, followed by a progressive declining in the following three years. In one study, the decline was estimated at 14% per year in white men who received treatment regimens containing zidovudine/lamivudine or stavudine/lamivudine plus protease inhibitor or non-nucleoside reverse transcriptase inhibitor. In contrast, trunk fat increases initially and then remains stable for two or three years, resulting in relative central adiposity. These changes are clinically evident in 20 to 35% of patients after about 12 to 24 months of combination antiretroviral therapy (Grinspoon & Carr, 2005).

The type, duration and current use or not of antiretroviral therapy are strongly associated with the lipoatrophy severity. Therapy based on two nucleoside analogue reverse transcriptase inhibitors and one protease inhibitor has strong association with severe lipoatrophy (Mallon et al., 2003).

Now, the mechanism by which the protease inhibitor causes lipodystrophy remains unknown. Several protease inhibitors prevent preadipocytes differentiation and mild to moderate apoptosis in subcutaneous adipose tissue. Adipose tissue of patients with lipodystrophy has reduced expression of mRNA of several key factors involved in adipogenesis, including Sterol regulatory element binding protein (SREBP1c) and Peroxisome proliferator-activated receptor gamma (PPARγ). *In vitro* studies have shown that protease inhibitors can inhibit lipogenesis and adipocyte differentiation, stimulate lipolysis and prevent nuclear localization of SREBP-1c (Garg, 2000; Grinspoon & Carr, 2005).

The nucleoside analog more strongly associated with lipoatrophy is stavudine, particularly when used in combination with didanosine. Lipoatrophy associated with nucleoside analogue may be due in part by mitochondrial injury caused by inhibition of the mitochondrial DNA polymerase γ within adipocyte and mitochondrial DNA depletion, although the extent and specificity of this effect remains unknown. The nucleoside analogue can inhibit adipogenesis and adipocyte differentiation, promote lipolysis and exert synergistic toxic effect with protease inhibitors *in vitro* and *in vivo* (Grinspoon & Carr, 2005).

In nine studies assessing risk factors for lipoatrophy, were statistically significant more common duration and exposure to thymidine analogues, most commonly stavudine (d4T) (6/9), age (5/9), markers of disease severity (CD4/HIV RNA) (5/9), duration of therapy (3/9) and Caucasian (3/9). A prospective nonrandomized study in 40 HIV-positive patients starting antiretroviral therapy for the first time resulted after an average of 96 weeks, using multivariate analysis, that treatment with d4T is an independent factor for lipoatrophy (Lichtenstein, 2005).

In eight studies assessing lipohypertrophy, the most significant risk factors were duration of therapy (3/8), a marker of disease severity (3/8), age (3/8) and protease inhibitor use (4/8). An additional study evaluating 2258 HIV-positive patients evaluated change in adipose tissue for both gender. Logistic regression showed that men have a significantly lower adjusted risk than women have (OR: 0.47, CI 95%: from 0.38 to 0.58) and a significantly lower risk of lipohypertrophy and mixed redistribution, while the risk of lipoatrophy was similar between genders. Therefore, a rigorous multivariate analysis controlling for numerous variables reveals multiple risk factors, suggesting that the pathogenic mechanism for fat redistribution seems to be the result of complex interactions between host, disease and drugs factors (Lichtenstein, 2005).

As for the diagnosis of HIVLS, there is not one standard pattern used to subjective body changes mentioned by the patients, anthropometric measurements and metabolic changes demonstrated in fasting laboratory tests (Diehl et al., 2008). Other tests that assist in conducting the HIVLS patients are: bone densitometry, for the investigation of osteopenia/osteoporosis; Dual-emission X-ray absorptiometry (DEXA), which allows an analysis of body composition, especially fat in the limbs, Computed Tomography, to observe presence of visceral fat deposits, and upper abdominal ultrasound for hepatic steatosis assessment (Mallon et al., 2003).

Therefore, the main consequences of HIVLS are increased cardiovascular risk and consequent development of hypertension, diabetes mellitus, atheromatous disease, stroke, myocardial infarction (Kramer et al., 2009). Psychological disorders as well as, like stress and low self-esteem by stigmatizing body changes (Santos et al., 2005; Seidl & Machado, 2008), which not cease to be risk factor for these events already mentioned by activation of sympathetic and glucocorticoids systems, and neuropeptide Y production potentiating the metabolic changes (Licht et al., 2010; Rasmusson et al., 2010).

3. Pathophysiology of dyslipidemia secondary to antiretroviral therapy

Since the implementation of antiretroviral therapy (HAART), in the 90s of last century, the treatment of AIDS has increased the mean life expectancy of HIV-infected population. Until then seen as a death sentence in a matter of short time, the disease have been faced like chronic, and with more optimism. However, despite a decrease in morbidity and mortality, HAART led to a problem that has become a major challenge that patients with AIDS must control: dyslipidemia (Cahn et al., 2010).

The dyslipidemia associated with HAART has been characteristic of elevated total cholesterol (TC), low-density lipoprotein (LDL-C) and triglycerides (TG), in addition to decreased high-density lipoprotein (HDL-C), which results in increased predisposition to the development of hypertension, insulin resistance, diabetes mellitus and cardiovascular complications. There are evidences that cardiovascular manifestations proportions in HIV-infected patients on HAART are higher than in general population (Almeida et al., 2009). This does not mean that the occurrence of dyslipidemia has emerged only with the implementation of antiretroviral drugs to treat AIDS. Before the existence of HAART had been reported lipid profile changes with high levels of triglycerides and low rate of VLDL-C and HDL-C (Sprinz et al., 2010; Grunfeld et al., 1992).

Several studies investigate ways of relating to HAART the effects of dyslipidemia like type of drug used by the patient and how the treatment regimen it has been implemented, but is still lacking a precise explanation for the lipid profile origin. Protease inhibitors (PI) are associated with dyslipidemia and insulin resistance for a considerable time, specifically ritonavir, and a variety of hypotheses (albeit not conclusive) it is presented to explain this association (Noor, 2007; Dubé et al., 2003).

One proposed mechanism to emergence of dyslipidemia is the lipoprotein lipase inhibition by PI, responsible for LDL-C increased, due to difficulty in capturing chylomicrons, resulting in lower hepatic clearance of triglycerides (Sprinz et al., 2010, as cited in Carr & Mooser, 2001). Another hypothesis is that PI has the ability to inhibit steps in lipid metabolism by binding to cellular retinoic acid binding protein type 1 (CRABP-1) and related protein receptor LDR-c, resulting in hyperlipidemia by higher release of lipids in the circulation. More specifically, the PI on CRABP-1 receptor leads to a reduction of 9-cis retinoic acid and dimerization with the receptor activated by peroxisome proliferator-activated receptor gamma (PPAR-γ), which is involved both in apoptosis of adipocytes and in differentiation between these two. (Sprinz et al., 2010; Carr et al., 1998). A third theory, restricted to ritonavir, antiretroviral therapy suggests it increases the activity of sterol regulatory element binding protein 1 (SREBP-1c), increasing lipogenesis, the rate of VLDL-C and apolipoprotein B liver. Thus, the increase in triglycerides caused by ritonavir that could be related to elevation in hepatic lipoprotein, inhibiting degradation mediated by apolipoprotein B and SREBP-1c in liver (Riddle et al., 2001; Liang et al., 2001).

As regard the insulin resistance promoted by PI, this class of antiretroviral drugs has been related to inhibition of GLUT-4 in the transmembrane transport of glucose, leading to reduced glucose uptake mediated by insulin in peripheral tissue (skeletal muscle and adipocytes), which can lead the modification of lipid levels (Noor, 2007). The fact that some patients had a clinical and laboratory profile more or less flowered depending on the effects that PI has on the lipids metabolism may be related to genetics, suggesting that certain people are more prone to PI effects through manifestation of certain genes so far not identified (Shahmanesh et al., 2001).

With regard to nucleoside reverse transcriptase inhibitors (NRTIs), it is speculated that can lead to reduced synthesis of mitochondrial DNA, leading to decreased oxidative phosphorylation, resulting in subcutaneous adipocyte apoptosis, dyslipidemia, and increased insulin resistance (Maagaard & Kvale, 2009). The reverse transcriptase inhibitor non-nucleoside (NNRTI), particularly Efavirenz, are also related to the onset of metabolic disorders, including dyslipidemia – but they have lower participation. When compared to patients receiving Nevirapine, patients who make use of Efavirenz have higher levels of triglycerides and HDL-C (Sprinz et al., 2010, as cited in Carr et al., 1998).

The type of antiretroviral used in HAART case amends significantly the lipid profile of patient it might be replaced. However, make use of a change in medication or combination of drugs (a strategy that appears more practical than prescription of lipid, at least at first glance) does not always result in improving lipid metabolism, considering the dyslipidemia in HIV infection is related to a multifactorial framework (Sprinz et al., 2010).

Although there are doubts considering the mechanisms linked to development of dyslipidemia in patients receiving HAART, and about assumptions not fully understood, this is still the most effective treatment in patients with AIDS and should not be proscribed for patients. To minimize risks that dyslipidemia implies to health, we recommend the same precautions, both dietary and behavioral (avoiding a sedentary lifestyle) and drug (statins/fibrates) for the general population. The use of fibrates is primarily indicated for reduction of hypertriglyceridemia, while statins are used to reverse the hypercholesterolemia. However, must be careful in prescribing of statins, since there is risk of drug interactions with HAART (Sprinz et al., 2010).

4. Treatment of dyslipidemia secondary to antiretroviral therapy

Hyperlipidemia is a major risk factor for developing of atherosclerosis. Epidemiological studies in adults show a direct association between high levels of total cholesterol and LDL and the incidence of mortality and morbidity in coronary artery disease (CAD) and is LDL-C a predictor of CAD risk at any age, besides low HDL and *diabetes mellitus* (Giddings, 1999).

Dyslipidemia in HIV infection is related to a multifactorial framework (Sprinz et al., 2010), so treatment should be done with non-pharmacological and pharmacological measures.

4.1 Hypercholesterolemia
4.1.1 Non-pharmacologic therapy
The HIV-infected patients with dyslipidemia they should be screened before using those drugs as therapy, with the implementation of the change of lifestyle of these patients through diet, exercise, tobacco control, diabetes mellitus and hypertension (Dubé et al., 2003). In one study, the diet associated with exercise in 11% reduced cholesterol levels of patients infected with HIV (Henry et al., 1998). In another study showed that diet accompanied by resistance exercise at least three times a week reduced the cholesterol level by 18% and triglycerides by 25% (Jones et al., 2001).

The first measure to be taken will always be non-pharmacologic therapy, unless there is urgent need for intervention, as patients at high risk for coronary artery disease (obesity, diabetes, family history of cardiovascular disease) and extremely high levels of LDL-C greater than 220 mg / dL (Dubé et al., 2003).

4.1.2 Pharmacological therapy
The pharmacological treatment for dyslipidemia it is performed with HMG-CoA reductase inhibitors, or statins, are the main representatives of pravastatin and atorvastatin groups. They have been used extensively in clinical practice as first-line treatment for hypercholesterolemia in the general population and in HIV-infected patients, promoting reduction of cardiovascular risk in patients without no history of coronary artery disease and of progression of coronary artery stenosis with decrease of cardiovascular events recurrence, working in primary and secondary, respectively (Dube et al., 2003).

In one study, patients with altered levels of total cholesterol (TC) and triglycerides (TG), using pravastatin 20 mg/day occurring 19% decrease in the level of TC and 37% in the level of TG (Baldini et al., 2000). In another study, diet was associated with therapy with pravastatin 40 mg/day in patients with TC levels greater than 240 mg/dL, indicating a 17% decline in the levels of TC and 19% in the level of LDL-C (Moyle, 2001). Therefore, Palacios et al., in 2002, analyzing a group of patients with TC levels greater than 240 mg/dL under atorvastatin 10 mg/day was found a 27% decrease in the level of TC, 41% of TG and 37% in the LDL-C.

Thus, statins are the first choice in the treatment of elevated LDL-C (> 220 mg / dL) and patients with high total cholesterol associated with hypertriglyceridemia (TG between 200 to 500 mg/dL), initial dose may be used 20-40 mg of pravastatin or atorvastatin 10 mg monitoring possible liver toxicity with laboratory tests (Dube et al., 2003). Protease inhibitors and non-nucleoside inhibitors of reverse transcriptase enzyme use in its metabolism the cytochrome P450 pathway (Smith et al., 2001), the same route used by simvastatin, lovastatin and atorvastatin, then the first two are proscribed to patients under antiretroviral therapy and the latter can be used with caution.

Fibrates are used as second choice in the treatment of hypercholesterolemia. In patients with normal TG and elevated LDL-C levels, a slight decrease in LDL-C ranging from 5 to 20% in the studies carried out. Therefore, the therapeutic fibrates use should be reserved for treatment of hypertriglyceridemia (TG> 500 mg/dL) in these patients (Dube et al., 2003).

4.2 Hypertriglyceridemia

4.2.1 Non-pharmacologic therapy

The non-pharmacologic therapy should be first applied to all patients with hypertriglyceridemia, through modification of lifestyle; diet should be instituted to reduce fat intake, weight reduction, reduction or elimination of alcohol intake, smoking cessation control of hyperglycemia and diabetes with insulin sensitizers such as metformin. In studies, it has been found that diets associated with exercise and resistance training promotes decrease of 21% and 27%, respectively, TG levels in HIV-infected patients (Henry et al., 1998; Yarashesky et al., 2001).

Patients who demonstrate extreme elevations in TG level (> 1000 mg / dL) and with a history of pancreatitis should be treated associating pharmacologic and non-pharmacologic therapy (Dube et al., 2003).

4.2.2 Pharmacologic therapy

Drug therapy should be instituted in all patients with TG levels greater than 500 mg/dL with the introduction of Gemfibrozil with starting dose of 600 mg half an hour before meals (lunch and dinner) or fibrates at a dose 54 to 160 mg/day (Dube et al., 2003). In a study carried out in patients with TG levels higher than 400 mg/dL using fibrate dose of 200 mg/day was observed 14% and 54% decrease of TC and TG levels, respectively (Palácios et al., 2002). Therefore, in another study, patients with TG levels higher than 266 mg/dL, using Gemfibrozil 600 mg/day associated with diet, evolved with a reduction of TG values in 18% (Miller et al., 2002).

The use of statins in general is not recommended for the treatment of hypertriglyceridemia (TG> 500 mg / dL) alone, is recommended when triglyceride levels are between 200 to 500 mg/dL associated with increased total cholesterol (Dubé et al., 2003).

5. Experience of the assistance service of metabolic diseases secondary to antiretroviral therapy for patients with dyslipidemia

Assistance Service of Metabolic Diseases Secondary to Antiretroviral Therapy (HAART) of the João de Barros Barreto University Hospital (HUJBB), Brazilian national reference in transmissible infectious diseases and AIDS, actually, assist about 99 HIV carriers' patients with lipodystrophy syndrome. Into this service, the authors develop a Project titled Lipodystrophy and Antiretroviral Therapy, financed by The State of Pará Research Foundation (FAPESPA), Research Program for the Unified Health System (PPSUS). One of the Project's purposes was the implantation of the lipodystrophy ambulatory care.

The HUJBB lipodystrophy ambulatory care works with team composed by an endocrinologist, a nutrition doctoral student, two medicine M.Sc students, four medical undergraduate students. The medical accompaniment is performed once a week. In the first service is diagnosed the clinical form of lipodystrophy and requested the proper tests (total cholesterol, HDL, LDL, triglycerides, fasting glucose test, oral glucose tolerance, insulin, abdominal ultrasonography to hepatic steatosis diagnostic and computed tomography for evaluation of visceral lipohypertrophy and electrocardiogram). The first patient's return is around 45 days and subsequently every three months for medical accompaniment. Each medical consultation is also performed medical history, measurement of blood pressure, heart auscultation, anthropometric evaluation (measurements of weight, height, skin folds) and bioimpedance. In addition, if need be the patient is referred to other professionals of the multidisciplinary team HUJBB.

Of the accompanied patients with lipodystrophy syndrome in this ambulatory care, 77% (n = 77) have dyslipidemia and presents the following profile: 67.9% were male, mean age of 44.5 years, average time of HIV infection of 8, 3 years, average time of use of antiretroviral therapy for 6.9 years and body mass index of 24.5 kg/m². Regarding risk factors, it is observed that 18.2% are smokers, 40.3% alcoholics, 71.4% sedentary and 45.5% had hepatic steatosis. Regarding the classification of nutritional status (WHO, 1995) 58.4% are eutrophic, thin 6.5% and 35.1% overweight/obesity. Among the co morbidities studied, it appears that 24.7% and 21.1% are hypertensive and diabetics, respectively. When stratifying the lipodystrophy syndrome, according to the clinical manifestations, 35.1%, 10.4% and 54.5% of patients had lipoatrophy, hypertrophy and mixed syndrome, respectively. Concerning average serum lipid levels, there is high levels blood of cholesterol and triglycerides, low HDL-C, and LDL-C within the normal range. In regard to dyslipidemia classification (Sposito et al., 2007), have been observed that 48.7% of patients have mixed hyperlipidemia, 32.9% hypertriglyceridemia, low HDL-C 10.5% and 7.9% isolated hypercholesterolemia (Table 1 and 2). In the assessment of cardiovascular risk by Framingham Risk Score was found that more than 30% of the sample had medium and high cardiovascular risk.

Variables	Total Sample	n	%
Male		52	67.5
Female		25	32.5
Smoking	77	14	18.2
Alcoholism	77	31	40.3
Sedentary	77	55	71.4
Diabetes mellitus	77	17	21.1
SH *	77	19	24.7
Family history			
Diabetes	77	37	48.1
Hypertension	77	55	71.4
Dyslipidemia	72	28	38.9
Hepatic steatosis	66	30	45.5
Nutritional status**	76		
Thinness**		05	6.6
Eutrophic		44	57.9
Overweight/Obesity		27	35.5
Lipodystrophy	77		
Lipoatrophy		27	35.1
Hypertrophy		8	10.4
Mixed		42	54.5
Classification of dyslipidemia***	76		
Mixed Hyperlipidemia		37	48.7
Hypertriglyceridemia		25	32.9
Low HDL		8	10.5
Isolated hypercholesterolemia		6	7.9

Legend: SH - systemic hypertension; ** WHO, 1995; *** Sposito et al., 2007

Table 1. Patients profile with lipodystrophy and dyslipidemia accompanied by the Assistance Service of Metabolic Diseases Secondary to Antiretroviral Therapy, João de Barros Barreto University Hospital, Pará, Brazil.

Variable	Total Sample	Mean ± SD	Median
Age (years)	77	44.5 ± 9.6	45.0
ART Time (years)	77	6.9 ± 4.1	7.0
Time of HIV (years)	77	8.3 ± 5.4	8.0
BMI (kg/m²)	76	24.5 ± 4.2	23.9
Fasting glucose (mg/dL)	72	103.4 ± 27.7	98.5
Total Cholesterol (mg/dL)	76	218.9 ± 59.7	220.0
Triglycerides (mg/dL)	76	373.3± 393.8	280.5
HDL-c (mg/dL)	60	40.8 ± 13.34	39
Male HDL-c	36	37.4 ± 11.7	37.0
Female HDL-c	24	46.0 ±14.2	46.5
LDL-c (mg/dL)	58	115.6 ± 45.4	117.9

Legend: ART – Antiretroviral Therapy, BMI – body mass index, SD standard deviation.

Table 2. Distribution of mean and median values of some variables in patients with lipodystrophy and dyslipidemia accompanied by the Assistance Service of Metabolic Diseases Secondary to Antiretroviral Therapy, João de Barros Barreto University Hospital, Pará, Brazil.

The ambulatory care authors conducted an intervention study with outpatient HIV-positive with lipodystrophy syndrome, in use of HAART in the period October 2006 to December 2007. Patients were evaluated every quarter for four visits. This study followed all the guidelines contained in Resolution 196/1996 of the National Committee for Ethics in Research (CONEP), being approved by the Ethics in Human Research of the Center for Tropical Medicine, Federal University of Para, according to opinion of approval No. 058/2006, to date of October 19, 2006. The sample consisted of patients with positive serology for HIV, use of HAART for at least 12 months, with clinical diagnosis of lipodystrophy. We selected only adult patients, aged 20 to 60 years, of both sexes. All were invited and agreed to participate by reading and signing the Free and Informed Consent Term - FICT.

We excluded all patients with mental illness, malignant tumors, and chronic users of glucocorticoids, Diabetes Mellitus and dyslipidemia diagnosed before starting HAART and those who did not achieve at least three follow-up visits clinical and nutritional care at the Ambulatory care of Lipodystrophy HUJBB.

To collect data we used a treatment protocol for metabolic evaluation, nutritional counseling and patient outcomes, among several details registered there were: patient identification, socio-economic, personal and family morbidity history, time of HIV diagnosis, time of HAART treatment, clinical history and biochemical tests. Among the lipodystrophy syndrome metabolic changes were required tests to total serum cholesterol, LDL-C, HDL-C and triglycerides for dyslipidemia analysis (Sposito et al., 2007).

We studied 29 patients, 17 (59%) and 12 (41%), male and females, respectively, with an average age of 46.07 (± 9.04) years. In males, the average age was 47.59 (± 7.66) years, median 46 years, whereas in females the mean age was 43.92 (± 10.67) years, median 44. The most prevalent age group for both sexes was 41 to 50 years.

In regarding to lipodystrophy syndrome classification, was observed that 11 (37.91%), 2 (6,9%) and 16 (55,17%) patients demonstrated lipoatrophy, lipohypertrophy and mixed syndrome, respectively. There is no sex association with lipoatrophy and mixed syndrome (p= 0.4138, OR= 0.3750, IC 95%= 0.0744 – 1.8891), whilst lipohypertrophy syndrome had predominance in females. It is assumed when calculating Odds Ratio to lipohypertrophy presence, was noted that female chance present lipohypertrophy is 2.66 times more, However, the results have not been significant (p=0.4130, IC 95% 0.5294 a 13.4334), data shown in Figure 2.

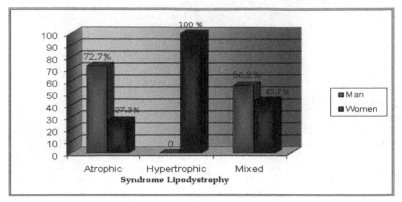

Fig. 2. Distribution of the lipodystrophy syndrome in relation to sex, Pará, Brazil 2006-2008.

The HAART temporal analysis showed that there was a growing evolution of lipoatrophy and lipohypertrophy presence in association with prolonged use of HAART (p = 0.0485, p = 0.0393, respectively).

Among the 29 patients, 6 were taking hypolipidemic. The lipid profile found in patient's evaluation, including those who had made use hypolipidemic therapy, was no statistically significant changes on the total cholesterol and LDL-C, however, for the HDL-C and triglycerides had significant differences between the first and last clinical follow-up nutritional (Figure 3).

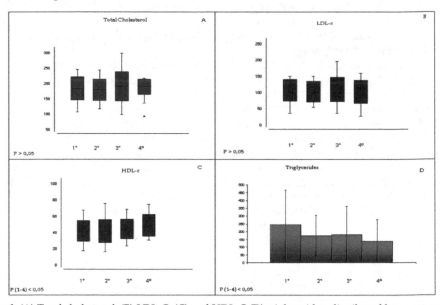

Legend: (A) Total cholesterol, (B) LDL-C, (C) and HDL-C (D) triglycerides, distributed by quarters. Dependent t-test for paired samples.

Fig. 3. HIV patients Serum lipids who did not use hypolipidemic, distributed by quarters, 2006-2008 Para-Brazil.

When analyzing only the sample of patients who were taking hypolipidemic (n = 7), there was no statistically significant changes in the levels of serum total cholesterol, LDL-C and triglycerides (Table 3).

Biochemical Tests	1°	2°	3°	4°	p value*
Cholesterol Total	207.7 (±40.2)	264.0 (±128.2)	216.7 (± 69.2)	219.3 (±60.9)	0.6626
LDL cholesterol	91.7 (±45.6)	136.6 (±56.3)	108.8 (±29.6)	89.7 (±46.04)	0.2539
Triglycerides	597.0 (±300.1)	996.0 (±1300.0)	488.3 (±637.6)	415.0 (±209.3)	0.0503

* Legend: *Friedman* test.

Table 3. Comparison of mean only of lipid profile of patients who were taking hypolipidemic therapy for the clinical follow-up of four nutritional consultations, Pará, Brazil 2006-2008.

In assessing relation between lipids and lipodystrophy syndrome, there was no significant association, as sample data in Table 4.

Lipodystrophy Syndrome				
	Lipoatrophy N (%)	Lipohypertrophy N (%)	Mixed N (%)	p value
Total Cholesterol				
Normal levels	3 (27.27)	0 (0.00)	7 (43.75)	0.3840
Abnormal levels	8 (72.73)	2 (100.00)	9 (56.25)	
LDL cholesterol				
Normal levels	9 (81.82)	1 (50.00)	14 (87.50)	0.4141
Abnormal levels	2 (18.18)	1 (50.00)	2 (12.50)	
HDL cholesterol				
Normal levels	1 (9.09)	0 (0.00)	5 (31.25)	0.2849
Abnormal levels	10 (90.91)	2 (100.00)	11 (68.75)	
Triglycerides				
Normal levels	3 (27.27)	1 (50.00)	5 (31.25)	0.3023
Abnormal levels	8 (72.73)	1 (50.00)	11 (68.75)	

Legend: N - number of patients. Test: Partitioning Chi-square.

Table 4. Association between lipid profile and lipodystrophy syndrome, Pará, Brazil 2006-2008.

In assessing comparison of mean of lipid profile of all patients before and after the clinical and nutritional intervention (first and fourth visit), there was a significant difference between the levels of total cholesterol, LDL-C, HDL-C and triglycerides between the lipoatrophy and mixed syndrome (p> 0.05) (Table 5). No analysis was performed on the lipohypertrophy syndrome due to be there of only two patients.

	Before			After		
	Lipoatrophy	Mixed	p-value	Lipoatrophy	Mixed	p-value
Total cholesterol	196.91 (±35.05)	183.00 (±41.84)	0.3744	198.14 (± 39.26)	185.58 (±45.97)	0.5538
LDL cholesterol	112.42 (±40.61)	94.54 (±34.67)	0.2308	110.37 (±50.44)	86.33 (±32.10)	0.2313
HDL cholesterol	37.91 (±11.65)	40.28 (±15.92)	0.6809	42.14 (±9.25)	44.92 (±14.64)	0.4504
Triglycerides	299.36 (±27.77)	310.75 (±259.21)	0.9133	220.86 (±193.46)	218.90 (±179.92)	0.9829

Table 5. Comparison of mean of lipid profile of all patients, including who were taking hypolipidemic therapy before and after the intervention in lipodystrophy syndrome, Pará, Brazil 2006-2008.

The manifestation of lipodystrophy syndrome with regard to gender did not present significant differences for lipoatrophy or mixed syndrome. However, the syndrome was related to female lipohypertrophy corroborating other studies (Galli et al., 2002; Heath et al., 2002) and disagreeing with most published data has been shown increased risk of lipoatrophy syndrome among women. Tien et al. (2003) in prospective study of lipodystrophy syndrome risk among HIV-infected women and non-infected observed a risk 2,1 times more of develop lipoatrophy in infected women with virus than non-infected, whereas it did not differ lipohypertrophy syndrome between the two groups and the most prevalent de form lipodystrophy was mixed syndrome (81%). Van Griensven et al. (2007) evaluated the lipodystrophy syndrome prevalence among patients using stavudine in antiretroviral therapy and found lipoatrophy syndrome prevalence in 9.8% of patients on stavudine and 4.9% with lipohypertrophy syndrome. The HAART temporal analysis showed that there was a growing evolution of the appearance of lipoatrophy and lipohypertrophy associated with HAART prolonged use, as demonstrated by studies of Lichtenstein et al. (2005) and Goujard et al. (2003).

As regards the evaluation of metabolic changes associated with use of HAART coupled with the treatment of nutritional guidance, it must be pointed out that some factors may have affected the outcome of this work as the low adherence to medical treatment, nutrition, failure to follow the previous recommendations for achieving of biochemical tests and the small sample size of patients available for this study. This difficulty in adhering to medical treatment and/or diet therapy was also found by other authors (Quintaes & Garcia, 1999; Ceccato et al. 2004; Parenti et al., 2005; Barros et al. 2007; Chencinski & Garcia, 2006). The reluctance of patients to nutritional treatment may be related to low purchasing power (Barros et al., 2007), cultural and dietary habits proper to the Amazon region, who abuse food that are rich in lipids. In addition to psychosocial factors of patients, where the prejudice, social isolation and emotional disorders such as anxiety and depression commonly observed in patients infected with HIV make it difficult to change lifestyle (personal and food) as suggested by Quintaes & Garcia (1999) Chencinski & Garcia (2006). There was also that patients profile evaluated before intervention reflected increase in serum total cholesterol and triglycerides, and lowering HDL-C as described in the literature (Caar et al. 1998; Hadigan et al. 2006; Having Hofstede et al., 2003; Abreu et al., 2006), disagreeing with main studies analyzed only about LDL-C, where most patients remained within normal range. Lipid disorders and association with lipodystrophy syndrome were common in all patients, especially in mixed syndrome, according to studies by Thiebaut et al. (2000) and Haugaard et al. (2005).

The lipid abnormalities evolution in patients after clinical and nutritional intervention during study noted significant changes of lowering triglycerides and increase in HDL-C, regardless of hypolipidemic use. The increased levels of HDL-C have been associated with decreased cardiovascular risk, as has been discussed in the work of Manninen et al. (1988). Where was reported that for every 1% increase in HDL-C was 3% reduction in coronary events and Pedersen et al. (1998) who said that for each 1% increase in HDL-C there was 1% reduction in coronary events, both independently of changes in LDL-C levels.

The lipid profile of patients before and after nutritional intervention clinically observed that patients who had shown serum levels of triglycerides, total cholesterol and fractions (LDL-C and HDL-C) normal at first, had increasing them at the end of treatment. These patients had borderline values facilitating risk of increased total cholesterol, LDL-C and triglycerides and decreased HDL-C associated with nutrition acceptance less than 75%. Other patients in the first consultation showed values above the reference levels for total cholesterol, LDL-C and triglycerides as well as lowering HDL-C, reaching normal values due to good acceptance to nutritional care. The remaining patients showed levels of total cholesterol, LDL-C fractions, HDL-C and triglycerides changed during the research; probably was not able to perceive the importance of nutritional treatment. There were also cases of patients who had their lipid profile within the normal range, suggesting that not only the use of HAART interfered with these metabolic changes, but also other factors may be implicated as genetic predisposition.

In regarding to lipodystrophy syndrome, the cholesterol and LDL-C means demonstrated it more significant in lipoatrophy than mixed syndrome compared before and after intervention. Triglyceride levels showed independent growing in despite to lipodystrophy syndrome, while HDL-C showed changed levels in mixed syndrome.

The physiopathology by which HAART determines HIV lipodystrophy syndrome, dyslipidemia therefore remains unknown. Second Andrade & Hutz (2002), the lipid serum levels are multifactorial characteristics, determinate by genetic and environmental factors, highlighting the genetic variability found in those genes that can affect the response to drugs used in hyperlipidemia treatment.

The authors of the lipodystrophy ambulatory care are developing a research paper about a case-control study conducted from December 2009 to July 2012. For data collection is being performed a clinical, epidemiological and nutritional evaluation where are registered information about patient identification, socio-economic conditions, personal and family history of morbidity, time of HIV diagnosis, HAART treatment duration, medication used - HAART, viral load, CD4 counts, clinical history, biochemical tests for dyslipidemia classification, anthropometric analysis and, APOAI and APOAV apolipoprotein polymorphism evaluation. This study aims to investigate these polymorphisms in an attempt to discover the main causes responsible for this metabolic disorder, the dyslipidemia.

6. Conclusion

The HAART has as one of its major collateral effect the lipodystrophy syndrome. There is necessity of more studies to deep into physiopathology of this syndrome; and metabolic and cardiovascular complications secondary to HAART. Dyslipidemia stands out as one of the most prevalent metabolic changes in patients with HIV, what makes it essential to feasibility of research in therapeutic care to clarifying of the clinical management. It is noted that nutritional guideline and/or hypolipidemic use, when have there been acceptance to treatment, takes place improvements of the lipid profile, can also there be normalization of those levels, in particular of the triglyceride levels. However, the adherence neither always takes place, what difficult the management of those patients.

7. References

Abreu, L., Escosteguy, C., Sodré, C., Godomiczer, A., Passoni, L., & Menezes, J. (2006). Tratamento anti-retroviral e hipercolesterolemia em população HIV positiva. *Revista da Sociedade de Cardiologia do Estado do Rio de Janeiro*, Vol. 19, No. 3, (Mai-Jun 2006), pp. (219-24), ISSN 2177-6024.

Almeida, L., Giudici, K., & Jaime, P. (2009). Consumo alimentar e dislipidemia decorrente da terapia antirretroviral combinada para infecção pelo HIV: uma revisão sistemática. *Arquivos Brasileiros de Endocrinologia & Metabologia*, Vol. 53, No. 5, (Jul 2009), pp. (519-527), ISSN 0004-2730.

American Heart Association. (2002). Third Report of the National Cholesterol Education Program (NCEP) Expert Panel on Detection, Evaluation, and Treatment of High Blood Cholesterol in Adults (Adult Treatment Panel III) Final Report. *Circulation*, Vol. 106, No. 25, (Dec 2002), pp. (3143-3421), ISSN 0009-7322.

Andrade, F., & Hutz, M. (2002). O componente genético da determinação dos lipídeos séricos. *Ciência & Saúde Coletiva*, Vol. 7, No. 1, (2002), pp. (175-182), ISSN 1413-8123.

Aouizerat, B., Kulkarni, M., Heilbron, D., Drown, D., Raskin, S., Pullinger, C., Malloy, M., & Kane, J. (2003). Genetic analysis of a polymorphism in the human apoA-V gene: effect on plasma lipids. *Journal of Lipid Research*, Vol. 44, No. 6, (Jun 2003), pp. (1167–1173), ISSN 1539-7262.

Assmann, G., Schmitz, G., Funke, H., & von Eckardstein, A. (1990) Apolipoprotein A-I and HDL deficiency. *Current Opinion in Lipidology*, Vol. 1, No. 1, (1990), pp. (110-115), ISSN: 0957-9672.

Baldini F, Di Giambenedetto S, Cingolani A, Murri R, Ammassari A, De Luca A (2000). Efficacy and tolerability of pravastatin for the treatment of HIV-1 protease inhibitor–associated hyperlipidaemia: a pilot study. *AIDS*, Vol. 14, No 11, (Jul 2000), pp. (1660–1662), ISSN: 0269-937.

Barros, E., Araujo, A., Freitas, M., & Liberato, E. (2007). Influencia da alimentação na lipodistrofia em portadores de HIV-Aids praticantes de atividade física regular. *Revista Brasileira de Prescrição e Fisiologia do Exercício*, Vol. 1, No. 2, (Mar-Abr 2007), pp. (13-18), ISSN 1981-9900.

Boccara, F., Auclair, M., Cohen, A., Lefèvre, C., Prot, M., Bastard, J.P., Capeau, J., & Caron-Debarle, M. (2010). HIV protease inhibitors activate the adipocyte renin angiotensin system. *Antiviral Therapy*, Vol. 15, No. 3, (2010), pp. (363-375).

Blanco Vaca, F., Ordóñez Llanos, J., Pérez Pérez, a., Sánchez Quesada, j. L., & Wägner Fahlin A. (2000). Lípidos, lipoproteínas y apolipoproteínas. Nuevas indicaciones en el diagnóstico, evaluación y prevención del riesgo cardiovascular. Roche Diagnóstica. S. L. In: Diaz, J. I.S. (2007). Guia practica. Marcadores Bioquimicos Cardiacos. Prologo, indice y presentacion. Acesso em 20 jun 2011. Disponível em: http://www.portalesmedicos.com/publicaciones/articles/828/2/Marcadores-cardiacos.-Factores-de-riesgo-cardiaco-en-la-aterosclerosis.-Recopilacion-de-datos-de-revisiones-bibliograficas-y-conclusiones

Caar, A., Sâmaras, K., Burton, S., Law, M., Freund, J., Chisholm, D., & Cooper, D. (1998). A syndrome of peripheral lipodystrophy, hyperlipidaemia and insulin resistance in patients receiving HIV protease inhibitors. AIDS, Vol. 12, No. 7, (Mai 1998), pp.51-58, ISSN: 0269-937.

Cahn, P., Leite, O., Rosales, A., Cabello, R., Alvarez, C., Seas, C., Carcamo, C., Cure-Bolt, N., L'Italien, G., Masntilla, P., Deibis, L., Zala, C., & Suffert, T. (2010). Metabolic profile and cardiovascular risk factors among Latin American HIV-infected patients receiving HAART . Brazilian Journal of Infectious Diseases, Vol. 14, No. 2, (Mar-Abr 2010), pp. (158-166), ISSN 1413-8670.

Carr, A., & Cooper, D. (2000). Adverse effects of antiretroviral therapy. The Lancet, Vol.356, No. 9232, (Oct 2000), pp. (1423-1430), INSS 0140-6736.

Ceccato, M., Acurcio, F., Bonolo, P., Rocha, G., & Guimarães, M. (2004). Compreensão de informações relativas ao tratamento anti-retroviral entre indivíduos infectados pelo HIV. Caderno de Saúde Pública, Vol. 20, No. 5, (Set-Out 2004), pp. (1388-1397), ISSN 0102-311X.

Chen, D., Misra, A., & Garg, A. (2002). Lipodystrophy in Human Immunodeficiency Virus-Infected Patients. The Journal of Clinical Endocrinology & Metabolism, Vol. 87, No. 11, (Nov 2002), pp. (4845-4856).

Chencinski, J., & Garcia, V. (Abr-Jun 2006). Dislipidemia em pacientes HIV/AIDS. In: Conselho Regional de Nutrição-3 Notícias. n.82, Acesso em 10 Mar 2008. Disponível em: <http://www.crn3.org.br/atualidades/revistas/arquivos/edicao_082_atualidades.pdf>.

Coté, H. (2007). Mechanisms of antiretroviral therapy-induced mitochondrial dysfunction. Current Opinion in HIV and AIDS, Vol. 2, No. 4, (Jul 2007), pp. (253-260), ISSN 1746-630X.

Diehl, L., Dias, J., Paes, A., Thomazini, M., Garcia, L., Cinagawa, E., Wiechmann, S., & Carrilho, A. (2008). Prevalência da Lipodistrofia Associada ao HIV em Pacientes Ambulatoriais Brasileiros: Relação com Síndrome Metabólica e Fatores de Risco Cardiovascular. Arquivos Brasileiros de Endocrinologia e Metabologia, Vol. 52, No. 4, (Jun 2008), pp. (658-667), ISSN 0004-2730.

Dubé, M., Stein, J., Aberg, J., Fichtenbaum, C., Gerber, J., Tashima, K., Henry, W., Currier, J., Sprecher, D., & Glesby, M. (2003). Guidelines for the evaluation and management of dyslipidemia in human immunodeficiency virus (HIV)-infected adults receiving antiretroviral therapy: Recommendations of the HIV Medicine Association of the Infectious Disease Society of America and the Adult AIDS Clinical Trials Group. Clinical Infectious Diseases, Vol. 37, No. 5, (Sep 2003), pp. (613-627), ISSN 378131.

Dutra, C. & Libonati, R. (2008). Perfil metabólico e nutricional de pacientes HIV positivos com lipodistrofia submetidos à terapia anti-retroviral: Orientação Nutricional. Dissertação de mestrado. Universidade Federal do Pará. Belém-Brazil. (Abr 2008), 151pp.

Eichenbaum-Voline S., Olivier, M., Jones, E., Naoumova, R., Jones, B., Gau, B., Patel, H., Seed, M., Betteridge, D., Galton, D., Rubin, E., Scott, J., Shoulders, C., & Pennacchio, L. (2004). Linkage and association between distinct variants of the APOAI/C3/A4/A5 gene cluster and familial combined hyperlipidemia. *Arteriosclerosis, Thrombosis and Vascular Biology*, Vol. 24, No. 1, (Jan 2004), pp. (167-174), ISSN 10795642.

Friis-M øller, N., Reiss, P., Sabin, C. A., Weber, R., Monforte, A., El-Sadr, W.,Thiebaut, R., De Wit, S., Kirk, O., Fontas, E., Law, M. G., Phillips, A., & Lundgren, J. D. (Mai 2003). Cardiovascular disease risk factors in HIV patients - association with antiretroviral therapy. In: *Official Journal of International AIDS Society*, Acesso em 06 Jun 2011, Disponível em: <http://discovery.ucl.ac.uk/6830/1/6830.pdf>

Friis-Møller, N; Weber, R., Reiss, P; Thiébaut, R., Kirk, O., Monforte, A., Pradier, C., Morfeldt, L., Mateu, S., Law, M., El-Sadr, W., De Wit, S., Sabin, C., Phillips, A., Lundgren, J. (2003). Cardiovascular disease risk factors in HIV patients - association with antiretroviral therapy. Results from the DAD study. *AIDS*, Vol 17, No 8,(May 2003), pp. (1179-1193), ISSN: 0269-937.

Furtado, J., Zambrini, H., Neto, D., Scozzafave, G., & Brasileiro, R. (2007). Ambulatório de Lipodistrofia do Hospital Heliópolis - Uma experiência com as correções cirúrgicas em dois anos de atendimento. *Prática hospitalar*, Vol. 58, No. 28, (Set-Out IX), pp. (28-32), ISSN 1679-5512.

Galli, M., Cozzi-Lepri, A., Ridolfo, A., Gervasoni, C., Ravasio, L., Corsico, L., Gianelli, E., Vaccarezza, M., Vullo, V., Cargnel, A., Minoli, L., Coronado, O., Giacometti, A., Antinori, A., Antonucci, G., D'Arminio Monforte, A., & Moroni, M. (2002). Incidence of adipose tissue alterations in first-line antiretroviral therapy: the LipolCoNa Study. *Archives of Internal Medicine*, Vol. 22, No. 162, (Dez 2002), pp. (2621-2628), ISSN 00039926.

Garg, A. (2000). Lipodystrophies. *The American Journal of Medicine*, Vol. 108, No. 2, (Feb 2000), pp. (143-152), ISSN: 0002-9343.

Gidding, S. S. Preventive pediatric cardiology(1999). *The Pediatric Clinics North America*. Vol. 46, No 2 (abr. 1999), pp. (253-262), ISSN:0031-3955.

Gkrania-Klotsas, E., & Klotsas, A. (2007). HIV and HIV treatment: effects on fats, glucose and lipids. *British Medical Bulletin*, Vol. 84, No. 1, (Nov 2007), pp. (49-68), ISSN 0007-1420.

Goujard, C., Vincent, I., Meynard, J., Choudet, N., Bollens, D., Rousseau, C., Demarles, D., Gillotin, C., Bidault, R., & Taburet, A. (2003). Steady-state pharmacokinetics of amprenavir coadministered with ritonavir in human immunodeficiency virus type 1-infected patients. *Antimicrobial agents and chemotherapy*, Vol. 47, No. 1, (Jan 2003), pp. (118-123), ISSN 0066-4804.

Grinspoon, S., & Carr, A. (2005) Cardiovascular Risk and Body-Fat Abnormalities in HIV-Infected Adults. *New England Journal of Medicine*, Vol. 352, No. 1, (Jan 2005), pp. (48-62), ISSN 0028-4793.

Grunfeld, C., Pang, M., Doerrler, W., Shigenaga, J., Jensen, P., & Feingold, K. (1992). Lipids, lipoproteins, triglyceride clearance, and cytokines in human immunodeficiency virus infection and the acquired immunodeficiency syndrome. *Journal of Clinical Endocrinology & Metabolism*, Vol. 74, No. 5, (May 1992), pp. (1045-1052), ISSN 0021-972X.

Hadigan, C., Kamin, D., Liebau, J., Mazza, S., Barrow, S., Torriani, M., Rubin, R., Weise, S., Fischman, A., & Grinspoon, S. (2006). Depot-specific regulation of glucose uptake and insulin sensitivy in HIV-lipodystrophy. *American Journal of Physiology, Endocrinology & Metabolism*, Vol. 2, No. 290, (Feb 2006), pp. 289-298, ISSN 0193-1849.

Haugaard, S., Andersen, O., Dela, F., Holst, J., Storgaard, H., Fenger, M., Iversen, J., & Madsbad, S. (2005). Defective glucose and lipid metabolism in human immunodeficiency virus-infected patients with lipodystrophy involve liver, muscle tissue and pancreatic beta-cells. *European Journal of Endocrinology*, Vol. 152, No. 1, (Jan 2005), pp. (103-112), ISSN 0804-4643.

Heath, K., Chan, K., Singer, J., O'shaughnessy, M., Montaner, J., & Hoogg, R. (2002). Incidence of morphological and lipid abnormalities: gender and treatment differentials after initiation of first antiretroviral therapy. *International Journal of Epidemiology*, Vol. 31, No. 5, (Oct 2002), pp.1016-1020, ISSN *0300-5771*.

Henry K, Melroe H, Huebesch J, Hermundson J, Simpson J. Atorvastatin and gemfibrozil for protease-inhibitor–related lipid abnormalities (1998). *Lancet.* Vol. 352, No 9133(Sep. 1998), pp. (1031–1032), ISSN 0140-6736.

Jones SP, Doran DA, Leatt PB, Maher B, Pirmohamed M (2001). Short-term exercise training improves body composition and hyperlipidaemia in HIV-positive individuals with lipodystrophy . *AIDS* . Vol. 15, No 15, pp. (2049–2051), , ISSN: 0269-937.

Kotler D. (2008). HIV and Antiretroviral Therapy: Lipid Abnormalities and Associated Cardiovascular Risk in HIV-Infected Patients. *Journal of Acquires Immune Deficiency Syndromes*, Vol. 53, No. 3, (Sep 2008), pp. (79-85), ISSN *1525-4135*.

Kramer, A., Lazzarotto, A., Sprinz, E., & Manfroi, W. (2009). Alterações metabólicas, terapia antirretroviral e doença cardiovascular em idosos portadores de HIV. *Arquivos Brasileiros de Cardiologia*, Vol. 93, No. 5, (Nov 2009), pp. (561-568), ISSN 0066-782X.

Liang, J., Distler, O., Cooper, D., Jamil, H., Deckelbaum, R., Ginsberg, H., & Sturley, S. (2001). HIV protease inhibitors protect apolipoprotein B from degradation by the proteasome: a potential mechanism for protease inhibitor-induced hyperlipidemia. *Nature Medicine*, Vol.7, No. 12, (Dec 2001), pp. (1327-1331), ISSN 1078-8956.

Licht, C., Vreeburg, S., van Reedt Dortland, A., Giltay, E., Hoogendijk, W., DeRijk, R., Vogelzangs, N., Zitman, F., de Geus, E., & Penninx, B. (2010) Increased sympathetic and decreased parasympathetic activity rather than changes in hypothalamic-pituitary-adrenal axis activity is associated with metabolic abnormalities *Journal of Clinical Endocrinology & Metabolism*, Vol. 95, No. 5, (May 2010), pp. (2458-2466), ISSN 0021-972X.

Lichtenstein, K. (2005) Redefining Lipodistrophy Syndrome: Risks and Impact on Clinical Decision Making. *Journal of Acquired Immune Deficiency Syndromes*, Vol. 39, No. 4, (Aug 2005), pp. (395-400), ISSN *1525-4135*.

Lihn, A., Richelsen, B., Pedersen, S., Haugaard, S., Rathje, G., Madsbad, S., & Andersen, O. (2003) Increased expression of TNF-α, IL-6, and IL-8 in HALS: implications for reduced adiponectin expression and plasma levels. *American Journal of Physiology Endocrinology & Metabology*, Vol. 285, No. 5, (Nov 2003), pp. (1072-1080), ISSN 0193-1849.

Maagaard, A., & Kvale, D. (2009). Mitochondrial toxicity in HIV-infected patients both off and on antiretroviral treatment: a continuum or distinct underlying mechanisms? *Journal of Antimicrobial Chemistry*, Vol. 64, No. 5, (Sep 2009), pp. (901-909), ISSN 0929-8673.

Mallewa, J., Wilkins, E., Vilar, J., Mallewa, M., Doran, D., Back, D., & Pirmohamed, M. (2008) HIV-associated lipodystrophy: a review of underlying mechanisms and therapeutic options. *The Journal of Antimicrobial Chemotherapy*, Vol. 62, No. 4, (Oct 2008), pp. (648-660), ISSN 0305-7453.

Mallon, P., Miller, J., Cooper, D., & Carr, A. (2003). Prospective evaluation of the effects of antiretroviral therapy on body composition in HIV-1-infected men starting therapy. *AIDS*, Vol. 17, No. 7, (May 2003), pp. (971–979), ISSN 0269-9370.

Manninen, V., Elo, M., Frick, M., Haapa, K., Heinonen, O., Heinsalmi, P., Helo, P., Huttunen, J., Kaitaniemi, P., & Koskinen, P. (1988). Lipid alterations and decline in the incidence of coronary heart disease in the Helsinki Heart Study, *The Journal of the American Medical Association*, Vol. 260, No. 1, (1988), pp. (641-651), ISSN 00987484.

Marshall, H., Morrison, L., Wu, L., Anderson, J., Corneli, P., Stauffer, D., Allen, A., Karagounis, L., & Ward, R. (1994). Apolipoprotein polymorphism fail to define risk of coronary artery disease. Results of a prospective, angiographically controlled study. *Circulation*, Vol. 89, No. 2, (Feb 1994), pp. (567-577), ISSN 0009-7322.

Mello, A., Reis, E., & Ribeiro, R. (2008). Lipodistrofia no uso da Terapia Antiretroviral com Inibidores da Protease no HIV. *Saúde & Ambiente em Revista*, Vol. 3, No. 1, (Jan-jun 2008), pp. (66-75), ISSN 1980-2676.

Miller J, Brown D, Amin J, et al (2002). A randomized, double-blind study of gemfibrozil for the treatment of protease inhibitor–associated hypertriglyceridaemia. *AIDS*. Vol 16, No 16 (Nov. 2002), pp. (2195–2200), ISSN: 0269-937.

Ministério da Saúde do Brasil. (2008). Recomendações para terapia anti-retroviral em adultos infectados pelo HIV: manual de bolso. In: *Série A. Normas e Manuais Técnicos*, Data de acesso: Jun 2011, Disponível em: http://www.crt.saude.sp.gov.br/resources/crt_aids/arquivos_transmissao_vertic al/transmissao_vertical_hiv/portarias_manuais_recomendacoes_outros/consenso _adulto_2008.pdf>.

Moyle GJ, Lloyd M, Reynolds B, Baldwin C, Mandalia S, Gazzard BG (2001). Dietary advice with or without pravastatin for the management of hypercholesterolemia associated with protease inhibitor therapy. *AIDS*. Vol. 15, No 12 (Aug 2001), pp. (503–508), , ISSN: 0269-937.

Mooser, V. & Carr, A. (2001). Antiretroviral therapy-associated hyperlipidaemia in HIV disease. *Current Opinion in Lipidology.*, Vol. 12, No. 3, (Jun 2001), pp. 313-319, ISSN 0957-9672.

Mulligan, K. (2003). Metabolic Abnormalities in Patient with HIV Infection. *Journal of the International Association of Physicians in Aids Care (Chicago)*, Vol. 2, No. 2, (Apr-Jun 2003), pp. (66-74), ISSN 1545-1097.

Noor, M. (2007). The role of protease inhibitors in the pathogenesis of HIV-associated insulin resistance: cellular mechanisms and clinical implications. *Current HIV/AIDS Reports*, Vol.4, No. 3, (Dec 2007), pp. 126-134, ISSN 1548-3568.

Palacios R, Santos J, Gonzalez M, et AL (2002). Efficacy and safety of atorvastatin in the treatment of hypercholesterolemia associated with antiretroviral therapy. *Journal of Acquired Immune Deficiency Syndromes*. Vol. 30, No 5 (Aug. 2002), pp. (536–537), ISSN 1525-4135.

Parenti, C., Pereira, L., Brandão, Z., & Silvério, A. (2005). Perfil dos pacientes com AIDS acompanhados pelo Serviço de Assistência Domiciliar Terapêutica do Município de Contagem, Estado de Minas Gerais, Brasil, 2000-2003. *Epidemiologia e Serviços de Saúde*, Vol. 14, No. 2, (Jun 2005), pp. (91-96), ISSN 1679- 4974.

Pedersen, T., Olsson, A., Faergeman, O., Kjekshus, J., Wedel, H., Berg, K., Wilhelmsen, L., Haghfelt, T., Thorgeirsson, G., Pyörälä, K., Miettinen, T., Christophersen, B., Tobert, J., Musliner, T., & Cook, T. (1998). Lipoprotein changes and reduction in the incidence of coronary heart disease events in the Scandinavian Simvastatin Survival Study (4S). *Circulation*, Vol. 97, No. (1), (1998), pp. (1453-1461), ISSN 0009-7322.

Quintaes, D., & Garcia, R. (1999). Adesão de pacientes HIV positivos à dietoterapia ambulatorial. *Revista de Nutrição*, Vol. 12, No. 2, (Mai-Ago 1999), pp. (175-181).

Rasmusson, A., Schnurr, P., Zukowska, Z., Scioli, E., & Forman, D. (2010). Adaptation to extreme stress: post-traumatic stress disorder, neuropeptide Y and metabolic syndrome. *Experimental Biology and Medicina (Maywood)*, Vol. 235, No. 10, (Oct 2010), pp. (1150-1162), ISSN 1535-3702.

Riddle, M., Kuhel, D., Woollett, L., Fichtenbaum, C., & Hui, D. (2001). HIV protease inhibitor induces fatty acid and sterol biosynthesis in liver and adipose tissues due to the accumulation of activated sterol regulatory element-binding proteins in the nucleus. *Journal of Biological Chemistry*, Vol. 276, No. 40, (Oct 2001), pp. 37514-37519, ISSN 0021-9258.

Samaras, K., Wand, H., Law, M., Emery, S., Cooper, D., & Carr, A. (2009). Dietary intake in HIV-infected men with lipodystrophy: relationships with body composition, visceral fat, lipid, glucose and adipokine metabolism. *Current HIV Research*, Vol. 7, No. 4, (Jul 2009), pp. (454-461), ISSN 1570-162X.

Santos, C., Felipe, Y., Braga, P., Ramos, D., Lima, R., & Segurado, A. (2005). Self-perception of body changes in persons living with HIV/AIDS: prevalence and associated factors. AIDS, Vol. 4, No. 1, (Oct 2005), pp. (14-21), , ISSN: 0269-937, ISSN: 0269-937.

Sattler, F. (2008). Pathogenesis and Treatment of Lipodystrophy: What Clinicians Need To Know. *Topics in HIV Medicine*, Vol. 16, No. 4, (Oct-Nov 2008), pp. (127-133), ISSN 1542-8826.

Segarra-Newnham, M. (2002). Hyperlipidemia in HIV-positive patients receiving antiretrovirals. *The Annals of Pharmacotherapy*, Vol. 36, No. 4, (Apr 2002), pp. (592-595), ISSN 1060-0280.

Seidl, E., & Machado, A. (2008). Bem-estar psicológico, enfrentamento e lipodistrofia em pessoas vivendo com HIV/aids. *Psicologia em estudo*, Vol. 13, No. 2, (Apr-Jun 2008), pp. (239-247), ISSN 1413-7372.

Shahmanesh, M., Jaleel, H., DeSilva, Y., Ross, J., Caslake, M. & Cramb, R. (Jun 2001) Protease inhibitor related type III hyperlipoproteinaemia is common and not associated with apolipoprotein-E E2/E2 phenotype. In: *Sexually Transmitted Infections,* Acesso em 04 Jun 2011, Disponível em: < http://sti.bmj.com/content/77/4/283.abstract>

Smith P, DiCenzo R, Morse G (2001). Clinical pharmacokinetics of nonnucleosidereverse transcriptase inhibitors. *Clinical Pharmacokinetics*, Vol. 40, No 12, (2001), pp. (893–905), ISSN 0312-5963.

Sposito, A., Caramelli, B., Fonseca, F., & Bertolami, M. (2007). IV Diretriz Brasileira sobre Dislipidemias e Prevenção da Aterosclerose: Departamento de Aterosclerose da Sociedade Brasileira de Cardiologia. *Arquivos Brasileiros de Cardiologia*, Vol. 88, No. 1, (Abr 2007), pp. (2-19), ISSN 1678-4170.

Sprinz, E., Lazzaretti, R., Kuhmmer, R., & Ribeiro, J. (2010). Dyslipidemia in HIV-infected individuals. *Brazilian Journal of Infectious Diseases*, Vol. 14, No. 6, (Nov 2010), pp. (575-588), ISSN 1413-8670.

Stankov, M., & Behrens, G. (2010) Contribution of Inflammation to Fat Redistribution and Metabolic Disturbances in HIV-1 Infected Patients. *Current Pharmaceutical Design*, Vol. 16, No. 30, (Out 2010), pp. (3361-3371), ISSN 1381-6128.

Tall, A. (1990) Plasma high density lipoproteins. Metabolism and relationship to atherogenesis. *The Journal of Clinical Investigation*, Vol. 86, No. 2, (Aug 1990), pp. (379-384), ISSN 00219738.

Ter Hofstede, H., Burger, D., & Koopmans, P. (2003). Antiretroviral therapy in HIV patients: aspects of metabolic complications and mitochondrial toxicity. *The Netherlands Journal of Medicine*, Vol. 61, No. 12, (Dec 2003), pp. (393-403), ISSN 0300-2977.

The HIV/Aids Treatment Information Service (ATIS). (Sep 2002). *Glossary of HIV/AIDS-Related Terms*, The HIV/Aids Treatment Information Service (ATIS), Retirado de <http://www.hiv.gov.gy/edocs/glossary.pdf>.

Thiébaut, R., Daucourt, V., Mercié, P., Ekouévi, D. K., Malvy, D., Morlat, P., Dupon, M., Neau, D., Farbos, S., Marimoutou, C., & Dabis, F. (2000). Lipodystrophy, metabolic disorders, and human immunodeficiency virus infection: Aquitaine cohort, France, 1999. Groupe d'Epidémiologie Clinique du Syndrome d'Immunodéficience Acquise en Aquitaine. *Clinical Infectious Diseases*. Vol. 31, No. 6 (Dec 2000), pp. (1482-7), ISSN 1058-4838.

Tien, P., Cole, S., Williams, C., Li, R., Justman, J., Cohen, M., Young, M., Rubin, N., Augenbraun, M., & Grunfeld, C. (2003). Incidence of lipoatrophy and lipohypertrophy in the women's interagency HIV study. *Journal of Acquired Immune Deficiency Syndromes*, Vol. 34, No. 5, (Dec 2003), pp. (461-466), ISSN 1077-9450.

Tovar, J., & Schering, D. (2006) Management of Dyslipidemia in Special Populations. *Journal of Pharmacy Practice*, Vol. 19, No. 2, (Apr 2006), pp. (63-78), ISSN 0897-1900.

Valente, A., & Valente, O. (2007). Síndrome Lipodistrófica do HIV: Um Novo Desafio para o Endocrinologista. *Arquivos Brasileiros de Endocrinologia e Metabologia*, Vol. 51, No. 1, (Fev 2007), pp. (3-4), ISSN 0004-2730.

Van Griensven, J., De Naeyer, L., Mushi, T., Ubarijoro, S., Gashumba, D., Gazielle, C., & Zachariah, R. (2007). High prevalence of lipoatrophy among patients on stavudine-containing first-line antiretroviral therapy regimens in Rwanda. *Transactions of the Royal Society of Tropical Medicine and Hygiene*, Vol. 101, No. 8, (Ago 2007), pp. (793-798), ISSN 0035-9203.

World Health Organization (CH), United Nations Programme on HIV/Aids - UNAIDS (CH). (2009). Aids epidemic update: November 2009, In: *WHO Library Cataloguing-in-Publication Data*, Date of access: Jun 2011, Available from: <http://data.unaids.org/pub/Report/2009/jc1700_epi_update_2009_en.pdf>.

World Health Organization. (1995). Physical Status: The Use and Interpretation of Antropometry. In: *WHO Technical Report Series 854*, Date of Access: May 2011, Available from: <http://whqlibdoc.who.int/trs/WHO_TRS_854.pdf>.

Yarasheski KE, Tebas P, Stanerson B, et al (2001). Resistance exercise training reduces hypertriglyceridemia in HIV-infected men treated with antiviral therapy. *Journal of Applied Physiology*; Vol. 90, No. 1 (april 2001),. pp. (133–138), ISSN 8750-7587.

Yu, P., Calderaro, D., Lima, E. & Caramelli, B. (2005). Terapia hipolipemiante em situações especiais – Síndrome de Imunodeficiência Adquirida. *Arquivos Brasileiros de Cardiologia*, Vol. 85, No. 5, (Oct 2005), pp. (58-61).

9

Lipids in the Pathogenesis of Benign Prostatic Hyperplasia: Emerging Connections

Ajit Vikram and Poduri Ramarao
Central University of Punjab
India

1. Introduction

Benign prostatic hyperplasia (BPH) is a common melody of the aging men characterized by noncancerous enlargement of the prostate gland and is often associated with lower urinary tract symptoms (LUTS) (Berry et al., 1984). Approximately, 60 percent of men aged over 50 years have histological evidence of BPH and, after the age of 70, the proportion increases to 80 percent (Berry et al., 1984). It is a chronic, progressive and highly prevalent disease, clinically manifests as LUTS, posing a socioeconomic burden to the patients (Saigal and Joyce, 2005). Recently, Stranne et al., reported that one-third of the Swedish male population aged over 50 years have LUTS, which is often associated with BPH (Stranne et al., 2009). BPH is rarely fatal, but affects the quality of life, and if left untreated, serious life-threatening complications may arise. Prostatic growth and development are governed by the genetic (Sanda et al., 1994), hormonal (Marker et al., 2003) and dietary factors (Bravi et al., 2006). Although, its etiology is not well understood, several theories have been proposed to explain the pathogenesis of BPH (Alberto et al., 2009; Bosch, 1991; Srinivasan et al., 1995). Augmented steroidal signaling and mesenchymal-epithelial interactions are required for the normal as well as pathological growth of the prostate gland (Marker et al., 2003). However, current literature indicates that apart from steroids, peptides and lipids are also playing a crucial role in the pathogenesis of BPH (Cai et al., 2001; Culig et al., 1996; Escobar et al., 2009; Kaplan-Lefko et al., 2008; Rahman et al., 2007; Rick et al., 2011; Story, 1995; Vikram and Jena, 2011a; Vikram et al., 2010c). Even if the effects of peptides and lipids on the growth of the gland is milder as compared to that of steroids, chronic change in their levels either due to dietary habit or genetic predispositions can significantly contribute to the initiation and/or progression of the disease over a period of time. Existing clinical/epidemiological and preclinical studies provide convincing evidence for the association between insulin-resistance, metabolic disorder and type 2 diabetes with the BPH (Francisco and Francois, 2010; Vikram et al., 2010a; Wang and Olumi, 2011). Previous experimental studies in our laboratory suggested that insulin-resistance associated secondary rise in the plasma insulin level plays a central role in the prostatic enlargement (Vikram and Jena, 2011b; Vikram et al., 2010a; b; 2011a; Vikram et al., 2010c; Vikram et al., 2011b). Other peptides such as insulin-like growth factor-I (IGF-I), IGF-I binding proteins (IGFBPs), growth hormone (GH), transforming growth factor-β (TGF-β) family proteins are reported to have important implications in the prostatic growth (Culig et al., 1996; Ikeda et al., 2000; Rick et al., 2011; Vikram et al., 2010c). However, information on the role of lipids in the prostatic growth is scarce and there is a need of further research in this area. Nevertheless, existing in-vitro, in-vivo and clinical/epidemiological studies suggests that apart from contributing to the development of insulin-resistance and secondary hyperinsulinemia, lipids has a direct role in the normal prostatic growth and pathogenesis of the BPH.

2. Role of lipids in transcriptional regulation

Lipids are conventionally known as an important constituent of the biological membranes and as a signaling molecule in the cytoplasm. The presence of lipids in the nucleus and identification of phosphotidylinositol (PtdIns)-4-kinse activity in the preparation that were enriched in nuclear membranes (Smith and Wells, 1983a; b), and identification of PtdIns-4-phosphate and PtdIns-4,5-bisphosphate that were differentially metabolized from lipids in the cytoplasm provided early evidence for the nuclear lipid signaling (Irvine, 2003). A recent study by Lee et al., explores the nuclear activities of lipids, showing that dilauroyl phosphotidlycholine controls transcriptional program through nuclear-receptor dependent pathway (Ingraham, 2011; Lee et al., 2011). The study was of particular interest as phosphotidylcholine reversed some of the consequences of high-fat diet feeding (Lee et al., 2011), which is known to promote the cellular proliferation, contractility and overall enlargement of the prostate in rodents (Vikram et al., 2010c). The nuclear signaling and transcriptional regulation by lipids implies that targeting nuclear lipid signaling might be of value in finding the answers for the diseases associated with dietary habit and sedentary lifestyle such as insulin-resistance, type 2 diabetes, several cancers and BPH.

3. Insulin-resistance and BPH

The main function of insulin includes regulation of glucose uptake, glycogenesis and tight control of the plasma glucose level (Vikram and Jena, 2010). Insulin-resistance is a condition in which normal level of insulin elicits subnormal response. It is a condition which is associated with a group of disorders such as obesity, dyslipidemia, elevated fasting glucose level, hyperinsulinemia and hypertension. In addition to the type 2 diabetes and cardiovascular diseases, patients with insulin-resistance syndrome are at higher risk of BPH (Kasturi et al., 2006). Possible implications of the diabetes, insulin-resistance and insulin-resistance associated disorders in the pathogenesis of BPH have been previously reviewed, and interested readers are encouraged to read the concerned articles for more information (Vikram et al., 2010a; Wang and Olumi, 2011).

4. Fatty acids, dietary fat and BPH

Strong appetite for the sugar, fat, and salt might have been adaptive for our ancestors, as they had very little access to sweet, fatty and salty foods. We have inherited these appetites and have easy access to these foods. As a consequence many of us suffer from obesity, high blood level of lipids, insulin-resistance, diabetes, hypertension, heart disease, several types of cancer and other aging-related disorders, including BPH. Sedentary lifestyle and fat-rich diets are considered as major contributor to the rise in the incidences of metabolic disorders. Over the past 60 years in USA, the ratio of dietary intake of ω-6-FA verses ω-3-FA has increased from 2:1 to 25:1 (Simopoulos, 1999), and animal fat is a major source of ω-6-FAs which has been found to be associated with the higher risk of LUTS and BPH (Maserejian et al., 2009; Suzuki et al., 2002). Considering the rise in the incidence of LUTS/BPH in the obese and insulin-resistant individuals, it becomes increasingly important to understand the role of lipids in the pathogenesis of disease.

4.1 Evidence from in-vitro experiments

Limited information is available on the direct role of fatty acids (FAs) in the growth of normal and benign prostatic cells, as most of the studies have been conducted on the prostate cancer cell lines. However, cancer cell lines studies have indicative value for the potential effects of these FAs, as like prostate cancer, BPH is also associated with the pathological increase in the cell proliferation. A recent report indicating dominant uptake of FAs by the prostate cells [non-malignant (RWPE-1) as well as malignant (LnCaP and PC-3)] suggests their important role in the growth and development of the gland (Liu et al., 2010). Pandalai et al., reported growth promoting effects of ω-6-FAs on the rat non metastatic epithelial cell lines (EPYP1 & EPYP2), rat metastatic cell line (Met-Ly-Lu), and human metastatic prostate cancer cells (PC-3, LnCaP & TSU) (Pandalai et al., 1996). Arachidonic acid, a ω-6-FA treatment led to accelerated growth of the PC-3 cells in-vitro (Ghosh and Myers, 1997). Further, Rose et al., reported concentration-dependent stimulation of PC-3 cells by the linolenic acid (ω-6-FA) and inhibition with the eicosapentanoic acid and docosahexanoic acid (ω-3-FAs) (Rose and Connolly, 1991). Further, long term eicosapentanoic acid treatment has been found to inhibit the metastatic activities of the PC-3 cells (Rose and Connolly, 1991). Recently, we investigated the effects of the serum of high-fat diet-fed (saturated animal fat-lard) rats on the growth of PC-3 cells, and a significant acceleration in the growth was observed (Vikram and Jena, 2011a). The serum characteristics of these rats indicated a rise in the glucose, triglyceride, cholesterol and insulin levels. Although, rise in the insulin level appears to be the primary cause for the accelerated growth of the cells owing to the mitogenic effects of the hormone, the possibility of direct growth promoting effects of lipids cannot be denied. Taken together, these studies suggest that at least ω-6-FAs have a growth stimulating effects on the prostatic cells, and thus represent a potential risk factor for BPH.

4.2 Evidence from in-vivo experiments

The study by Cai et al., provided first evidence for the prostatic growth promoting effects of dietary fat in rats (Cai et al., 2001). Similarly, Rahman et al., observed enlargement of the ventral prostate and increased expression of alpha-adrenergic receptors in the hyperlipidemic rats (Rahman et al., 2007). Further, inclusion of the saturated animal fat (lard) in the diet induced prostatic enlargement and changed the expression of androgen receptor and peroxysome proliferator activated receptor γ (PPARγ) (Escobar et al., 2009). Polyunsaturated FAs are ligands for the PPARγ, which is involved in the regulation of cell differentiation and proliferation (Morales-Garcia et al., 2011; Parast et al., 2009), and therefore appears to represent a possible link between diet and prostatic growth (Escobar et al., 2009). Prostatic atrophy and increased apoptosis in the hypoinsulinemic rats (induced by selective β-cell toxins, either streptozotocin or alloxan) further supports the view that insulin plays a central role in the prostatic growth and development (Arcolino et al., 2010; Ikeda et al., 2000; Suthagar et al., 2009; Vikram et al., 2011b; Vikram et al., 2008; Yono et al., 2008;

Yono et al., 2005). Increased cell proliferation and enlargement of ventral prostate in rats kept on the diet rich in saturated fat was observed (Vikram et al., 2010b; 2011a; Vikram et al., 2010c). Interestingly, pioglitazone (a synthetic PPARγ receptor agonist) treatment led to decreased cell proliferation, increased apoptosis and restoration of prostatic weight in the diet-induced insulin-resistant rats (Vikram et al., 2010b; Vikram et al., 2010c). This observation can be explained on the basis of the restoration of insulin-sensitivity and secondary hyperinsulinemia as pioglitazone is known to improve the insulin-sensitivity (Vikram and Jena, 2010). Further, increased oxidative stress and incidence of prostatic adenocarcinoma and hyperplasia was observed in the rats kept on high-cholesterol diet for long time (80 – 100 weeks) (Homma et al., 2004). Increased expression of NADPH oxidase subunits, activation of NF-kB signaling and decreased expression of glutathione peroxidase 3 clearly indicated the increased oxidative stress and activation of inflammatory response in ventral prostate of the HFD-fed rats (Sekine et al., 2011; Vykhovanets et al., 2011). Inflammation has been greatly implicated as a risk factor for the development of BPH (Abdel-Meguid et al., 2009; Chughtai et al.; Donnell, 2011; Kim et al., 2011a; Wang et al., 2008). Despite a marginal decrease in the weight of the prostate in ACI/seg rats an significant increase in the expression of 5-α-reductase 2 mRNA level was observed in the high-fat diet-fed rats (Cai et al., 2006). Based on these evidences from animal studies it appears that (i) insulin-resistance associated secondary hyperinsulinemia, (ii) activation of PPARγ signaling by FAs and (iii) increased prostatic inflammation are the important nodes for further investigative studies.

4.3 Evidence from clinical/epidemiological studies
Presence of dyslipidemia in the BPH patients is a frequently noted condition under clinical setups (Nandeesha et al., 2006). High level of total cholesterol, LDL-cholesterol, triglyceride, decreased level of HDL-cholesterol increases the risk of BPH, and cholesterol-lowering medication may reduce the risk (Moyad and Lowe, 2008). Yang et al., compared FA profiles in the serum of patients with prostate cancer and BPH and proposed that polyunsaturated FAs have certain relation with BPH and prostate cancer (Yang et al., 1999). Higher serum LDL is associated with greater risk of BPH (Parsons et al., 2008), and physical activity, which is known to decrease the serum lipid level is associated with the decreased risk for BPH (Parsons and Kashefi, 2008). Hyperlipidemia is closely associated with the obesity, higher body mass index (BMI), and these parameters show a positive correlation with the BPH (Dahle et al., 2002; Hammarsten and Hogstedt, 1999; Hammarsten et al., 1998; Parsons et al., 2006; Parsons et al., 2009). Kim et al., reported that the patients with more BMI tend to have larger prostate volume and higher International Prostate Symptom Score (Kim et al., 2011b). Several studies indicate that obesity and sedentary lifestyle substantially increases the risk for BPH (Dahle et al., 2002; Parsons, 2011; Parsons et al., 2006; Parsons et al., 2009). Recently, it has been reported that the central obesity is a better predictor of LUTS (Kim et al.; Lee et al., 2009). In a health professionals follow up study a moderate association between FAs intake and risk of BPH was observed (Suzuki et al., 2002). A cross-sectional study of 1545 men aged 30-79 years in the Boston Area Community Health Study the associations between dietary intakes of total energy, carbohydrates, protein, fat, cholesterol and LUTS in men was examined (Maserejian et al., 2009). Results indicated that high-energy intake was associated with higher LUTS symptoms and the storage symptoms increased with the higher fat intake

(Maserejian et al., 2009). Further, Kristal et al., reported significant increase in the symptomatic BPH with higher total fat intake and polyunsaturated fats, and showed a significant decrease in the symptomatic BPH with high-protein intake and alcohol consumption (Kristal et al., 2008). Leptin and adiponectin are closely associated with the obesity, and effort has been made to identify the relationship, if any, between these mediators and the risk of BPH. Although, no association has been observed between plasma leptin level and BPH (Hoon Kim et al., 2008; Lagiou et al., 1998), high plasma adiponectin concentrations were found to be associated with the reduced risk of symptomatic BPH (Schenk et al., 2009). Few independent studies indicate that obesity is associated with hyperinsulinemia, which in turn promotes the prostatic growth and risk for BPH (Becker et al., 2009; Kogai et al., 2008; Vogeser et al., 2009). In contrast, few reports argue that, obesity is associated with increased estrogen/androgen ratio and sympathetic activity, both individually hypothesized to promote the development of BPH (Giovannucci et al., 1994). Obesity can augment prostatic growth either by (i) promoting the development of insulin-resistance and secondary hyperinsulinemia or by (ii) increasing the estrogen/androgen ratio. In contrast, isolated report indicates an inverse association between obesity and BPH owing to reduced testosterone level in the obese people (Zucchetto et al., 2005). However, further studies investigating the relationship between plasma FAs level, obesity, BMI and prostatic growth are needed to shed light on the pathogenesis of BPH. Although, systematic clinical studies have not been performed to evaluate the effect of lifestyle modifications on the BPH outcomes, number of studies supports the view that heart-healthy lifestyle changes would have beneficial effect on the prostatic health and will eventually improve the quality of life of patients.

5. Emerging mechanistic connections

5.1 Autotaxin-lysophosphatidic acid pathway

Lysophophatidic acid (LPA) is a small water soluble phospholipid, which binds to its G-protein coupled receptors and activates several downstream signaling pathways (Berdichevets et al., 2010; Rancoule et al., 2011). It is primarily produced by the activity of the phospholipase autotaxin (ATX) (Van Meeteren and Moolenaar, 2007). Excessive fat intake is associated with adiposity, development of insulin-resistance and obesity, and these conditions are known to increase the expression of ATX, and therefore the LPA levels (Ferry et al., 2003). Recent study indicating the expression of LPA-related molecules in the prostate (Zeng et al., 2009) suggests that LPA might have an important role in the normal prostatic growth and pathogenesis of the BPH (Sakamoto et al., 2004). Kulkarni et al., proposed ATX-LPA axis as a possible link between excessive dietary fat intake and prostatic hyperplasia (Kulkarni and Getzenberg, 2009). LPA is involved in the inflammatory responses and experimental studies indicating increased oxidative stress and NF-kB activation in the ventral prostate of high-fat diet-fed rodents (Sekine et al., 2011; Vykhovanets et al., 2011), which are known to develop prostatic enlargement (Vikram et al., 2010b; 2011a; Vikram et al., 2010c) supports the hypothesis. Further, clinical studies indicate that systemic inflammation or lower level of soluble receptors that bind to the inflammatory cytokines increase the BPH risk (Schenk et al., 2010). The pharmacological inhibitors of ATX such as S32826 (Ferry et al., 2008) and ongoing efforts of medicinal chemists (North et al., 2010; North et al., 2009; Parrill and Baker, 2010) in this direction might provide an answer to therapeutic management of the BPH.

5.2 PPARγ signaling

PPARs are ligand activated transcription factors, which includes polyunsaturated FAs, eicosanoids, prostaglandins, docosahexaenoic acid, thiozolidinediones, and non-steroidal anti-inflammatory drugs. A recent study by Jiang et al., showed that conditional prostatic epithelial knockout of PPARγ resulted in the inflammation and focal hyperplasia which developed into prostatic intraepithelial neoplasia (Jiang et al.). Increased expression of PPARγ and overall enlargement of the prostate was observed in the rats kept on diet rich in saturated fat (Escobar et al., 2009). We also observed increased cell proliferation and prostatic enlargement in rodents kept on high-fat diet (Vikram et al., 2010b; 2011a; Vikram et al., 2010c). Moreover, pioglitazone (a PPARγ agonist) treatment restored prostate size in these rats (Vikram et al., 2010b; Vikram et al., 2010c). A recent study indicating the dominant uptake of FAs (as compared to glucose) by the malignant as well as non-malignant prostatic cells (Liu et al., 2010) underlines the possible role of PPARγ in the prostatic growth and development. These findings suggest that PPARγ represents a potential link between dietary fat and prostatic growth. However, further studies are needed to characterize its role in the normal and pathological growth of the prostate.

5.3 Hyperinsulinemia: Altered insulin/IGF signaling

Hyperinsulinemia generally develops as a compensatory response to the decreased insulin mediated actions under the insulin-resistant conditions (McKeehan et al., 1984). Experimental (Cai et al., 2001; Escobar et al., 2009; Rahman et al., 2007; Vikram et al., 2010a; b; 2011a; Vikram et al., 2010c) and clinical/epidemiological (Hammarsten et al., 2009; Hammarsten and Hogstedt, 2001; Nandeesha et al., 2006) studies indicate that the hyperinsulinemia is an independent contributor to the prostatic cell proliferation and pathogenesis of the BPH. Further, hyperinsulinemic condition can contribute to the augmented prostatic growth by several ways such as (i) increasing the serum level of IGF-I (Chokkalingam et al., 2002; Nam et al., 1997), (ii) possibility of the binding of insulin with the IGF-I receptor (IGF-IR) under the hyperinsulinemic conditions and (iii) binding of IGF-I to the insulin receptor (IR) (Belfiore and Frasca, 2008; Li et al., 2005). Further, IR has two isoforms, A and B, the former is having metabolic as well as mitogenic effects while B is mainly concerned with the metabolic effects. IR isoforms exhibit difference in the binding affinities to the ligand(s) and downstream signaling cascade (Giudice et al., 2011; Kosaki et al., 1995; Leibiger et al., 2001; Sciacca et al., 2003; Uhles et al., 2003; Vogt et al., 1991). IGF-II binds to the IR-A and mediates its growth promoting effects but not with IR-B (Frasca et al., 1999; Morrione et al., 1997). This means that insulin, IGF-I and IGF-II competes to bind with the IR-A, while only insulin binds with the IR-B. The hybrid receptors, IR-A/IR-B and IR/IGF-I further complicates the molecular diversification of the insulin signaling system. IR-A/IR-B hybrid receptors were found to bind to both insulin and IGF-II and therefore, resemble IR-A homodimers rather IR-B homodimers (Blanquart et al., 2008). The IR/IGF-IR hybrid receptors (Pandini et al., 2002; Soos et al., 1990) are activated by both insulin as well as IGF-I, but the IGF-I effect is predominant, and it resembles IGF-1R homodimers rather IR homodimers (Langlois et al., 1995). The IGF and insulin signaling system has been summarized in figure 1. Prostate is known to have both isoforms of the IR (Cox et al., 2009). Experimental studies investigating the effect of dietary habits (particularly dietary fat) on the expression of IR isoforms and signaling kinetics might provide valuable insight in the understanding of the pathogenesis of the BPH under the insulin-resistant, obese and diabetic conditions.

5.4 Estrogen/androgen ratio

Androgen deprivation leads to rapid apoptosis of the luminal secretory cells and atrophy of the prostate gland (Ikeda et al., 2000; Vikram et al., 2010c; Vikram et al., 2008). However, with the re-administration of the androgens prostate regains its normal size, and is capable of more than 15 rounds of the regression / regeneration cycle (Wang et al., 2009). Further, administration of either estrogen or dihydrotestosterone leads to hyperproliferation and induction of prostatic hyperplasia in the experimental animals. These simple experiments highlights the crucial role of steroidal hormones in the growth and development of the gland. Aromatase is a CYP450 enzyme which irreversibly converts testosterone to the estradiol, and obesity is associated with increased aromatase activity (Subbaramaiah et al., 2011). Increased aromatase activity in the obese people may lead to rise in the estrogen/androgen ratio and hence the susceptibility for developing BPH. These aspects have been recently reviewed by Nicholson et al., and readers are encouraged to read the review (Nicholson and Ricke, 2011).

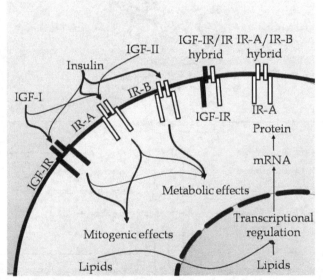

Fig. 1. The IGF and insulin receptor signaling system. To avoid confusion, the binding affinity of the ligands and relative effects of hybrid receptors (metabolic and mitogenic) are not depicted in the figure. However, the IGF-IR/IR hybrid resembles IGF-IR homodimer and IR-A/IR-B resembles IR-A homodimers. Lipids are involved in nuclear signaling and can influence transcriptional regulation and thus growth and differentiation. IGF-I/II; insulin-like growth factor-I/II, IGF-IR; insulin-like growth factor-I receptor, IR-A/B; insuln receptor isoform-A/B.

6. Summary

BPH is a highly prevalent condition of prostate in the aging men population. The worldwide increase in the prevalence of BPH has been thought to be associated with obesity and lifestyle changes such as excessive intake of fat-rich diet and physical inactivity. Considering the changing dietary habits and rising incidences of BPH, it becomes increasingly important to delineate the precise roles of lipids in the normal as well as pathological growth of the prostate. Although, experimental and clinical/epidemiological studies suggest that these conditions contribute to the pathogenesis of both insulin-resistance and BPH, the direct role of lipids in the pathogenesis of prostatic enlargement is far from complete understanding. Role of lipids in the progression of insulin-resistance and other disorders and indirect effect on the prostatic growth owing to compensatory rise in the plasma insulin level is essentially correct, but what has emerged is that the lipids might have a direct influence on the normal as well as pathological growth of the prostate.

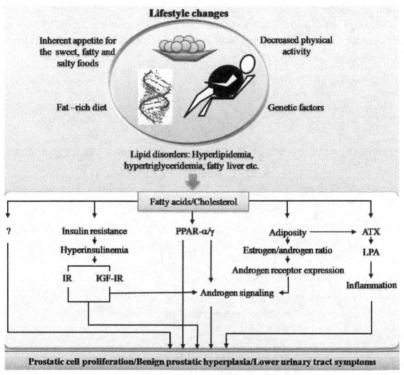

Fig. 2. Modern lifestyle associated changes including increased consumption of fat-rich diets and decreased physical activities contributes to the development of lipid-disorders and obesity. The present illustration demonstrates the possible influence of these factors on the prostatic growth and development. IR; insulin receptor, IGF-IR; insulin-like growth factor-1 receptor, PPAR-α/γ; peroxisome-proliferator activated receptor alpha/gamma, ATX; autotaxin, LPA, lysophosphatidic acid.

7. Conclusion

In addition to the genetic factors, environmental factors such as physical inactivity and excessive intake of dietary fat contribute to the increased incidence of lipid-disorders and obesity worldwide. These factors directly as well as indirectly promote the prostatic growth and contractility of the prostate gland, and represent important risk factors for the development of symptomatic LUTS / BPH (Fig. 2). ATX-LPA axis, PPARγ signaling, hyperinsulinemia/IGF signaling and steroidal signaling are the emerging mechanisms which explains the association between dietary fat intake, obesity and BPH. However, further mechanistic as well as epidemiology based studies are required to delineate the role of lipids in the pathogenesis of BPH. Future research to investigate the direct effect of different types of FAs on the prostatic growth and isoforms specific characterization of insulin and IGF-IR signaling in response to dietary habit is warranted.

8. Acknowledgements

We are thankful to the Central University of Punjab (CUP), Bathinda, Punjab 151 001, India for providing necessary resources to complete the review work.

9. References

Abdel-Meguid, T.A., Mosli, H.A., Al-Maghrabi, J.A., 2009. Prostate inflammation. Association with benign prostatic hyperplasia and prostate cancer. *Saudi Med J*, 30, 1563-1567.

Alberto, B., Umberto, C., Nazareno, S., Andrea, G., Andrea, S., Marco, B., Manuela, T., Valerio, D.G., Giorgio, G., Patrizio, R., Francesco, M., 2009. Benign prostatic hyperplasia and Its aetiologies. *Eur Urol Suppl*, 8, 865-871.

Arcolino, F.O., Ribeiro, D.L., Gobbo, M.G., Taboga, S.R., Goes, R.M., 2010. Proliferation and apoptotic rates and increased frequency of p63-positive cells in the prostate acinar epithelium of alloxan-induced diabetic rats. *Int J Exp Pathol*, 91, 144-154.

Becker, S., Dossus, L., Kaaks, R., 2009. Obesity related hyperinsulinaemia and hyperglycaemia and cancer development. *Arch Physiol Biochem*, 115, 86-96.

Belfiore, A., Frasca, F., 2008. IGF and insulin receptor signaling in breast cancer. *J Mammary Gland Biol Neoplasia*, 13, 381-406.

Berdichevets, I.N., Tyazhelova, T.V., Shimshilashvili Kh, R., Rogaev, E.I., 2010. Lysophosphatidic acid is a lipid mediator with wide range of biological activities. Biosynthetic pathways and mechanism of action. *Biochemistry*, 75, 1088-1097.

Berry, S.J., Coffey, D.S., Walsh, P.C., Ewing, L.L., 1984. The development of human benign prostatic hyperplasia with age. *J Urol*, 132, 474-479.

Blanquart, C., Achi, J., Issad, T., 2008. Characterization of IRA/IRB hybrid insulin receptors using bioluminescence resonance energy transfer. *Biochem Pharmacol*, 76, 873-883.

Bosch, R.J., 1991. Pathogenesis of benign prostatic hyperplasia. *Eur Urol*, 20, 27-30.

Bravi, F., Bosetti, C., Dal Maso, L., Talamini, R., Montella, M., Negri, E., Ramazzotti, V., Franceschi, S., La Vecchia, C., 2006. Macronutrients, fatty acids, cholesterol, and risk of benign prostatic hyperplasia. *Urology*, 67, 1205-1211.

Cai, L.Q., Imperato-McGinley, J., Zhu, Y.S., 2006. Regulation of prostate 5alpha-reductase-2 gene expression and prostate weight by dietary fat and caloric intake in the rat. *Prostate*, 66, 738-748.

Cai, X., Haleem, R., Oram, S., Cyriac, J., Jiang, F., Grayhack, J.T., Kozlowski, J.M., Wang, Z., 2001. High fat diet increases the weight of rat ventral prostate. *Prostate*, 49, 1-8.

Chokkalingam, A.P., Gao, Y.T., Deng, J., Stanczyk, F.Z., Sesterhenn, I.A., Mostofi, F.K., Fraumeni, J.F., Jr., Hsing, A.W., 2002. Insulin-like growth factors and risk of benign prostatic hyperplasia. *Prostate*, 52, 98-105.

Chughtai, B., Lee, R., Te, A., Kaplan, S., Inflammation and benign prostatic hyperplasia: clinical implications. *Curr Urol Rep*, 12, 274-277.

Cox, M.E., Gleave, M.E., Zakikhani, M., Bell, R.H., Piura, E., Vickers, E., Cunningham, M., Larsson, O., Fazli, L., Pollak, M., 2009. Insulin receptor expression by human prostate cancers. *Prostate*, 69, 33-40.

Culig, Z., Hobisch, A., Cronauer, M.V., Radmayr, C., Hittmair, A., Zhang, J., Thurnher, M., Bartsch, G., Klocker, H., 1996. Regulation of prostatic growth and function by peptide growth factors. *Prostate*, 28, 392-405.

Dahle, S.E., Chokkalingam, A.P., Gao, Y.T., Deng, J., Stanczyk, F.Z., Hsing, A.W., 2002. Body size and serum levels of insulin and leptin in relation to the risk of benign prostatic hyperplasia. *J Urol*, 168, 599-604.

Donnell, R.F., 2011. Benign prostate hyperplasia: a review of the year's progress from bench to clinic. *Curr Opin Urol*, 21, 22-26.

Escobar, E.L., Gomes-Marcondes, M.C., Carvalho, H.F., 2009. Dietary fatty acid quality affects AR and PPARgamma levels and prostate growth. *Prostate*, 69, 548-558.

Ferry, G., Moulharat, N., Pradere, J.P., Desos, P., Try, A., Genton, A., Giganti, A., Beucher-Gaudin, M., Lonchampt, M., Bertrand, M., Saulnier-Blache, J.S., Tucker, G.C., Cordi, A., Boutin, J.A., 2008. S32826, a nanomolar inhibitor of autotaxin: discovery, synthesis and applications as a pharmacological tool. *J Pharmacol Exp Ther*, 327, 809-819.

Ferry, G., Tellier, E., Try, A., Gres, S., Naime, I., Simon, M.F., Rodriguez, M., Boucher, J., Tack, I., Gesta, S., Chomarat, P., Dieu, M., Raes, M., Galizzi, J.P., Valet, P., Boutin, J.A., Saulnier-Blache, J.S., 2003. Autotaxin is released from adipocytes, catalyzes lysophosphatidic acid synthesis, and activates preadipocyte proliferation. Up-regulated expression with adipocyte differentiation and obesity. *J Biol Chem*, 278, 18162-18169.

Francisco, C., Francois, D., 2010. New concepts and pathophysiology of lower urinary tract symptoms in men. *Eur Urol Suppl*, 9, 472-476.

Frasca, F., Pandini, G., Scalia, P., Sciacca, L., Mineo, R., Costantino, A., Goldfine, I.D., Belfiore, A., Vigneri, R., 1999. Insulin receptor isoform A, a newly recognized, high-affinity insulin-like growth factor II receptor in fetal and cancer cells. *Mol Cell Biol*, 19, 3278-3288.

Ghosh, J., Myers, C.E., 1997. Arachidonic acid stimulates prostate cancer cell growth: critical role of 5-lipoxygenase. *Biochem Biophy Res Commun*, 235, 418-423.

Giovannucci, E., Rimm, E.B., Chute, C.G., Kawachi, I., Colditz, G.A., Stampfer, M.J., Willett, W.C., 1994. Obesity and benign prostatic hyperplasia. *Am J Epidemiol*, 140, 989-1002.

Giudice, J., Leskow, F.C., Arndt-Jovin, D.J., Jovin, T.M., Jares-Erijman, E.A., 2011. Differential endocytosis and signaling dynamics of insulin receptor variants IR-A and IR-B. *J Cell Sci*, 124, 801-811.

Hammarsten, J., Damber, J.E., Karlsson, M., Knutson, T., Ljunggren, O., Ohlsson, C., Peeker, R., Smith, U., Mellstrom, D., 2009. Insulin and free oestradiol are independent risk factors for benign prostatic hyperplasia. *Prostate Cancer Prostatic Dis*, 12, 160-165.

Hammarsten, J., Hogstedt, B., 1999. Clinical, anthropometric, metabolic and insulin profile of men with fast annual growth rates of benign prostatic hyperplasia. *Blood Press*, 8, 29-36.

Hammarsten, J., Hogstedt, B., 2001. Hyperinsulinaemia as a risk factor for developing benign prostatic hyperplasia. *Eur Urol*, 39, 151-158.

Hammarsten, J., Hogstedt, B., Holthuis, N., Mellstrom, D., 1998. Components of the metabolic syndrome-risk factors for the development of benign prostatic hyperplasia. *Prostate cancer and prostatic dis*, 1, 157-162.

Homma, Y., Kondo, Y., Kaneko, M., Kitamura, T., Nyou, W.T., Yanagisawa, M., Yamamoto, Y., Kakizoe, T., 2004. Promotion of carcinogenesis and oxidative stress by dietary cholesterol in rat prostate. *Carcinogenesis*, 25, 1011-1014.

Hoon Kim, J., Lee, S.Y., Myung, S.C., Kim, Y.S., Kim, T.H., Kim, M.K., 2008. Clinical significance of the leptin and leptin receptor expressions in prostate tissues. *Asian J Androl*, 10, 923-928.

Ikeda, K., Wada, Y., Foster, H.E., Jr., Wang, Z., Weiss, R.M., Latifpour, J., 2000. Experimental diabetes-induced regression of the rat prostate is associated with an increased expression of transforming growth factor-beta. *J Urol*, 164, 180-185.

Ingraham, H.A., 2011. Metabolism: A lipid for fat disorders. *Nature*, 474, 455-456.

Irvine, R.F., 2003. Nuclear lipid signalling. *Nat Rev Mol Cell Biol*, 4, 349-360.

Jiang, M., Fernandez, S., Jerome, W.G., He, Y., Yu, X., Cai, H., Boone, B., Yi, Y., Magnuson, M.A., Roy-Burman, P., Matusik, R.J., Shappell, S.B., Hayward, S.W., Disruption of PPARgamma signaling results in mouse prostatic intraepithelial neoplasia involving active autophagy. *Cell Death Differ*, 17, 469-481.

Kaplan-Lefko, P.J., Sutherland, B.W., Evangelou, A.I., Hadsell, D.L., Barrios, R.J., Foster, B.A., Demayo, F., Greenberg, N.M., 2008. Enforced epithelial expression of IGF-1 causes hyperplastic prostate growth while negative selection is requisite for spontaneous metastogenesis. *Oncogene*, 27, 2868-2876.

Kasturi, S., Russell, S., McVary, K.T., 2006. Metabolic syndrome and lower urinary tract symptoms secondary to benign prostatic hyperplasia. *Curr Urol Rep*, 7, 288-292.

Kim, B.H., Kim, C.I., Chang, H.S., Choe, M.S., Jung, H.R., Kim, D.Y., Park, C.H., 2011a. Cyclooxygenase-2 overexpression in chronic inflammation associated with benign prostatic hyperplasia: is it related to apoptosis and angiogenesis of prostate cancer? *Korean J Urol*, 52, 253-259.

Kim, G.W., Doo, S.W., Yang, W.J., Song, Y.S., 2010. Effects of obesity on prostate volume and lower urinary tract symptoms in korean men. *Korean J Urol*, 51, 344-347.

Kim, J.M., Song, P.H., Kim, H.T., Moon, K.H., 2011b. Effect of obesity on prostate-specific antigen, prostate volume, and international prostate symptom score in patients with benign prostatic hyperplasia. *Korean J Urol*, 52, 401-405.

Kogai, M.A., Lutov, U.V., Selyatitskaya, V.G., 2008. Hormonal and biochemical parameters of metabolic syndrome in male patients with body weight excess and obesity. *Bull Exp Biol Med*, 146, 806-808.

Kosaki, A., Pillay, T.S., Xu, L., Webster, N.J., 1995. The B isoform of the insulin receptor signals more efficiently than the A isoform in HepG2 cells. *J Biol Chem*, 270, 20816-20823.

Kristal, A.R., Arnold, K.B., Schenk, J.M., Neuhouser, M.L., Goodman, P., Penson, D.F., Thompson, I.M., 2008. Dietary patterns, supplement use, and the risk of symptomatic benign prostatic hyperplasia: results from the prostate cancer prevention trial. *Am J Epidemiol*, 167, 925-934.

Kulkarni, P., Getzenberg, R.H., 2009. High-fat diet, obesity and prostate disease: the ATX-LPA axis? *Nat Clin Pract Urol*, 6, 128-131.

Lagiou, P., Signorello, L.B., Trichopoulos, D., Tzonou, A., Trichopoulou, A., Mantzoros, C.S., 1998. Leptin in relation to prostate cancer and benign prostatic hyperplasia. *Int J Cancer*, 76, 25-28.

Langlois, W.J., Sasaoka, T., Yip, C.C., Olefsky, J.M., 1995. Functional characterization of hybrid receptors composed of a truncated insulin receptor and wild type insulin-like growth factor 1 or insulin receptors. *Endocrinology*, 136, 1978-1986.

Lee, J.M., Lee, Y.K., Mamrosh, J.L., Busby, S.A., Griffin, P.R., Pathak, M.C., Ortlund, E.A., Moore, D.D., 2011. A nuclear-receptor-dependent phosphatidylcholine pathway with antidiabetic effects. *Nature*, 474, 506-510.

Lee, S.H., Kim, J.C., Lee, J.Y., Kim, J.H., Oh, C.Y., Lee, S.W., Yoo, S.J., Chung, B.H., 2009. Effects of obesity on lower urinary tract symptoms in Korean BPH patients. *Asian J Androl*. 11, 663-668.

Leibiger, B., Leibiger, I.B., Moede, T., Kemper, S., Kulkarni, R.N., Kahn, C.R., de Vargas, L.M., Berggren, P.O., 2001. Selective insulin signaling through A and B insulin receptors regulates transcription of insulin and glucokinase genes in pancreatic beta cells. *Mol Cell*, 7, 559-570.

Li, G., Barrett, E.J., Wang, H., Chai, W., Liu, Z., 2005. Insulin at physiological concentrations selectively activates insulin but not insulin-like growth factor I (IGF-I) or insulin/IGF-I hybrid receptors in endothelial cells. *Endocrinology*, 146, 4690-4696.

Liu, Y., Zuckier, L.S., Ghesani, N.V., 2010. Dominant uptake of fatty acid over glucose by prostate cells: a potential new diagnostic and therapeutic approach. *Anticancer Res*, 30, 369-374.

Marker, P.C., Donjacour, A.A., Dahiya, R., Cunha, G.R., 2003. Hormonal, cellular, and molecular control of prostatic development. *Dev Biol*, 253, 165-174.

Maserejian, N.N., Giovannucci, E.L., McKinlay, J.B., 2009. Dietary macronutrients, cholesterol, and sodium and lower urinary tract symptoms in men. *Eur Urol*, 55, 1179-1189.

McKeehan, W.L., Adams, P.S., Rosser, M.P., 1984. Direct mitogenic effects of insulin, epidermal growth factor, glucocorticoid, cholera toxin, unknown pituitary factors and possibly prolactin, but not androgen, on normal rat prostate epithelial cells in serum-free, primary cell culture. *Cancer Res*, 44, 1998-2010.

Morales-Garcia, J.A., Luna-Medina, R., Alfaro-Cervello, C., Cortes-Canteli, M., Santos, A., Garcia-Verdugo, J.M., Perez-Castillo, A., 2011. Peroxisome proliferator-activated receptor gamma ligands regulate neural stem cell proliferation and differentiation in vitro and in vivo. *Glia*, 59, 293-307.

Morrione, A., Valentinis, B., Xu, S.Q., Yumet, G., Louvi, A., Efstratiadis, A., Baserga, R., 1997. Insulin-like growth factor II stimulates cell proliferation through the insulin receptor. *Proc Natl Acad Sci U S A*, 94, 3777-3782.

Moyad, M.A., Lowe, F.C., 2008. Educating patients about lifestyle modifications for prostate health. *Am J Med*, 121, S34-42.

Nam, S.Y., Lee, E.J., Kim, K.R., Cha, B.S., Song, Y.D., Lim, S.K., Lee, H.C., Huh, K.B., 1997. Effect of obesity on total and free insulin-like growth factor (IGF)-1, and their relationship to IGF-binding protein (BP)-1, IGFBP-2, IGFBP-3, insulin, and growth hormone. *Int J Obes Relat Metab Disord*, 21, 355-359.

Nandeesha, H., Koner, B.C., Dorairajan, L.N., Sen, S.K., 2006. Hyperinsulinemia and dyslipidemia in non-diabetic benign prostatic hyperplasia. *Clin Chim Acta*, 370, 89-93.

Nicholson, T.M., Ricke, W.A., 2011. Androgens and estrogens in benign prostatic hyperplasia: Past, present and future. *Differentiation*, (In-press).

North, E.J., Howard, A.L., Wanjala, I.W., Pham, T.C., Baker, D.L., Parrill, A.L., 2010. Pharmacophore development and application toward the identification of novel, small-molecule autotaxin inhibitors. *J Med Chem*, 53, 3095-3105.

North, E.J., Osborne, D.A., Bridson, P.K., Baker, D.L., Parrill, A.L., 2009. Autotaxin structure-activity relationships revealed through lysophosphatidylcholine analogs. *Bioorg Med Chem*, 17, 3433-3442.

Pandalai, P.K., Pilat, M.J., Yamazaki, K., Naik, H., Pienta, K.J., 1996. The effects of omega-3 and omega-6 fatty acids on in vitro prostate cancer growth. *Anticancer Res*, 16, 815-820.

Pandini, G., Frasca, F., Mineo, R., Sciacca, L., Vigneri, R., Belfiore, A., 2002. Insulin/insulin-like growth factor I hybrid receptors have different biological characteristics depending on the insulin receptor isoform involved. *J Biol Chem*, 277, 39684-39695.

Parast, M.M., Yu, H., Ciric, A., Salata, M.W., Davis, V., Milstone, D.S., 2009. PPARgamma regulates trophoblast proliferation and promotes labyrinthine trilineage differentiation. *PLoS One*, 4, e8055.

Parrill, A.L., Baker, D.L., 2010. Autotaxin inhibitors: a perspective on initial medicinal chemistry efforts. *Expert Opin Ther Pat*, 20, 1619-1625.

Parsons, J.K., 2011. Lifestyle factors, benign prostatic hyperplasia, and lower urinary tract symptoms. *Curr Opin Urol*, 21, 1-4.

Parsons, J.K., Bergstrom, J., Barrett-Connor, E., 2008. Lipids, lipoproteins and the risk of benign prostatic hyperplasia in community-dwelling men. *BJU Int*, 101, 313-318.

Parsons, J.K., Carter, H.B., Partin, A.W., Windham, B.G., Metter, E.J., Ferrucci, L., Landis, P., Platz, E.A., 2006. Metabolic factors associated with benign prostatic hyperplasia. *J Clin Endocrinol Metab*, 91, 2562-2568.

Parsons, J.K., Kashefi, C., 2008. Physical activity, benign prostatic hyperplasia, and lower urinary tract symptoms. *Eur Urol*, 53, 1228-1235.

Parsons, J.K., Sarma, A.V., McVary, K., Wei, J.T., 2009. Obesity and benign prostatic hyperplasia: clinical connections, emerging etiological paradigms and future directions. *J Urol*, 182, S27-31.

Rahman, N.U., Phonsombat, S., Bochinski, D., Carrion, R.E., Nunes, L., Lue, T.F., 2007. An animal model to study lower urinary tract symptoms and erectile dysfunction: the hyperlipidaemic rat. *BJU Int*, 100, 658-663.

Rancoule, C., Pradere, J.P., Gonzalez, J., Klein, J., Valet, P., Bascands, J.L., Schanstra, J.P., Saulnier-Blache, J.S., 2011. Lysophosphatidic acid-1-receptor targeting agents for fibrosis. *Expert Opin Investig Drugs*, 20, 657-667.

Rick, F.G., Schally, A.V., Block, N.L., Nadji, M., Szepeshazi, K., Zarandi, M., Vidaurre, I., Perez, R., Halmos, G., Szalontay, L., 2011. Antagonists of growth hormone-releasing hormone (GHRH) reduce prostate size in experimental benign prostatic hyperplasia. *Proc Natl Acad Sci U S A*, 108, 3755-3760.

Rose, D.P., Connolly, J.M., 1991. Effects of fatty acids and eicosanoid synthesis inhibitors on the growth of two human prostate cancer cell lines. *Prostate*, 18, 243-254.

Saigal, C.S., Joyce, G., 2005. Economic costs of benign prostatic hyperplasia in the private sector. *J Urol*, 173, 1309-1313.

Sakamoto, S., Yokoyama, M., Zhang, X., Prakash, K., Nagao, K., Hatanaka, T., Getzenberg, R.H., Kakehi, Y., 2004. Increased expression of CYR61, an extracellular matrix signaling protein, in human benign prostatic hyperplasia and its regulation by lysophosphatidic acid. *Endocrinology*, 145, 2929-2940.

Sanda, M.G., Beaty, T.H., Stutzman, R.E., Childs, B., Walsh, P.C., 1994. Genetic susceptibility of benign prostatic hyperplasia. *J Urol*, 152, 115-119.

Schenk, J.M., Kristal, A.R., Neuhouser, M.L., Tangen, C.M., White, E., Lin, D.W., Kratz, M., Thompson, I.M., 2010. Biomarkers of systemic inflammation and risk of incident, symptomatic benign prostatic hyperplasia: results from the prostate cancer prevention trial. *Am J Epidemiol*, 171, 571-582.

Schenk, J.M., Kristal, A.R., Neuhouser, M.L., Tangen, C.M., White, E., Lin, D.W., Thompson, I.M., 2009. Serum adiponectin, C-peptide and leptin and risk of symptomatic benign prostatic hyperplasia: results from the Prostate Cancer Prevention Trial. *Prostate*, 69, 1303-1311.

Sciacca, L., Prisco, M., Wu, A., Belfiore, A., Vigneri, R., Baserga, R., 2003. Signaling differences from the A and B isoforms of the insulin receptor (IR) in 32D cells in the presence or absence of IR substrate-1. *Endocrinology*, 144, 2650-2658.

Sekine, Y., Osei-Hwedieh, D., Matsuda, K., Raghavachari, N., Liu, D., Furuya, Y., Koike, H., Suzuki, K., Remaley, A.T., 2011. High fat diet reduces the expression of glutathione peroxidase 3 in mouse prostate. *Prostate*, (In-Press).

Simopoulos, A.P., 1999. Essential fatty acids in health and chronic disease. *Am J Clin Nutr*, 70, 560S-569S.

Smith, C.D., Wells, W.W., 1983a. Phosphorylation of rat liver nuclear envelopes. I. Characterization of in vitro protein phosphorylation. *J Biol Chem*, 258, 9360-9367.

Smith, C.D., Wells, W.W., 1983b. Phosphorylation of rat liver nuclear envelopes. II. Characterization of in vitro lipid phosphorylation. *J Biol Chem*, 258, 9368-9373.

Soos, M.A., Whittaker, J., Lammers, R., Ullrich, A., Siddle, K., 1990. Receptors for insulin and insulin-like growth factor-I can form hybrid dimers. Characterisation of hybrid receptors in transfected cells. *Biochem J*, 270, 383-390.

Srinivasan, G., Campbell, E., Bashirelahi, N., 1995. Androgen, estrogen, and progesterone receptors in normal and aging prostates. *Microsc Res Tech*, 30, 293-304.

Story, M.T., 1995. Regulation of prostate growth by fibroblast growth factors. *World J Urol*, 13, 297-305.

Stranne, J., Damber, J.E., Fall, M., Hammarsten, J., Knutson, T., Peeker, R., 2009. One-third of the Swedish male population over 50 years of age suffers from lower urinary tract symptoms. *Scandinavian J Urol Nephrol*, 43, 199-205.

Subbaramaiah, K., Howe, L.R., Bhardwaj, P., Du, B., Gravaghi, C., Yantiss, R.K., Zhou, X.K., Blaho, V.A., Hla, T., Yang, P., Kopelovich, L., Hudis, C.A., Dannenberg, A.J., 2011. Obesity is associated with inflammation and elevated aromatase expression in the mouse mammary gland. *Cancer Prev Res (Phila)*, 4, 329-346.

Suthagar, E., Soudamani, S., Yuvaraj, S., Ismail Khan, A., Aruldhas, M.M., Balasubramanian, K., 2009. Effects of streptozotocin (STZ)-induced diabetes and insulin replacement on rat ventral prostate. *Biomed Pharmacother*, 63, 43-50.

Suzuki, S., Platz, E.A., Kawachi, I., Willett, W.C., Giovannucci, E., 2002. Intakes of energy and macronutrients and the risk of benign prostatic hyperplasia. *Am J Clin Nutr*, 75, 689-697.

Uhles, S., Moede, T., Leibiger, B., Berggren, P.O., Leibiger, I.B., 2003. Isoform-specific insulin receptor signaling involves different plasma membrane domains. *J Cell Biol*, 163, 1327-1337.

Van Meeteren, L.A., Moolenaar, W.H., 2007. Regulation and biological activities of the autotaxin-LPA axis. *Prog Lipid Res*, 46, 145-160.

Vikram, A., Jena, G., 2010. S961, an insulin receptor antagonist causes hyperinsulinemia, insulin-resistance and depletion of energy stores in rats. *Biochem Biophy Res Commun*, 398, 260-265.

Vikram, A., Jena, G., 2011a. Diet-induced hyperinsulinemia accelerates growth of human androgen independent PC-3 cells. *Nut Cancer*, (In-Press).

Vikram, A., Jena, G., 2011b. Role of insulin and testosterone in prostatic growth: who is doing what? *Med Hypotheses*, 76, 474-478.

Vikram, A., Jena, G., Ramarao, P., 2010a. Insulin-resistance and benign prostatic hyperplasia: the connection. *Eur J Pharmacol*, 641, 75-81.

Vikram, A., Jena, G., Ramarao, P., 2010b. Pioglitazone attenuates prostatic enlargement in diet-induced insulin-resistant rats by altering lipid distribution and hyperinsulinaemia. *Brit J Pharmacol*, 161, 1708-1721.

Vikram, A., Jena, G., Ramarao, P., 2011a. Insulin-resistance reduces botulinum neurotoxin-type A induced prostatic atrophy and apoptosis in rats. *Eur J Pharmacol*, 650, 356-363.

Vikram, A., Jena, G.B., Ramarao, P., 2010c. Increased cell proliferation and contractility of prostate in insulin resistant rats: linking hyperinsulinemia with benign prostate hyperplasia. *Prostate*, 70, 79-89.

Vikram, A., Kushwaha, S., Jena, G.B., 2011b. Relative influence of testosterone and insulin in the regulation of prostatic cell proliferation and growth. *Steroids*, 76, 416-423.

Vikram, A., Tripathi, D.N., Ramarao, P., Jena, G.B., 2008. Intervention of D-glucose ameliorates the toxicity of streptozotocin in accessory sex organs of rat. *Toxicol Appl Pharmacol*, 226, 84-93.

Vogeser, M., Schwandt, P., Haas, G.M., Broedl, U.C., Lehrke, M., Parhofer, K.G., 2009. BMI and hyperinsulinemia in children. *Clin Biochem*, 42, 1427-1430.

Vogt, B., Carrascosa, J.M., Ermel, B., Ullrich, A., Haring, H.U., 1991. The two isotypes of the human insulin receptor (HIR-A and HIR-B) follow different internalization kinetics. *Biochem Biophy Res Commun*, 177, 1013-1018.

Vykhovanets, E.V., Shankar, E., Vykhovanets, O.V., Shukla, S., Gupta, S., 2011. High-fat diet increases NF-kappaB signaling in the prostate of reporter mice. *Prostate*, 71, 147-156.

Wang, L., Yang, J.R., Yang, L.Y., Liu, Z.T., 2008. Chronic inflammation in benign prostatic hyperplasia: implications for therapy. *Med Hypotheses*, 70, 1021-1023.

Wang, X., Kruithof-de Julio, M., Economides, K.D., Walker, D., Yu, H., Halili, M.V., Hu, Y.P., Price, S.M., Abate-Shen, C., Shen, M.M., 2009. A luminal epithelial stem cell that is a cell of origin for prostate cancer. *Nature*, 461, 495-500.

Wang, Z., Olumi, A.F., 2011. Diabetes, growth hormone-insulin-like growth factor pathways and association to benign prostatic hyperplasia. *Differentiation*, (In-Press).

Yang, Y.J., Lee, S.H., Hong, S.J., Chung, B.C., 1999. Comparison of fatty acid profiles in the serum of patients with prostate cancer and benign prostatic hyperplasia. *Clin Biochem*, 32, 405-409.

Yono, M., Mane, S.M., Lin, A., Weiss, R.M., Latifpour, J., 2008. Differential effects of diabetes induced by streptozotocin and that develops spontaneously on prostate growth in Bio Breeding (BB) rats. *Life Sci*, 83, 192-197.

Yono, M., Pouresmail, M., Takahashi, W., Flanagan, J.F., Weiss, R.M., Latifpour, J., 2005. Effect of insulin treatment on tissue size of the genitourinary tract in BB rats with spontaneously developed and streptozotocin-induced diabetes. *Naunyn Schmiedebergs Arch Pharmacol*, 372, 251-255.

Zeng, Y., Kakehi, Y., Nouh, M.A., Tsunemori, H., Sugimoto, M., Wu, X.X., 2009. Gene expression profiles of lysophosphatidic acid-related molecules in the prostate: relevance to prostate cancer and benign hyperplasia. *Prostate*, 69, 283-292.

Zucchetto, A., Tavani, A., Dal Maso, L., Gallus, S., Negri, E., Talamini, R., Franceschi, S., Montella, M., La Vecchia, C., 2005. History of weight and obesity through life and risk of benign prostatic hyperplasia. *Int J Obes*, 29, 798-803.

10

Predictors of the Common Adverse Drug Reactions of Statins

Hadeer Akram AbdulRazzaq[1], Noorizan Abd Aziz[2], Yahaya Hassan[2],
Yaman Walid Kassab[1] and Omar Ismail[3]
[1]Department of Clinical Pharmacy, School of Pharmaceutical Sciences,
Universiti Sains, Penang,
[2]Faculty of Pharmacy, UiTM, Puncak Alam Campus,
Bandar Puncak Alam, Selangor DE,
[3]Department of Cardiology, Hospital Pulau Pinang, Penang,
Malaysia

1. Introduction

Statins are common lipid lowering agents to reduce elevation of cholesterol or as prophylaxis against other cardiac diseases. It estimated that 62.5% to 91.7% of dyslipidemic patients in United State of America are using statins[1] These agents widely used among cardiovascular patients in Malaysia[2]. In other countries, for example in UK, it has found that most patients who use statins are older than 35 years old and more of them are males (56%)[3]. In Canada, about 90% of cardiac patients are using statin, while in US, at least one third of all cardiac patients are using statins[4]. About 60% of American patients who older than 60 years old are using statin[5]. Thus, high number of users contributed to increase the risk of adverse drug reactions (ADRs).

The Food and Drug Administration (FDA) has determined that common statin-associated ADRs are fatigue, muscle pain, joints pain, back pain, visual disturbance and insomnia[6,7]. Previous studies have examined the incidence of these ADRs, and their results showed that more than half of the reported cases of muscle pain were related to statin use[8,9]. Clearfield et al found that fatigue, muscle pain, and bone pain were common and frequent ADRs in UK, and related to atorvastatin and rosuvastatin use[10]. Other studies exploring ADRs in patients using atorvastatin and lovastatin in the US found that muscle pain and fatigue were the most common statin-related ADRs[11]. The UK Committee on Safety of Medicines, as well as other studies, have reported that these symptoms should consider as early signs for more serious ADRs[8,12-15]. However, from our knowledge, no data available on the common ADRs statin-related and their predictors for Asian patients. Only a few studies (not related with Asian patients) have found out the predictors of the statin-related ADRs[8,9,10,16,17]. As health care professional, they should find methods to ensure patients not only receive effective medication but also feel comfortable with the therapy. Thus, the objectives of this study was to determine the common statin-related ADRs and their predictors in one of the referral hospital in Malaysia (one of country in South East Asia).

2. Method

Cross-sectional with convenient sampling study conducted for volunteer outpatients from the cardiac clinic of Penang Hospital in Pulau Pinang State of Malaysia. Study protocol was approved by Clinical Research Committee of Penang General Hospital, and signed consent forms were obtained from all participants. The patients included in this study were at least 18 years old and voluntarily to participate in this study. They have to used statins and could understand Malay Language (the National Language of Malaysia) or English Language, since Malaysia is a multiracial country. Patients who allergies to statin, pregnant or lactating women, or changing in types or dosage of statin used were excluded from this study. These types of patients excluded because their conditions may affected outcomes of the study. The study period was 5 months, and 1900 patients presented in the cardiac clinic within this study period. Depending on inclusion and exclusion criteria, 500 patients voluntarily agreed to participate in this study. A validated questionnaire form (Cronbach's alpha is 0.853) were used for reporting of ADRs. The patients were asked whether they have experience of common statin-related ADRs while they were on statin therapy and give their answers on the self-report questionnaire forms. This questionnaire form has some questions on demographic data and undesired symptoms that patients had during statin therapy. There were 27 ADRs of statin listed in the questionnaire form. They were required to tick yes or no on these listed ADRs. They can tick more than one ADR. In order to ensure these ADRs really related with statin therapy these patients had to indicate in the questionnaire form that these ADRs occurred while they were receiving statin therapy and these symptoms should continuously occurred at least for 3 months.

3. Statistics

Statistical Package for Social Science software (SPSS) version 18 used to analyze the data for this study. Odd ratio and Chi-square and logistic regression tests were used to ensure these ADRs were related with stain therapy and to determine their predictors. The results with p value less than 0.05 was considered statistically significant.

4. Results

Male patients (70%) were the more frequent users of statins, with mean age 60±10 years. The most frequent race that used statins was Chinese (37.6%), followed by Malays (34.4%), Indians (26.6%) and foreigners (1.4%). Small numbers of patients were cigarette smoker (12%) and alcohol consumers (9%).

Higher number of patients had dyslipidemia with primary type (51.5%) based on the Friedewald et al[18] and Stone et al[19] classifications. For primary subtypes of dyslipidemia, the most common subtype was IIa (50.6%), while common subtype of secondary dyslipidemia was diabetes (86.3%). The common type of statin used was lovastatin (81%), followed by simvastatin (9.4%) and atorvastatin (8%). The low dose (20 mg) of statin was the common prescribed to these patients. The mean duration of statin therapy was 3.5 years and the most frequent range of duration was 1-5 years (52.5%), as shown in Table 1.

Statistical regression analysis was used to exclude symptoms related to other medications and diseases. It found only few symptoms from 27 ADRs that correlated significantly with statins were; fatigue (59.4%), muscle pain (53.6%), joint pain (53.4%), back pain (47.8%), insomnia (44.8%) and visual disturbances (44.2%).

Demographics	Variables	No (%)
Gender	Male	351 (70%)
	Female	149 (30%)
Race	Malay	172 (34.4%)
	Chinese	188 (37.6%)
	Indian	133 (26.6%)
	Foreign	7 (1.4%)
Age (mean 60±10)year	28-50 year	94 (19%)
	51-65 year	258 (51%)
	66-92 year	148 (30%)
Smoke	Yes	59 (12%)
	No	441 (88%)
Alcohol consuming	Yes	47 (9%)
	No	453 (91%)
Dyslipidiemia type	Primary	247 (51.5%)
	Secondary	233 (48.5%)
Primary dyslipidemia subtype	I	13 (5.3%)
	IIa	125 (50.6%)
	IIb	59 (23.9%)
	III	7 (2.8%)
	IV	32 (13%)
	V	11 (4.5%)
Secondary dyslipidemia subtype	Renal	17 (7.3%)
	Diabetes	201 (86.3%)
	Nephrotic syndrome	1 (0.4%)
	Liver	1 (0.4%)
	Drugs	2 (0.9%)
	Hypothyroidism	11 (4.7%)
Type of statin	Atorvastatin	40 (8%)
	Simvastatin	47 (9.4%)
	Lovastatin	405 (81%)
	others	8 (1.6)
Combination therapy	Yes	35 (7%)
	No	465 (93%)
Duration of therapy Mean (3.5±3.0) year	3months or less	16 (3.2%)
	3months -1 year	133 (26.7%)
	1-5 years	262 (52.5%)
	5-20 years	89 (17.6%)

Table 1. Demographic data of 500 cardiac outpatients in Penang General Hospital

Predictors	ADRs (percentage, P value, OR, CI)					
	Fatigue	Muscle pain	Joint pain	Back pain	Insomnia	Visual disturbances
Gender (female)	NS	NS	61.74%, P=0.007, OR= 1.864, CI= 1.18-2.94	56.38%, P= 0.02, OR= 1.73, CI= 1.09-2.75	NS	NS
Race (Indian)	68.42%, P=0.027, OR= 1.81, CI= 2.14-2.75)	66.92%, P= 0.016, OR=1.94, CI= 1.13-3.32)	NS	62.4%, P=0.007, OR= 2.18, CI= 1.23-3.72	NS	49.62%, P=0.016, OR= 1.74, CI= 1.11-2.73)
Smokers	NS	NS	NS	NS	NS	NS
Alcoholic	76.60%, P= 0.011, OR= 3.0 CI= 1.29-7.01)	NS	NS	65.96%, P= 0.003, OR= 3.58, CI= 1.53-8.38	59.57%, P=0.006, OR= 2.89, CI= 1.36-6.15	NS
Age	NS	NS	NS	NS	NS	NS
Duration More than 5 years	53.41%, P=0.036, OR= 1.83, CI= 1.04-3.23)	60.23%, P=0.016, OR=1.96, CI= 1.133-3.39	NS	57.95%, P=0.001, OR=2.61, CI= 1.50-4.54)	NS	NS
Primary subtypes (type IIb)	NS	NS	NS	33.90%, P= 0.014, OR= 2.50, CI= 1.21-5.19)	NS	NS
Secondary subtypes (renal disease)	NS	NS	NS	NS	64.71%, P= 0.33, OR= 3.7, CI= 1.11-12.33	NS
Statin types	NS	NS	NS	NS	NS	NS
Atorvastatin doses (20mg)	NS	NS	NS	NS	NS	NS

Simvastatin dose (40mg)	NS	NS	NS	NS	NS	NS
Lovastatin doses (60mg)	72.73%, P=0.003, OR= 1.90, CI= 1.25-2.89)	NS	NS	NS	NS	NS
Combination therapy	NS	NS	NS	NS	NS	NS

NS= no significant

Table 2. Relationship between statin related ADRs and predictors

In term of predictor, females significantly had joint pain (61.74%, OR = 1.864) and back pain (56.38%, OR = 1.73). However, there was no significant relation between gender with fatigue, muscle pain, insomnia and visual disturbance. Indian patients had significantly higher incidence of fatigue (68.42%, OR= 1.81), muscle pain (66.92%, OR =1.94), back pain (62.4 %, OR = 2.18), and visual disturbances (49.62 %, OR = 1.738) when compared to other races. No significant relationship found between smoking and statin related-ADRs. Patients who consumed alcohol significantly had fatigue (76.6%, OR = 3.0), back pain (65.96%, OR = 3.584) and insomnia (59.57%, OR = 2.893). Age was without effect on incidence of statin related-ADRs. Patients used statins for more than 5 years significantly had fatigue (53.41%, OR = 1.83) and muscle pain (60.23%, OR =1.958), as shown in Table 2.

For secondary dyslipidemia types, renal induced dyslipidemia significantly caused higher incidence of insomnia when compared to the other secondary subtypes (64.71%, OR = 3.7). For subtypes of primary dyslipidemia, subtype IIb patients had significantly back pain (81.82%, OR = 2.5).

No significant relationship found between statin related-ADRs and statin types, the patients used simvastatin had a higher incidence of fatigue (65.96%), joint pain (57.45%), back pain (55.32%) and visual disturbance (53.19%). Patients used lovastatin had insomnia (45.68%), while patients used atorvastatin had higher incidence of muscle pain (52.17%). No significant relationship found between doses of statins and other ADRs except for lovastatin dose. Patients used 60 mg dose of lovastatin had significantly fatigue than patients used lower doses (72.73%, OR = 1.904). No significant relation found between the combination with other lipid lowering agents and incidence of ADRs (as shown in Table 2).

5. Discussion

After two decades of statin marketing, significant incidences of adverse drug reactions still presented during therapy. Number of studies of medications' ADRs always increased after first years of launching, but it found this matter is different with type of statin used[20]. Most of previous studies focused on serious ADRs of statin like muscle toxicity, elevation of liver enzymes, renal toxicity and polyneuropathy[21,22]. Although serious ADRs caused mortalities and death to patients, but their incidences are lower than other adverse reactions of statin symptomatic related ADRs. Kashani A. et al. [23] found that incidences of patients discontinued their therapy because of symptomatic ADRs of statin (5.6%) were higher than patients had rhabdomyolysis (0.2%), hepatotoxicity (1.4%), and creatine kinase (CK) elevations (0.9%). Therefore, self-reporting of ADRs are useful to determine and predict the toxicities induced by medication[24]. There are few studies done on the common statin-related ADRs that use patient self-report. There was a previous study that focused on the common ADRs during statin therapy and their predictors in cardiac outpatients. They reported the use of a self-report questionnaire form is suitable approach to assess the common undesired symptoms found during statin therapy[25]. In the real-life practice, doctors are more focusing on dyslipidemia and its complications than statin-related ADRs of their patients. Furthermore, self-report approach allows the patients to express directly their unwanted problems associated with statin therapy. In addition, patients sometimes feel uncomfortable or inappropriate telling their doctor about these undesired symptoms of statin[26,27]. The finding in this study showed a higher incidence of fatigue and muscle pain in this cardiac outpatients setting, which consistent with previous studies[8,10].

In this study, females reported having back and joint pain significantly more than males did. Female patients are more sensitive to ADRs than males possibly because of pharmacokinetic and pharmacodynamic differences between genders[28]. Not all ADRs of statin related to gender, this finding supported by FDA, Bayer reports and previous studies[29-32]. When compared to other races, Indian patients had significantly higher incidence of some common ADRs (fatigue, muscle pain, back pain and visual disturbance). This is because genetics also has contributed in adverse drug reactions[23]. This result was supported by FDA reports in which ADRs were different among races[7]. Cigarette smokers had increased incidence of these ADRs than nonsmokers, however this finding was not statistically significant. Alcohol consumers had significant problems with fatigue, back pain and insomnia, and increased incidence of ADRs in general[30]. This is because alcohol causes mitochondrial dysfunction, which would increase the risk of muscle disorders caused by statins[33]. There was no relationship between age and ADRs, as shown in Table 2, which supported by Kucukarslan et al study[34]. There was a relationship between duration of statin used and ADRs in previous studies[29,35,36]. Their finding were consistent with this present finding, where the duration of statin therapy has related to fatigue, muscle pain and back pain.

Based on our knowledge, no previous studies reported the relationship between dyslipidemia types and the common ADRs. Significant relationship was found in this study between dyslipidemia type (primary and secondary) and common ADRs. Patients who had secondary dyslipidemia type had increase frequency of insomnia than with primary type. Patients with subtype IIb and renal induced dyslipidemia were significantly more likely to have back pain and insomnia than other subtypes.

Although statins differ in their pharmacokinetic properties[37,38], there is no significant relationship found between statin types and common ADRs. However, simvastatin was more likely to cause fatigue, joint pain, back pain and visual disturbance than other statins. Although there is no significant relation found between atorvastatin and common ADRs. Atorvastatin found to cause muscle pain more often than other statin types, this finding also proved by Clearfield et al. and Golomb et al. [10,11]. Patients on lovastatin therapy had higher incidence of insomnia than other types of statin. Higher doses for all types of statins have resulted in a higher incidence of ADRs. The higher dose of lovastatin (60 mg) significantly associated with fatigue. The dose of statins used did not have significant relationship with other symptoms of common ADRs. This result is consistent with other studies[12,39]. Finally, there was no significant relationship between combination therapy and ADRs. This relationship could not be seen possibly due to small number of patients receiving more than one type of antilipidemic agent.

The finding of this study showed that significant number of patients feel undesired effects of statin therapy and their predictors. Adjustment or manipulating of these preventable predictors such as to change type of statin used, reduce dose and duration are recommended to the prescribers. For example, based on the odd ratio, fatigue was the highest for patients who are alcohol consumers, followed by lovastatin dosage, duration and race. Therefore, steps needed to reduce the incidence of fatigue by avoiding or reducing the preventable predictors that related to these common ADRs like cessation of alcohol and changing in type or dose of statin used.

6. Conclusion

This paper explained that significant number of cardiac outpatients were experienced common ADRs related-statin through self-report approach and their predictors. Common ADRs of statin were fatigue, muscle pain, joint pain, back pain, insomnia and visual disturbances. The main predictors or contributing factors of common statin-related ADRs were gender, race, alcohol consumption, duration of statin used, renal induced-secondary dyslipidemia, subtype IIb of primary dyslipidemia and lovastatin dose. These predictors are useful in clinical practice to determine the likelihood of ADRs and to manage the common ADRs of statin in cardiac outpatients. Finding from this study was suggested appropriate dose and type of statin use and also adjustment of the preventable predictors may minimize common ADRs of statin in cardiac outpatients. Appropriate prospective study design with multicenter sites recommended determining the actual effects of these preventable predictors on common ADRs of statin.

7. References

[1] Avorn J, Monette J, Lacour A, Bohn RL, Monane M, Mogun H, LeLorier J.(1998). Persistence of Use of Lipid-Lowering Medications: a cross-national study. Journal of the American Medical Association 279:1458-1462

[2] National Cardiovascular Disease Database (NCVD) (2006), Malaysia

[3] Dewilde S, Carey IM, Bremner SA, Richards N, Hilton SR, Cook DG (2003). Evolution of statin prescribing 1994–2001: a case of agism but not of sexism? Heart 89:417–421

[4] National Cholesterol Education Program (NCEP) (2002). Expert panel on detection, evaluation, and treatment of high blood cholesterol in adults (adult treatment panel III). Third report of the national cholesterol education program (NCEP) expert panel on detection, evaluation, and treatment of high blood cholesterol in adults (Adult Treatment Panel III) final report 106:3143–3421

[5] Farahani P, Gaebel K, Lelorier J, Perrault S, Gillis J, Soon J, Levine M (2005). Assessment of patient characteristics associated with statin use. The Canadian Journal of Clinical Pharmacology 12: e41-e149: 31

[6] AHFS (2007). HMG-CoA Reductase Inhibitors (Statins) – Safety Overview. Drug Information Service, University of Utah.

[7] U.S food and drug administration: Rosuvastatin Calcium (marketed as Crestor) Information Patient information sheet. (2005) [Online]. [10th March 2008] available from World Wide Web:

http://www.fda.gov/cder/drug/ infopage/rosuvastatin/default.htm

[8] Thompson PD, Clarkson P, Karas RH. (2003). Statin associated Myopathy. Journal of the American Medical Association 289:1681–1690

[9] Ballantyne CM, Corsini A, Davidson MH, Holdaas H, Jacobson TA, Lieitersdorf E, Marz W., Reckless, J PD, Stein EA (2003). Risk for myopathy with statin therapy in high-risk patients. Archive of Internal Medicine 163: 553-564.

[10] Clearfield MB, Amerena J, Bassand JP, Hernández García HR, Miller SS, Sosef FF, Palmer MK and Bryzinski BS (2006). Comparison of the efficacy and safety of rosuvastatin 10 mg and atorvastatin 20 mg in high-risk patients with hypercholesterolemia – prospective study to evaluate the use of low doses of the statins atorvastatin and rosuvastatin (PULSAR). Licensee Biomed Central Ltd. Trial 7:35

[11] Golomb BA, Yang E, Denenberg J, Criqui M (2003). Statin-associated adverse events. Circulation 107; e7001-e7039, 95

[12] Pasternak RC, Smith SCJ, Bairey-Merz CN, Grundy SM, Cleeman JI, Lenfant C (2002). ACC/AHA/NHLBI Clinical advisory on the use and safety of statins. Journal of the American College of Cardiology 106: 567–572

[13] Hamilton CI (2003). Statins and muscle damage. Australian Prescriber 26:74-75

[14] Gaist D, Jeppesen U, Andersen M, García Rodríguez LA, Hallas J, Sindrup SH (2002). Statins and risk of polyneuropathy: a case-control study. Neurology 14; 58(9):1321-2.

[15] Committee on safety of medicines (2001). Cerivastatin (lipobay) withdrawn. Current Problem in Pharmacovigillance 27: 9

[16] Shepherd J, Cobbe SM, Ford I, Isles CG, Lorimer AR, MacFarlane PW, McKillop JH, Packard CJ (1995). Prevention of coronary heart disease with pravastatin in men with hypercholesterolemia. West of Scotland Coronary Prevention Study Group (WOSCOPS). The New England Journal of Medicine 333:1301-1307

[17] Cheryl A (2007). HMG-CoA Reductase Inhibitors/Statins, PHARMD, UCSF School of Pharmacy, University of California at San Francisco.

[18] Friedewald WT, Levy RI, Fredrickson DS (1972). Estimation of the concentration of low-density lipoprotein cholesterol in plasma without use of the preparative ultracentrifuge. Clinical Chemistry 18:499-502.

[19] Stone NJ and Blum CB (2008). Management of Lipids in Clinical Practice. Professional Communications p80

[20] Brown WV (2008). Safety of statins. Curr Opin Lipidol 19(6):558-62

[21] Zipes DP, Zvaifler NJ, Glassock RJ, Gilman S, Muñoz A, Gogolak V, Gordis L, Dedon PC, Guengerich FP, Wasserman SI, Witztum JL, Wogan GN (2006). Rosuvastatin: an independent analysis of risks and benefits. MedGenMed 8(2):73.

[22] Silva MA, Swanson AC, Gandhi PJ, Tataronis GR (2006). Statin-related adverse events: a meta-analysis. Clin Ther 28(1):26-35.

[23] Kashani A, Phillips CO, Foody JM, Wang Y, Mangalmurti S, Ko DT, Krumholz HM (2006). Risks associated with statin therapy: a systematic overview of randomized clinical trials. Circulation 114(25):2788-97.

[24] Grundy SM (2005). The issue of statin safety: where do we stand? Circulation 111:3016-3019

[25] Gholami K., Ziaie S., and Shalviri G (2008). Adverse drug reactions induced by cardiovascular drugs in outpatients. Pharmacy Practice 6(1):51-55.

[26] Golomb BA, Kane T and Dimsdale JE (2004). Severe irritability associated with statin cholesterol-lowering agents. The Quarterly Journal of Medicine 97:229-235.

[27] Golomb BA, Mcgraw JJ, Evans MA and Dimsdale JE (2007). Physician response to patient reports of adverse drug effects. Drug Safety 30(8): 669-675.

[28] Sigonda N (2003). guidelines for monitoring and reporting adverse drug reactions (ADRs) made under section 5 (c) of the Tanzania food, drugs and cosmetics Act 2003

[29] Alsheikh-Ali AA, Ambrose MS, Kuvin JT, Karas RH (2005). The safety of rosuvastatin as used in common clinical practice: a postmarketing analysis. Circulation 111:3051-3057.

[30] Hanston PD, and Horn JR (1998). Drug interactions with HMG CoA reductase inhibitors. Drug Interactions Newsletter 103-6

[31] EMEA (2002) Scientific conclusion and ground for withdrawal of the marketing authorization presented, CPMP/811/02

[32] Gray SL, Mahoney JE, Blough DK (1999). Adverse drug events in elderly patients receiving home health services following hospital discharge. The Annals of Pharmacotherapy 33:1147-1153

[33] Mabuchi H, Nohara A, Kobayashi J, Kawashiri MA, Inazu A (2007). Coenzyme Q10 Reduction with Statins: Another Pleiotropic Effect Current Drug Therapy 2: 39-51

[34] Kucukarslan SN, Peters M, Mlynarek M, Nafziger DA (2003). Pharmacists on rounding teams reduce preventable adverse drug events in hospital general medicine units. Arch Intern Med 22;163(17):2014-8.

[35] Corrao G, Zambon A, Bertù L, Botteri E, Leoni O, Contiero P (2004). Lipid lowering drugs prescription and the risk of peripheral neuropathy: an exploratory case-control study using automated databases. Journal of Epidemiology Community Health 58:1047–1051.

[36] Agostini JV, Tinetti ME, Ling H, Mcavay G, Foody JM and Concato J (2007). Effects of Statin use on muscle strength, Cognition, and Depressive Symptoms In older adults. The American Journal of Geriatric Cardiology in Society 55:420–425

[37] Jones P, Kafonek S, Laurora I, Hunninghake D (1998). Comparative dose efficacy study of atorvastatin versus simvastatin, pravastatin, lovastatin, and fluvastatin in patients with hypercholesterolemia (The Curves Study). The American Journal of Cardiology 81:582–587

[38] Corsini A, Bellosta S, Baetta R, Fumagalli R, Paoletti R, Bernini F (1999). New insights into the pharmacodynamic and pharmacokinetic properties of statins. Pharmacology and Therapeutic 84:413-428

[39] Ravnskov U, Rosch PJ, Sutter MC, Houston MC (2006). Should we lower cholesterol as much as possible? BMJ 332(7553):1330-1332.

Fenofibrate: Panacea for Aging-Related Conditions?

Makoto Goto

Division of Anti-Ageing & Longevity Sciences, Faculty of Medical Technology, Department of BioMedical Engineering, Toin University of Yokohama, Japan

1. Introduction

Fenofibrate, a selective peroxisome proliferator-activated receptors alpha (PPAR-α) activator, has been primarily developed to treat human dyslipidemia. PPAR modulate the expression of genes involved in lipid metabolism through peroxisome proliferator response elements (Willson et al., 2000). Although fenofibrate became commercially available in 1974 (Fournier, Inc., France), its lipid-lowering action mechanism has not been clarified until the late 1990's, contributing to open new research doors. With respect to the mechanisms of action, the drug with pleiotropic activity may be regarded as a "21st-century agent" (Staels et al., 1995).

Fenofibrate as a ligand of PPAR-α exhibits lipid-lowering effects by activating PPAR-α.

PPAR-α activators stimulate the β-oxidation of fatty acids in the liver resulting in a decreased availability of fatty acids for triglyceride (TG) synthesis (Schoonjans et al., 1995, 1996a, 1996b). In addition, fenofibrate enhances the production of apo-AI and apo-AII: the major component of HDL by activating PPAR-α and increases plasma level of HDL-C directly (Vu-Dac, 1994, 1995). Thus, the lipid-lowering action mechanism of fenofibrate involves potent TG-reducing and HDL-C-increasing actions. Statins, another type of lipid-lowering agent do not show such actions, though statins can inhibit hydroxymethylglutaryl (HMG)-CoA reductase (Endo A, 1992).

Furthermore, fenofibrate decreased the level of low-density lipoprotein cholesterol (LDL-C), especially "small dense LDL", which may be a powerful metabolic contributor to arteriosclerosis (Superko, 2000).

PPAR-α regulates the transcription of lipid-associated genes and various genes involved in homeostasis, suggesting the PPAR-α-mediated pleiotropic activities of fenofibrate. The reports on the pleiotropic activities of fenofibrate has been accumulated in a variety of large-scale, randomized, controlled trials (RCTs).

The studies presumably associated with the anti-aging actions of fenofibrate are reviewed in this article.

2. Clinical efficacy

The pleiotropic activities other than the lipid-lowering actions reported in clinical practice: the anti-inflammatory, antioxidant, and serum uric acid-reducing actions of fenofibrate are reviewed in this section. These activities may be tightly associated with anti-aging actions of fenofibrate. Three large-scale, randomized, comparative clinical studies of fenofibrate ("DAIS", "FIELD" and "ACCORD"), in which intervention was performed in patients with type II diabetes mellitus (DM), were published since 2000.

2.1 Anti-aging activities

Previous studies reported the involvement of various clinical parameters in anti-aging actions of fenofibrate (Schlesinger et al., 2009). In particular, chronic, systemic, silent, low-grade inflammation, named inflammaging is the target for intensive research in aging study (Goto, 2008b). Ross et al. defined arteriosclerosis as "chronic vascular inflammation" resulting from an interaction between oxidized lipid and macrophages (Ross, 1999). Inflammation is involved in the onset of arteriosclerotic disorders and acute coronary syndrome. Furthermore, oxidative stress that can induce a vicious cycle of chronic inflammation has been believed to be the major driving force to promote aging (Yu & Chung, 2001; Romano et al., 2010).

Uric acid has recently been considered to be a prognostic factor for the onset of DM and dementia that may accelerate aging (Hikita et al., 2007; Abate et al., 2004; Martinon et al., 2006), although an excess level of uric acid is the primary incite for gouty attack (Schlesinger et al., 2009).

2.1.1 Anti-inflammatory actions

The anti-inflammatory actions of fenofibrate were reported in Nature in 1998 (Staels et al., 1998). PPAR-α ligand: fenofibrate inhibited cyclooxygenase-2 (COX-2) expression and prostaglandin production by suppressing the transcription of COX-2 genes through the inhibition of nuclear factor κB (NF-κB: transcription factor) signals. Fenofibrate administration decreased the inflammatory parameters including serum levels of IL-6, fibrinogen, and C-reactive protein (CRP) in coronary disease patients and the patients with hypertriglyceridemia (Tsimihodimos et al., 2004; Muhlestein et al., 2006).

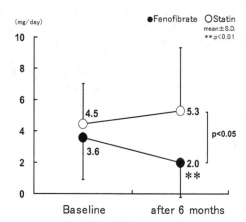

Closed circles represent fenofibrate; open circles represent statins. mean ± S.D.
Wilcoxon signed rank test versus baseline, ** P <0.01, Mann-Whitney U test versus group

Fig. 1. Changes in prednisolone (PSL) dosage.

We compared the anti-inflammatory effects of fenofibrate and statins in 44 patients with a chronic inflammatory disorder: rheumatoid arthritis (RA) (Goto, 2010). Japanese patients with RA and dyslipidemia were randomly divided into 2 groups: fenofibrate (Lipidil, Kaken Pharmaceutical Co., Ltd., micronized fenofibrate at 200 mg/day, n=23) and statins (n=21) groups. After 6-month administration, the laboratory data were compared, and pain was evaluated using the visual analogue scale (VAS) and dose change of prednisolone (PSL) was monitored. The VAS scores significantly decreased in the fenofibrate (from 49.1 to 14.7 mm, p<0.0001) and statin (from 47.4 to 20.2 mm, p<0.001) groups. The dose of PSL significantly reduced only in the fenofibrate group (from 3.58 to 2.00 mg/day, p<0.01). The reduction rate was also significantly better than in the statin group (Fig. 1).

In the fenofibrate group, a significant correlation was between the rate of change in the ΔVAS score and that in the ΔCRP level (Fig.2. p<0.05). The results suggest that, in patients with RA, fenofibrate exhibits more potent anti-inflammatory effects compared to statins.

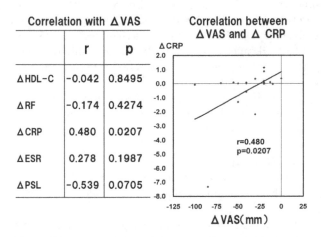

Correlation with ΔVAS		
	r	p
ΔHDL-C	-0.042	0.8495
ΔRF	-0.174	0.4274
ΔCRP	0.480	0.0207
ΔESR	0.278	0.1987
ΔPSL	-0.539	0.0705

Spearman rank correlation coefficient

VAS visual analogue scale; HDL-C high-density lipoprotein-cholesterol; RF rheumatoid factor; CRP C-reactive protein; ESR erythrocyte sedimentation rate; PSL prednisolone

Fig. 2. Fenofibrate administration group: correlation between anti-inflammatory markers and ΔVAS.

2.1.2 Antioxidant actions

Oxidative stress has been considered to promote aging (Harman, 1978; Yu & Chung, 2001; Romano et al., 2010). As for oxidative stress markers that can be measured on clinical examination, serum lipids, MDA-LDL and Ox-LDL, and urinary lipids, 8-OHdG and 15-isoprostane F2t: 8-epi-PGF2α/8-isoPGF2α, are employed (Harman, 1978; Yu& Chung, 2001). Coenzyme Q10 (CoQ10), also known as ubiquinone shows antioxidant actions and has been monitored as an in vivo marker of oxidative stress.

CoQ10 is biosynthesized from mevalonic acid in the liver. As the pathway of CoQ10 biosynthesis is partially overlapped with that of cholesterol synthesis, the administration of an HMG-CoA reductase inhibitor, statins, reduces the production of CoQ10. Therefore, statins, represented by atorvastatin, also inhibit CoQ10 biosynthesis in vivo, leading to the increase in oxidative stress (Mabuchi et al., 2005).

The administration of standard fenofibrate at 150 mg/day to 18 Japanese type II DM with dyslipidemia for 12 weeks significantly decreased the triglyceride (TG) level (from 232±109 to 145±74 mg/dL, -37%, p<0.01), and significantly improved the HDL-C level (from 45±8.7 to 52±9.8 mg/dL, +14%, p<0.01) (Asano et al., 2006).

The plasma ubiquinol-10 level in fenofibrate group increased significantly after 8 weeks (from 768±265 to 886±310 nM, p<0.05) and after 12 weeks (from 768±265 to 894±336 nM, p<0.05). However, total plasma CoQ10 level (ubiquinol-10 plus ubiquinone-10) as an oxidative stress marker, decreased in statin group, elevated in fenofibrate group after 12 weeks administration (from 1010±296 to 1070±285 nM, +6%). In addition, plasma ubiquinone-10 in fenofibrate group decreased insignificantly. Fenofibrate treatment elevates plasma CoQ10, especially plasma ubiquinol-10 level.

In the wild-type mice administered by diethylhexylphthalate (DEHP: PPAR-α activator), elevation of plasma ubiquinone was significant, but the elevation was not observed in the PPAR-α-null mice (Turunen et al., 2000). In addition, the expression of PPAR-α gene was regulated in the liver of SAMP1 (senescence accelerated mouse prone 1) mice given ubiquinol for long term (Schmelzer et al., 2010a, 2010b). Although the antioxidant action mechanisms of fenofibrate remained unclear in human, mice studies suggested the direct interaction between CoQ10 and PPAR-α.

Fenofibrate not only restores the serum lipid profiles, but also suppresses oxidative stress. Fenofibrate with a variety of pleiotropic activities may protect the pathogenesis and progression of aging-associated atherosclerosis.

2.1.3 Serum uric acid-reducing actions

Hyperuricemia, a common co-morbidity in the patients with metabolic syndrome and dyslipidemia has recently been emphasized as an independent risk factor for cardiovascular disease (Lippi et al., 2008).

Kodama et al. performed a meta-analysis of 11 clinical studies, and reported that a 1-mg/dL increase in the serum uric acid level significantly elevated the relative risk of type II DM by 1.17-fold (Kodama et al., 2009). Schretlen et al. investigated 96 persons aged 60 to 92 years, and indicated that the information-processing capacity and memory were reduced in persons with high uric acid level, suggesting that the serum uric acid level may be a prognostic factor for dementia (Schretlen et al., 2007). Thus, hyperuricemia may play a role not only in the onset of cardiovascular disease but also in the promotion of dementia and aging.

Fenofibrate has been known to reduce the serum levels of lipids and also uric acid (Schlesinger et al., 2009). The serum uric acid-reducing action mechanism of fenofibrate, independent of lipid-profile changes, involves the promotion of uric-acid excretion (Liamis et al., 1999).

Urate Transporter 1 (URAT1), the target molecule of uric acid-reducing agents such as benzbromarone was identified which is responsible for the reabsorption of uric acid in the proximal uriniferous tubule (Enomoto et al., 2002). Furthermore, URAT1 inhibition was involved in the serum uric acid-reducing action mechanism of fenofibrate (Uetake et al., 2010). According to their study, the single-dose administration of standard fenofibrate at 300 mg to healthy adults decreased the serum uric acid level by approximately 1.5 mg/dL. In Japan, fenofibrate has been administered to metabolic syndrome patients with hyperuricemia, leading to the decrease in the serum uric acid level by approximately 2 mg/dL.

2.2 Randomized controlled trial (RCT)

Large-scale, randomized, controlled clinical trials of fenofibrate involving type II DM, that is, high-risk patients for arteriosclerosis, were conducted. The representative 3 studies were reviewed in this section: "DAIS" study, regarding coronary arteriosclerosis retraction, "FIELD" study, in which the inhibitory effects on cardiovascular events were examined, and "ACCORD" study, in which the inhibitory effects of lipid-intensified therapy with statins on cardiovascular events were investigated.

2.2.1 Diabetes Atherosclerosis Intervention Study (DAIS)

The DAIS is a placebo-controlled, double-blind, comparative study to verify whether the deterioration of coronary arteriosclerosis can be prevented by restoring abnormal lipid metabolism with fenofibrate in type II diabetics employing quantitative coronary angiography (DAIS investigators, 2001). This international, interventional study was conducted based on the World Health Organization (WHO)'s request and cooperation. This study is the first interventional study in which it was prospectively evaluated whether the correction of disturbance of lipid metabolism in type II DM prevents the deterioration of arteriosclerosis. It was carried out in Canada, Finland, Sweden, and France. Four-hundred and eighteen patients with type II diabetes in whom blood sugar control was favourable were randomly divided into fenofibrate (micronized fenofibrate, 200 mg/day, n=207) and placebo (n=211) groups to evaluate the deterioration of coronary arteriosclerosis using quantitative coronary angiography after 38-month (mean duration) administration.

In the fenofibrate group, a decrease in the minimum lumen diameter and an increase in the percent stenosiswere significantly suppressed in comparison with the placebo group (by 40%), confirming the inhibitory effects of fenofibrate on the deterioration of coronary arteriosclerosis in type II DM.

In the continuing study of DAIS, fenofibrate reduced the small dense LDL level, leading to the inhibition of the deterioration of diabetic nephropathy (DAIS investigators, 2003, 2005), confirming that fenofibrate inhibited the deterioration of macro- and micro-angiopathy in type II DM.

2.2.2 Fenofibrate Intervention and Event Lowering in Diabetes Study (FIELD)

The FIELD is a study to verify the inhibitory effects of fenofibrate on cardiovascular events involving approximately 10,000 patients with type II DM (FIELD investigators, 2005). It was conducted in Finland, Australia, and New Zealand. The subjects were 9,795 type II diabetics with mild dyslipidemia. They were randomly divided into fenofibrate (micronized fenofibrate, 200 mg/day, n=4,895) and placebo (n=4,900) groups. Each agent was administered for 5 years.

In the fenofibrate group, this agent inhibited the incidence of coronary events by 11% in comparison with the placebo group. Unfortunately, there was no significant difference between two groups. This was possibly because statins were combined with the placebo/fenofibrate in 32% of patients receiving the placebo and in 16% of patients receiving fenofibrate, reducing the effects of fenofibrate alone. Fenofibrate decreased the incidence of non-fatal myocardial infarction by 24% (p<0.05) and that of total cardiovascular events by 11% (p<0.05), confirming its efficacy.

In primary prevention patients without a history of cardiovascular disease, accounting for approximately 80%, fenofibrate significantly inhibited the incidences of coronary (by 25%) and total cardiovascular (by 19%) events in comparison with the placebo group. Furthermore, in the FIELD, fenofibrate inhibited the onset of diabetic nephropathy, deterioration of diabetic retinopathy, proportion of patients undergoing lower-limb amputation, and deterioration of diabetic neuropathy (FIELD investigators, 2005, 2007, 2009, 2010, 2011). As fenofibrate reduced DM-associated 3 major complications (retinopathy, nephropathy and neuropathy), this agent may be useful for treating diabetic complications.

Study name	Micro/macro-angiopathy	Rate of decrease in the relative risk	p value	Reference
DAIS	Diabetic nephropathy	progression in albumin excretion fenofibrate 8%, Placebo 18%	p<0.05	DAIS investigators, 2005
FIELD	Diabetic nephropathy	-14%	p=0.002	FIELD investigators, 2005, 2011
	Diabetic retinopathy	-31%	p<0.001	FIELD investigators, 2007
	Lower-limb amputation	-36%	p=0.02	FIELD investigators, 2009
	Diabetic neuropathy	-40%	p=0.009	FIELD investigators, 2010
ACCORD-Lipid	Diabetic nephropathy	incidence of microalbuminuria fenofibrate 38.2%, Placebo 41.6%	p=0.01	ACCORD Study Group, 2010
		incidence of macroalbuminuria fenofibrate 10.5%, Placebo 12.3%	p=0.04	
ACCORD-EYE	Diabetic retinopathy	-40%	p=0.006	ACCORD Study Group; ACCORD Eye Study Group, 2010

Table 1. Inhibitory effects of fenofibrate on diabetic angiopathy in a large-scale clinical study involving type II DM

2.2.3 ACCORD-Lipid & ACCORD-EYE study

In the ACCORD-Lipid study, the inhibitory effects of 3 intensified/standard medicinal therapies (blood sugar, blood pressure, lipids) on compound cardiovascular events were investigated in approximately 10,000 type II diabetics with mild dyslipidemia and the high risk of cardiovascular disease (CVD) under the auspices of the National Institutes of Health (NIH). Lipid intervention was performed in 5,518 patients: intensified (simvastatin 20mg + micronized fenofibrate 200mg) and standard (simvastatin 20mg + placebo) therapies. The mean follow-up was 4.7 years. In the fenofibrate-combined group, the incidence of cardiovascular events was inhibited by 8%, although there was no significant difference. In patients with a pre-treatment TG level of 204 mg/dL or more and HDL-C level of 34 mg/dL or less, significant inhibitory effects on events were confirmed (-31% ($p<0.05$), NNT=20) (ACCORD Study Group et al., 2010).

In the ACCORD–EYE study, the deterioration of diabetic retinopathy was evaluated in 2,856 patients from whom informed consent was obtained (lipid intervention: 1,593 patients) among type II DM who participated in the ACCORD-Lipid study (ACCORD Study Group; ACCORD Eye Study Group et al., 2010). In the fenofibrate-combined group, intensified therapy significantly inhibited the deterioration of diabetic retinopathy (by 40%) in comparison with the simvastatin group ($p=0.006$). The ACCORD–EYE study, the second large-scale clinical study following the FIELD, demonstrated the inhibitory effects of fenofibrate on the deterioration of diabetic retinopathy, supporting its efficacy for diabetic retinopathy.

The inhibitory effects of fenofibrate on diabetic microangiopathy are summarized below (Table 1). In a large-scale clinical study of lipid-lowering agents, no statin exhibited any inhibitory effects on diabetic microangiopathy. Only fenofibrate inhibited the complication. Thus, fenofibrate should be recognized as a "prophylactic drug for diabetic complications", and not solely as a lipid-lowering agent.

3. Conclusion

Fenofibrate is a generalized, PPAR-α-mediated, serum lipid-lowering agent. In this chapter, the pleiotropic effects of fenofibrate other than serum lipid-lowering actions were primarily reviewed. Concerning to the anti-inflammatory actions, we examined the effects of fenofibrate in patients with a representative inflammatory disorder, RA. Although there were no significant changes in inflammation parameters including CRP and ESR, improvement in the ΔVAS and PSL dose was achieved in patients receiving fenofibrate. In particular, improvement in the ΔVAS was significantly correlated with a reduction in the ΔCRP level, suggesting that the anti-inflammatory effects of fenofibrate may contribute the improvement in the patient's quality of life (QOL).

In Japan, infectious diseases have been the major causes of death in patients with RA (Souen, 2007; Shinomiya et al., 2008). However, the proportion of cardiovascular events represented by cerebral/myocardial infarction has been increasing, probably because of the changes in life-style (Goto et al., 2008a). So, fenofibrate with lipid-lowering, anti-inflammatory and anti-oxidant actions may be appropriate for reducing disturbances of lipid metabolism and also homeostasis in Japanese patients with RA.

With respect to antioxidant actions, fenofibrate, but not statin increased the plasma level of ubiquinol-10: a family of CoQ10. As fenofibrate exhibits antioxidant actions, combination therapy with fenofibrate and statins may be useful for achieving anti-aging effects and reducing oxidative stress. However, the evaluation methods for antioxidant activity in human should be strictly reviewed in the near future.

The serum uric acid-reducing actions of fenofibrate are regarded as one of its characteristic pleiotropic effects. The action mechanism may be mediated by a uric acid transporter, URAT1, but not by PPAR-α. This may suggest that among fibrate preparations fenofibrate may be favorably administered to the patients with high serum TG and high uric acid levels, as no other fibrate preparations can reduce the serum level of uric acid.

The large-scale clinical study of fenofibrate (FIELD) showed that early administration to "primary prevention" diabetics without a history of cardiovascular events inhibited the onset of cardiovascular events. Furthermore, the DAIS, FIELD, and ACCORD-EYE studies suggested that early fenofibrate administration to all diabetics with dyslipidemia should inhibit the deterioration of diabetic complications regardless of the duration of disease or risk of events.

Fenofibrate shows pleiotropic actions, especially a variety of clinical effects that may not be achieved by statins. This agent may be useful for inhibiting the deterioration of arteriosclerosis, and may play a role as an anti-aging panacea if properly used.

4. References

Abate, N., Chandalia, M., Cabo-Chan, A.V. Jr., Moe, O.W. & Sakhaee, K. (2004). The metabolic syndrome and uric acid nephrolithiasis: novel features of renal manifestation of insulin resistance. *Kidney Int,* Vo.65, No.2, (Feb 2004), pp.386-392, ISSN 0085-2538

ACCORD Study Group. (2010). Effects of combination lipid therapy in type 2 diabetes mellitus. *N Engl J Med,* Vol.362, No.17, (Apr 2010), pp.1563-1574, ISSN 0028-4793

ACCORD Study Group, ACCORD Eye Study Group. (2010). Effects of medical therapies on retinopathy progression in type 2 diabetes. *N Engl J Med,* Vol.363, No.3, (Jul 2010), pp.233-244, ISSN 0028-4793

Asano, A., Kobayashi, J., Murase, Y., Nohara, A., Kawashiri, M.A., Inazu, A., Shimizu, M. & Mabuchi, H. (2006). Effects of fenofibrate therapy on plasma ubiquinol-10 and ubiquinone-10 levels in Japanese patients with hyperlipidemia and type 2 diabetes mellitus. *Pharmacotherapy,* Vol.26, No.4, (Apr 2006), pp.447-451, ISSN 0277-0008

DAIS investigators. (2001). Effect of fenofibrate on progression of coronary-artery disease in type 2 diabetes: the Diabetes Atherosclerosis Intervention Study, a randomised study. *Lancet,* Vol.357, No.9260, (Mar 2001), pp.905-910, ISSN 0140-6736

DAIS investigators. (2003). Relationships between low-density lipoprotein particle size, plasma lipoproteins, and progression of coronary artery disease: the Diabetes Atherosclerosis Intervention Study (DAIS). *Circulation,* Vol.107, No.13, (Apr 2003), pp.1733-1737, ISSN 0009-7322

DAIS Investigators. (2005). Fenofibrate reduces progression to microalbuminuria over 3 years in a placebo-controlled study in type 2 diabetes: results from the Diabetes Atherosclerosis Intervention Study (DAIS). *Am J Kidney Dis,* Vol.45, No.3, (Mar 2005), pp.485-493, ISSN 0272-6386

Endo, A. (1992). The discovery and development of HMG-CoA reductase inhibitors. *J Lipid Res*, Vol.33, No.11, (Nov 1992), pp.1569-1582, ISSN 0022-2275

Enomoto, A., Kimura, H., Chairoungdua, A., Shigeta, Y., Jutabha, P., Cha, S.H., Hosoyamada, M., Takeda, M., Sekine, T., Igarashi, T., Matsuo, H., Kikuchi, Y., Oda, T., Ichida, K., Hosoya, T., Shimokata, K., Niwa, T., Kanai, Y., & Endou, H. (2002). Molecular identification of a renal urate anion exchanger that regulates blood urate levels. *Nature*, Vol.417, No.6887, (May 2002), pp.447-452, ISSN 0028-0836

FIELD study investigators. (2005). Effects of long-term fenofibrate therapy on cardiovascular events in 9795 people with type 2 diabetes mellitus (the FIELD study): randomised controlled trial. *Lancet*, Vol.366, No.9500, (Nov 2005), pp.1849-1861, ISSN 0140-6736

FIELD study investigators. (2007). Effect of fenofibrate on the need for laser treatment for diabetic retinopathy (FIELD study): a randomised controlled trial. *Lancet*, Vol.370, No.9600, (Nov 2007), pp.1687-1697, ISSN 0140-6736

FIELD study investigators. (2009). Effect of fenofibrate on amputation events in people with type 2 diabetes mellitus (FIELD study): a prespecified analysis of a randomised controlled trial. *Lancet*, Vol.373, No.9677, (May 2009), pp.1780-1788, ISSN 0140-6736

FIELD study investigators. (2010). Fenofibrate reduces peripheral neuropathy in type 2 diabetes: The frnofibrate intervention and event lowering in diabetes (FIELD) study. *Atherosclerosis Supplements*, Vol.11, No.2, (Jun 2010), pp.219-220, ISSN 1567-5688

FIELD study investigators. (2011). Effects of fenofibrate on renal function in patients with type 2 diabetes mellitus: the Fenofibrate Intervention and Event Lowering in Diabetes (FIELD) Study. *Diabetologia*, Vol.54, No.2, (Feb 2011), pp.280-290, ISSN 0012-186X

Goto, M. & Matsuura, M. (2008a). Secular trends towards delayed onsets of pathologies and prolonged longevities in Japanese patients with Werner syndrome. *Biosci Trends*, Vol.2, No.2, (Apr 2008), pp.81-87, ISSN 1881-7815

Goto, M. (2008b). Inflammaging (inflammation-aging): A driving force for human aging based on an evolutionarily antagonistic pleiotropy theory? *Biosci Trends*, Vol.2, No.6, (Dec 2008), pp.218-230, ISSN 1881-7815

Goto, M. (2010). A comparative study of anti-inflammatory and antidyslipidemic effects of fenofibrate and statins on rheumatoid arthritis. *Mod Rheumatol*, Vol.20, No.3, (Jun 2010), pp. 238-243, ISSN 1439-7595

Harman, D. (1978). Free radical theory of aging: nutritional implications. *Age*, Vol.1, No.4, (Oct 1978), pp.143-150, ISSN 0161-9152

Hikita, M., Ohno, I., Mori, Y., Ichida, K., Yokose, T. & Hosoya, T. (2007). Relationship between hyperuricemia and body fat distribution. *Intern Med*, Vol.46, No.17, (Sep 2007), pp.1353-1358, ISSN 0918-2918

Kodama, S., Saito, K., Yachi, Y., Asumi, M., Sugawara, A., Totsuka, K., Saito, A. & Sone, H. (2009). Association between serum uric acid and development of type 2 diabetes. *Diabetes Care*, Vol.32, No.9, (Sep 2009), pp.1737-1742, ISSN 0149-5992

Liamis, G., Bairaktari, E.T. & Elisaf, M.S. (1999). Effect of fenofibrate on serum uric acid levels. *Am J Kidney Dis*, Vol.34, No.3, (Sep 1999), pp.594, ISSN 0272-6386

Lippi, G., Montagnana, M., Franchini, M., Favaloro, E.J. & Targher, G. (2008). The paradoxical relationship between serum uric acid and cardiovascular disease. *Clin Chim Acta*, Vol.392, No.1-2, (Jun 2008), pp.1-7, ISSN 0009-8981

Mabuchi, H., Higashikata, T., Kawashiri, M.,Katsuda, S., Mizuno, M., Nohara, A., Inazu, A., Koizumi, J. & Kobayashi, J. (2005). Reduction of serum ubiquinol-10 and ubiquinone-10 levels by atorvastatin in hypercholesterolemic patients. *J Atheroscler Thromb*, Vol.12, No.2, (Jun 2005), pp.111-119, ISSN 1340-3478

Martinon, F., Pétrilli, V., Mayor, A., Tardivel, A. & Tschopp, J. (2006). Gout-associated uric acid crystals activate the NALP3 inflammasome. *Nature*, Vol.440, No.7081, (Mar 2006), pp.237-241, 0028-0836

Muhlestein, J.B., May, H.T., Jensen, J.R., Home, B.D., Lanman, R.B., Lavasani, F., Wolfert, R.L., Pearson, R.R., Yannicelli, H.D. & Anderson, J.L. (2006). The reduction of inflammatory biomarkers by statin, fibrate, the combination therapy among diabeteic patients with mixed dyslipidemia: the DIACOR (Diabetes and Combined Lipid Therapy Regimen) study. *J Am Coll Cardiol*, Vol.48, No.2, (Jul 2006), pp.396-401, ISSN 0735-1097

Romano, A.D., Serviddio, G., de Matthaeis, A., Bellanti, F. & Vendemiale, G. (2010). Oxidative stress and aging. *J Nephrol*, Vol.23, No.suppl 15, (Sep-Oct 2010), pp.S29-S36, ISSN 1121-8428

Ross, R. (1999). Atherosclerosis--an inflammatory disease. *N Engl J Med*, Vol.340, No.2, (Jan 1999), pp.115-126, ISSN 0028-4793

Schlesinger, N., Dalbeth, N. & Perez-Ruiz, F. (2009). Gout-what are the treatment options? *Expert Opin Pharmacother*, Vol.10, No.8, (Jun 2009), pp.1319-1328, ISSN 1465-6566

Schmelzer, C., Kubo, H., Mori, M., Sawashita, J., Kitano, M., Hosoe, K., Boomgaarden, I.,Döring, F. & Higuchi, K. (2010a). Supplementation with the reduced form of Coenzyme Q10 decelerates phenotypic characteristics of senescence and induces a peroxisome proliferator-activated receptor-alpha gene expression signature in SAMP1 mice. *Mol Nutr Food Res*, Vol.54, No.6, (Jun 2010), pp.805-815, ISSN 1613-4133

Schmelzer, C., Okun, JG., Haas, D., Higuchi, K., Sawashita, J., Mori, M. & Döring, F. (2010b). The reduced form of coenzyme Q10 mediates distinct effects on cholesterol metabolism at the transcriptional and metabolite level in SAMP1 mice. *IUBMB Life*, Vol.62, No.11, (Nov 2010), pp.812-818, ISSN 1521-6551

Schoonjans, K., Watanabe, M., Suzuki, H., Mahfoudi, A., Krey, G., Wahli, W., Grimaldi, P., Staels, B., Yamamoto, T. & Auwerx, J. (1995). Induction of the acyl-coenzyme A synthetase gene by fibrates and fatty acids is mediated by a peroxisome proliferator response element in the C promoter. *J Biol Chem*, Vol.270, No.33, (Aug 1995), pp.19269-19276, ISSN 0021-9258

Schoonjans, K., Peinado-Onsurbe, J., Lefebvre, A.M., Heyman, R.A.; Briggs, M., Deeb, S., Staels, B. & Auwerx, J. (1996a). PPARalpha and PPARgamma activators direct a distinct tissue-specific transcriptional response via a PPRE in the lipoprotein lipase gene. *EMBO J*, Vol.15, No.19, (Oct 1996), pp.5336-5348, ISSN 0261-4189

Schoonjans, K., Staels, B. & Auwerx, J. (1996b). Role of the peroxisome proliferator-activated receptor (PPAR) in mediating the effects of fibrates and fatty acids on gene expression. *J Lipid Res*, Vol.37, No.5, (May 1996), pp.907-925. ISSN 0022-2275

Schretlen, D.J., Inscore, A.B., Jinnah, H.A., Rao, V., Gordon, B. & Pearlson, G.D. (2007). Serum uric acid and cognitive function in community-dwelling older adults. *Neuropsychology*. Vol.21, No.1, (Jan 2007), pp.136-140, ISSN 0894-4105

Shinomiya, F., Mima, N., Nanba, K., Tani, K., Nakano, S., Egawa, H., Sakai, T., Miyoshi, H. & Hamada, D. (2008). Life expectancies of Japanese patients with rheumatoid arthritis: a review of deaths over a 20-year period. *Mod Rheumatol*, Vo.18, No.2, (Apr 2008), pp.165-169, ISSN 1439-7595

Souen, S. (2007). Mortality and causes of death in RA patients. *Rheumatology*, Vol.37, No.2, (Feb 2007), pp.164-168, ISSN 0915-227X

Staels, B., Vu-Dac, N., Kosykh, V.A., Saladin, R., Fruchart, J.C., Dallongeville, J. & Auwerx, J. (1995). Fibrates downregulate apolipoprotein C-III expression independent of induction of peroxisomal acyl coenzyme A oxidase. A potential mechanism for the hypolipidemic action of fibrates. *J Clin Invest*, Vol.95, No.2, (Feb 1995), pp.705-712, ISSN 0021-9738

Staels, B., Koenig, W., Habib, A., Merval, R., Lebret, M., Torra, I.P., Delerive, P., Fadel, A., Chinetti, G., Fruchart, J.C., Najib, J., Maclouf, J. & Tedgui, A. (1998). Activation of human aortic smooth-muscle cells is inhibited by PPARalpha but not by PPARgamma activators. *Nature*, Vol.393, No.6687, (Jun 1998), pp.790-793, ISSN 0028-0836

Superko, H.R. (2000). Small, dense, low-density lipoprotein and atherosclerosis. *Curr Atheroscler Rep*, Vol.2, No.3, (May 2000), pp.226-231, ISSN 1523-3804

Tsimihodimos, V., Kostoula, A., Kakafika, A., Bairaktari, E., Tselepis, A.D., Mikhaikidis, D.P. & Elisaf, M. (2004). Effect of fenofibrate on serum inflammatory markers in patients with high triglyceride values. *J Cardiovasc Pharmacol Ther*, Vol.9, No.1, (Mar 2004), pp.27-33, ISSN 1074-2484

Turunen, M., Peters, J.M., Gonzalez, F.J., Schedin, S. & Dallner, G. (2000). Influence of peroxisome proliferator-activated receptor alpha on ubiquinone biosynthesis. *J Mol Biol*, Vol.297, No.3, (Mar 2000), pp.607-614, ISSN 0022-2836

Uetake, D., Ohno, I., Ichida, K., Yamaguchi, Y., Saikawa, H., Endou, H. & Hosoya, T. (2010). Effect of fenofibrate on uric acid metabolism and urate transporter 1. *Intern Med*, Vol.49, No.2, (Jan 2010), pp.89-94, ISSN 0918-2918

Vu-Dac, N., Schoonjans, K., Laine, B., Fruchart, J.C., Auwerx, J. & Staels, B. (1994). Negative regulation of the human apolipoprotein A-I promoter by fibrates can be attenuated by the interaction of the peroxisome proliferator-activated receptor with its response element. *J Biol Chem*, Vol.269, No.49, (Dec 1994), pp.31012-31018, ISSN ISSN 0021-9258

Vu-Dac, N., Schoonjans, K., Kosykh, V., Dallongeville, J., Fruchart, J.C., Staels, B. & Auwerx, J. (1995). Fibrates increase human apolipoprotein A-II expression through activation of the peroxisome proliferator-activated receptor. *J Clin Invest*, Vol.96, No.2, (Aug 1995), pp.741-750, ISSN 0021-9738

Willson, T.M., Brown, P.J., Sternbach, D.D. & Henke, B.R. (2000). The PPARs: from orphan receptors to drug discovery. *J Med Chem,* Vol.43, No.4, (Feb 2000), pp.527-550, ISSN 0022-2623

Yu, B.P. & Chung, H.Y. (2001). Oxidative stress and vascular aging. *Diabetes Res Clin Pract,* Vol.54, No.2, (Dec 2001), pp.S73-S80, ISSN 0168-8227

Permissions

The contributors of this book come from diverse backgrounds, making this book a truly international effort. This book will bring forth new frontiers with its revolutionizing research information and detailed analysis of the nascent developments around the world.

We would like to thank Prof. Roya Kelishadi, for lending her expertise to make the book truly unique. She has played a crucial role in the development of this book. Without her invaluable contribution this book wouldn't have been possible. She has made vital efforts to compile up to date information on the varied aspects of this subject to make this book a valuable addition to the collection of many professionals and students.

This book was conceptualized with the vision of imparting up-to-date information and advanced data in this field. To ensure the same, a matchless editorial board was set up. Every individual on the board went through rigorous rounds of assessment to prove their worth. After which they invested a large part of their time researching and compiling the most relevant data for our readers. Conferences and sessions were held from time to time between the editorial board and the contributing authors to present the data in the most comprehensible form. The editorial team has worked tirelessly to provide valuable and valid information to help people across the globe.

Every chapter published in this book has been scrutinized by our experts. Their significance has been extensively debated. The topics covered herein carry significant findings which will fuel the growth of the discipline. They may even be implemented as practical applications or may be referred to as a beginning point for another development. Chapters in this book were first published by InTech; hereby published with permission under the Creative Commons Attribution License or equivalent.

The editorial board has been involved in producing this book since its inception. They have spent rigorous hours researching and exploring the diverse topics which have resulted in the successful publishing of this book. They have passed on their knowledge of decades through this book. To expedite this challenging task, the publisher supported the team at every step. A small team of assistant editors was also appointed to further simplify the editing procedure and attain best results for the readers.

Our editorial team has been hand-picked from every corner of the world. Their multi-ethnicity adds dynamic inputs to the discussions which result in innovative outcomes. These outcomes are then further discussed with the researchers and contributors who give their valuable feedback and opinion regarding the same. The feedback is then collaborated with the researches and they are edited in a comprehensive manner to aid the understanding of the subject.

Apart from the editorial board, the designing team has also invested a significant amount of their time in understanding the subject and creating the most relevant covers. They scrutinized every image to scout for the most suitable representation of the subject and create an appropriate cover for the book.

The publishing team has been involved in this book since its early stages. They were actively engaged in every process, be it collecting the data, connecting with the contributors or procuring relevant information. The team has been an ardent support to the editorial, designing and production team. Their endless efforts to recruit the best for this project, has resulted in the accomplishment of this book. They are a veteran in the field of academics and their pool of knowledge is as vast as their experience in printing. Their expertise and guidance has proved useful at every step. Their uncompromising quality standards have made this book an exceptional effort. Their encouragement from time to time has been an inspiration for everyone.

The publisher and the editorial board hope that this book will prove to be a valuable piece of knowledge for researchers, students, practitioners and scholars across the globe.

List of Contributors

Dmitri Svistounov, Svetlana N. Zykova, Victoria C. Cogger, Alessandra Warren, Aisling C. McMahon and David G. Le Couteur
Centre for Education and Research on Ageing and ANZAC Research Institute, University of Sydney and Concord RG Hospital, Sydney, Australia

Svetlana N. Zykova
Department of Nephrology, University Hospital of Northern Norway, Tromsø, Norway

Robin Fraser
University of Otago, Christchurch, New Zealand

Hossein Fakhrzadeh and Ozra Tabatabaei-Malazy
Endocrinology & Metabolism Research Center, Tehran University of Medical Sciences, Tehran, Islamic Republic of Iran

Telmo Pereira
College of Health Technologies, Polytechnic Institute of Coimbra, Portugal

Fernanda Klein Marcondes, Vander José das Neves, Rafaela Costa, Andrea Sanches and Tatiana Sousa Cunha
Department of Physiological Sciences, Piracicaba Dental School, University of Campinas, Piracicaba, Brazil

Tatiana Sousa Cunha
Science and Technology Institute, Federal University of São Paulo, São José dos Campos, Brazil

Maria José Costa Sampaio Moura
Life Sciences Center, Pontifical Catholic University of Campinas, Campinas, Brazil

Ana Paula Tanno
Division of Pharmacy, Faculty of Americana, Americana, Brazil

Dulce Elena Casarini
Department of Medicine, Federal University of São Paulo, São Paulo, Brazil

D. Saravane
Head of Department Medicine and Specialists, Ville-Evrard Hospital Neuilly/Marne, France

Asma Ezzaher, Dhouha Haj Mouhamed, Fadoua Neffati, Wahiba Douki and Mohamed Fadhel Najjar
Laboratory of Biochemistry-Toxicology, Tunisia

Asma Ezzaher, Dhouha Haj Mouhamed, Anwar Mechri, Fadoua Neffati, Wahiba Douki and Lotfi Gaha
Research Laboratory "Vulnerability to Psychotic Disorders LR 05 ES 10", Department of Psychiatry/Monastir University Hospital, Tunisia

Romeo-Gabriel Mihăilă
"Lucian Blaga" University of Sibiu, Romania

Rosana Libonati, Cláudia Dutra, Leonardo Barbosa, Sandro Oliveira, Paulo Lisbôa and Marcus Libonati
Tropical Medicine Center, Federal University of the Pará, Pará, Brasil

Ajit Vikram and Poduri Ramarao
Central University of Punjab, India

Hadeer Akram AbdulRazzaq and Yaman Walid Kassab
Department of Clinical Pharmacy, School of Pharmaceutical Sciences, Universiti Sains, Penang, Malaysia

Noorizan Abd Aziz and Yahaya Hassan
Faculty of Pharmacy, UiTM, Puncak Alam Campus, Bandar Puncak Alam, Selangor DE, Malaysia

Omar Ismail
Department of Cardiology, Hospital Pulau Pinang, Penang, Malaysia

Makoto Goto
Division of Anti-Ageing & Longevity Sciences, Faculty of Medical Technology, Department of BioMedical Engineering, Toin University of Yokohama, Japan